Current Progress in Ophthalmology

Current Progress in Ophthalmology

Edited by **Danny Chapman**

hayle
medical

New York

Published by Hayle Medical,
30 West, 37th Street, Suite 612,
New York, NY 10018, USA
www.haylemedical.com

Current Progress in Ophthalmology
Edited by Danny Chapman

International Standard Book Number: 978-1-63241-390-1 (Hardback)

Printed in the United States of America.

Contents

Preface

Ophthalmology is the branch of medical science that deals with the study of eye and eye care. This discipline provides diagnosis and treatment of a wide range of eye diseases. Also, it has provisions for general medicines as well as surgeries. The various studies that are constantly contributing towards advancing technologies and evolution of this field are examined in detail. The aim of this book is to present researches that have transformed this discipline and aided its advancement. It is complied in such a manner, that it will provide in-depth knowledge about the theory and practice of opthalmology. With state-of-the-art inputs by acclaimed experts of this field, this book targets students and professionals.

All of the data presented henceforth, was collaborated in the wake of recent advancements in the field. The aim of this book is to present the diversified developments from across the globe in a comprehensible manner. The opinions expressed in each chapter belong solely to the contributing authors. Their interpretations of the topics are the integral part of this book, which I have carefully compiled for a better understanding of the readers.

At the end, I would like to thank all those who dedicated their time and efforts for the successful completion of this book. I also wish to convey my gratitude towards my friends and family who supported me at every step.

Editor

Conjunctival Foreign Body a Rare Presentation

Tarakeswararao Attada[1*] and V. V. L. Narasimha Rao[1]

[1]*Department of Ophthalmology, Andhramedical College, Govt. Regional Eye Hospital, Visakhapatnam, Andhra Pradesh, India.*

Authors' contributions

This work was carried out in collaboration between both authors. Both authors read and approved the final manuscript.

Editor(s):
(1) Li Wang, Department of Ophthalmology, Cullen Eye Institute, Baylor College of Medicine, USA.
Reviewers:
(1) Saka Eletu Sadiat, Department of Ophthalmology, Federal Medical Centre, Nigeria.
(2) Anonymous, University of Sao Paulo, Brazil.
(3) Anonymous, Ahi Evran University, Turkey.
(4) Sagili Chandarsekhara Reddy, Department of Ophthalmology, National Defence University of Malaysia, Malaysia.

ABSTRACT

Aim: Detection of subconjunctival or intra orbital wooden foreign bodies and its retrieval is important, because of severe blinding complications secondary to infection can occur. We describe, a case of post traumatic subconjunctival wooden foreign bodies retained in conjunctival culde-sac of upper fornix, presenting as conjunctival granuloma.

Case Report: A 50 year male patient was accidentally hit by a wooden stick on the right eye 25 days ago, while he was working in the paddy field. On examination, a granulomatous growth was present on the temporal side of the bulbar conjunctiva. Two wooden foreign bodies were removed from the conjunctival granulomatous mass.

Discussion: The superficial foreign bodies of the conjunctiva are common and the ocular protective mechanisms normally extrude superficial foreign bodies. The clinical course of orbital foreign bodies depends upon their composition. The organic foreign bodies like wood if left untreated results in sight threatening complications.

In our case, wooden foreign bodies penetrated subconjunctivally into the upper fornix and presented as conjunctival granuloma. Under topical anaesthesia (xylocaine 4%) two wooden foreign bodies were removed from conjunctival granuloma. The patient recovered uneventfully with antibiotic drops and oral analgesics and anti-inflammatory drugs.

Corresponding author: E-mail: tarakeye@gmail.com

Conclusion: In patients presenting with post traumatic conjunctival granuloma, we should strongly suspect a subconjunctival retained foreign body before initiating treatment.

Keywords: Conjunctiiva; granulation tissue; foreign body; growth; wood.

1. INTRODUCTION

Conjunctival foreign bodies of the eye are common. Wooden ocular foreign bodies are common in rural areas particularly in agricultural workers. Most of the times, foreign bodies are small particles of dust, stone piece, insect wing or small iron particles. Foreign bodies may settle on the bulbar conjunctiva, upper or lower fornix or on the cornea but most commonly retained in the upper conjunctival cul-de-sac. Sometimes wooden foreign bodies penetrate and are retained under the conjunctiva. In due course the foreign bodies are covered by granulation tissue which may simulate the cockscomb type of tuberculosis of conjunctiva [1]. This is a rare presentation of the conjunctival foreign body.

2. CASE REPORT

A 50 years male patient who is an agricultural worker, came with a complaint of redness, pain, foreign body sensation and discharge of right eye for the last 25 days. He was accidentally hit by a wooden stick on the right eye 25 days ago while he was working in the paddy field. Then he was treated by antibiotic eye drops and pain killers by local doctors for about 20 days, but the problem was not solved. He presented to our hospital outpatient Department.

On examination of the Right eye there was mild upper lid oedema. A pedunculated polyp like growth was present on the temporal side of the bulbar conjunctiva. The growth was not attached to the cornea. Cornea was clear and fluorescein stain was negative. Anterior chamber was of normal depth with clear contents, pupil was reacting to light. Fundus examination was within normal limits except a few lenticular opacities. Visual acuity was 6/18 in Right eye. The left eye was found normal and visual acuity was 6/9.

On careful examination of the right eye there were two small yellowish white spots noticed on the surface of the polyp like growth of the conjunctiva which appeared like pus points (Fig. 1). Under topical anaesthesia (4% lignocaine) the surface of the growth was manipulated with plain forceps by which it was found that those points are actually the tips of wooden foreign bodies (Fig. 2). Two pieces of wooden foreign bodies were removed from the pedunculated growth of the conjunctiva, one foreign body was measuring about 2cm and other one about 4 cm (Fig. 3. Fig. 4). There were no signs of perforation of the globe.

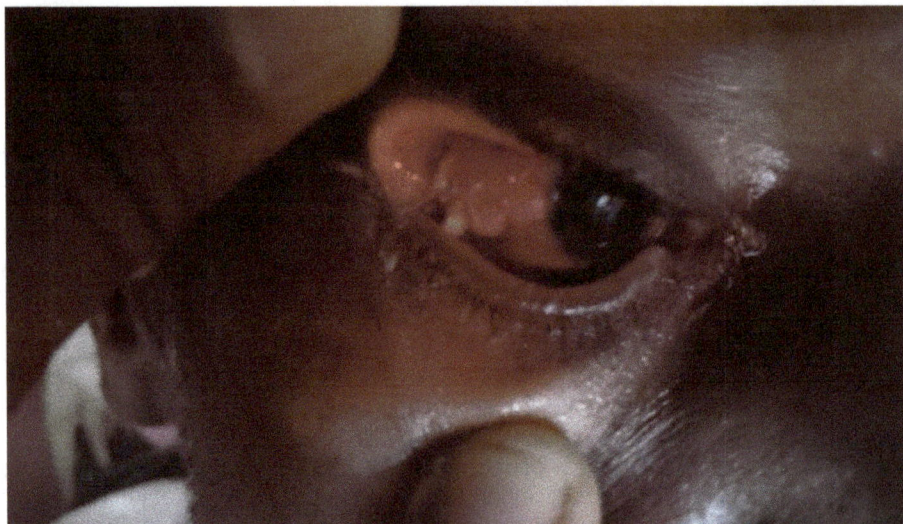

Fig. 1. Pus like points of foreign bodies

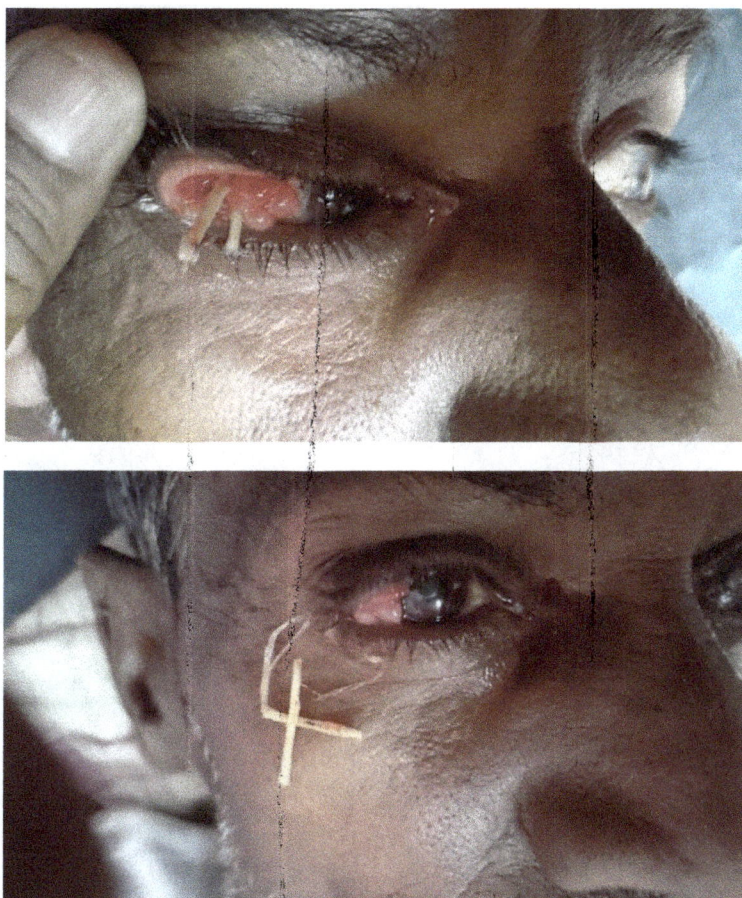

Fig. 2. Projected foreign bodies from conjunctivalgranuloma

Moxifloxacin eye drops 6times per day and tab aceclofen two times per day for 5 days was prescribed. All inflammatory signs and conjunctiva granulation markedly reduced within one week. Patient's vision in right eye improved to 6/9 by the end of one week.

3. DISCUSSION

The superficial foreign bodies of the conjunctiva are common, such as small particles of dust or steel and insect wings [2]. These foreign bodies impinge on the cornea or conjunctiva [1]. Ocular protective mechanisms which include blinking and tearing normally remove superficial foreign body that comes in contact with the ocular surface. [3]

The orbital foreign bodies are divided in to three types [4] 1. Metallic. 2. Non-organic like glass pieces. 3. Organic foreign bodies like wood. The clinical course of the foreign bodies depends upon their composition [5]. Some metallic foreign bodies remain quiescent for long period of time without causing any problems. But organic foreign bodies like wood cause sight threatening complications. They may remain asymptomatic for variable periods and manifest with delayed onset of conjunctival granuloma, cellulitis and abscess. When a foreign body with large surface area gets lodged in the conjunctiva, initially, there is an acute inflammatory response in the form of exudation of plasma and fibrin and the foreign body becomes embedded. This is followed by a chronic inflammatory response resulting in the formation of granuloma [2]

In our case, wooden foreign bodies penetrated subconjunctivally into the upper fornix and in due course covered by granulation tissue, presented as pedunculated conjunctival growth which simulated cockscomb type tuberculosis of the conjunctiva [1]. Occasionally, as in our case, foreign body retained in the fornix, encapsulated by mucus, embedded in the Underlying stroma may cause local inflammatory response. In case of conjunctival foreign bodies, we must search for signs of globe perforation.

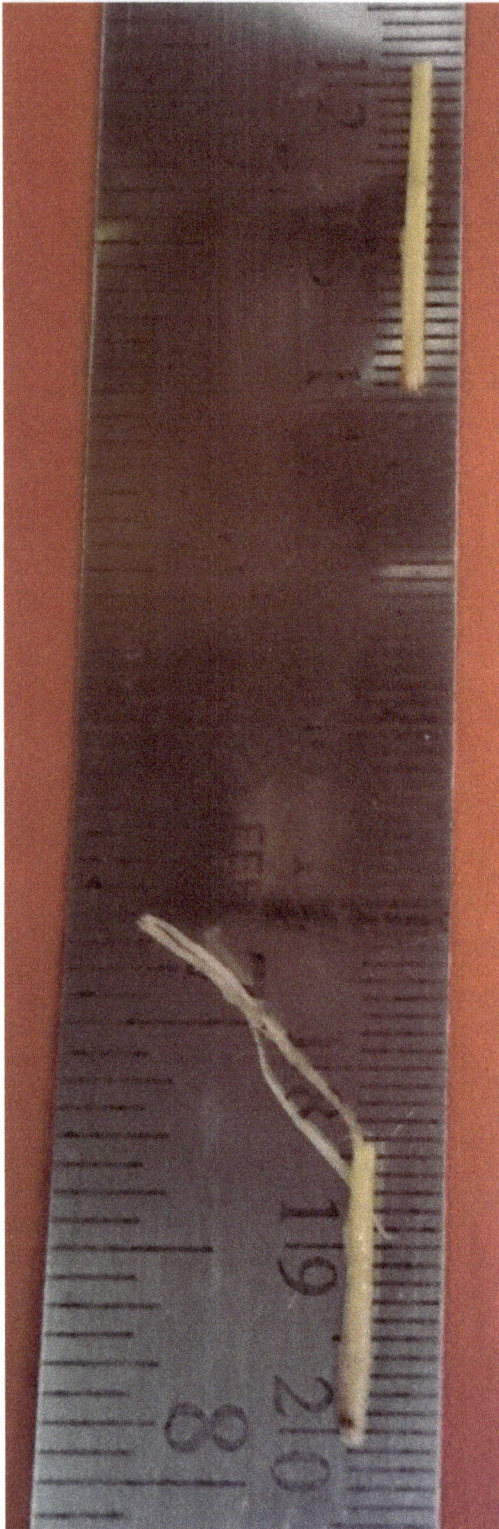

Fig. 3. Removed wooden foreign bodies　　　　Fig. 4. Measurement of foreign bodies

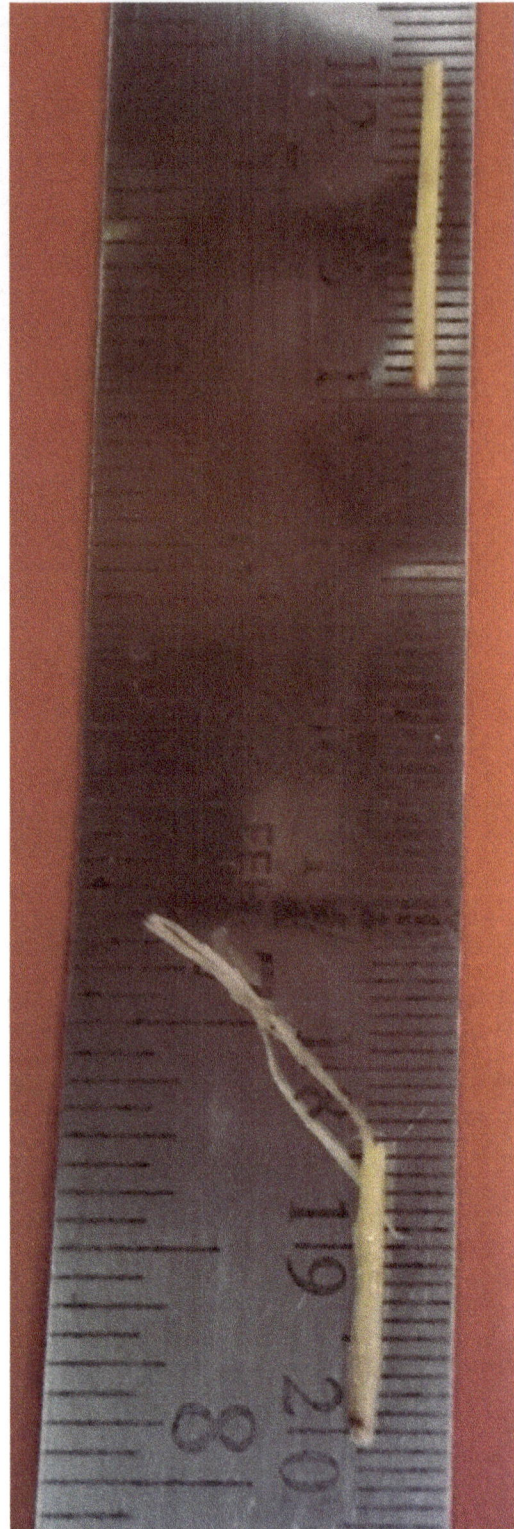

An intraorbital foreign body is an object that lies within the orbit but outside the ocular globe [4]. In the literature they reported evidence of orbital foreign body migration toward the cranium [6]. So, it is important to identify and remove intraorbital wooden foreign bodies as early as possible to prevent further complications.

Identification or localization and removal of Intra orbital wooden foreign body poses a challenge to the ophthalmologist. He has to use appropriate imaging modality for evaluation of intra orbital wooden foreign body. Plain X- ray has limited role in the diagnosis of intraorbital wooden foreign body. The detection rate of plain X-ray is very low (0-15%) [7]. B-scan Ultrasonography has a very limited role in localization of intraorbital wooden foreign body. The CT- Scan findings of intraorbital wooden foreign body are variable and may be similar to orbital fat and muscle. The MRI scan is better at demonstrating intra orbital wooden foreign bodies [8,9]. It can distinguish between air and wood easily.

In our case, there was definite history of injury with wooden stick present. The tips of wooden foreign bodies were visible on manipulation of conjunctival granulomatous mass. Therefore imaging investigation was not done to locate foreign body.

In our case, we identified retained intra orbital wooden foreign bodies immediately on presentation of the patient. The retained intraorbital foreign bodies were removed under topical anaesthesia (4% lignocaine). Double eversion of upper lid was done to locate any hidden foreign bodies in the fornix. But no foreign body was found.

Long and multiple foreign bodies in the orbit following an apparently trivial trauma is rare. In the literature, two pieces of wood measuring 5.1 cm and 4.5 cm, respectively were retained for six weeks have been reported [6]. In the present case, two pieces of wooden foreign bodies measuring 2cm and 4cm retained for 25 days. The possibility of such retained multiple foreign bodies in the orbit must be considered in an injury caused by organic material, particularly when signs of inflammation persist after routine therapy or with conjunctival granulation mass.

4. CONCLUSION

Patients presenting with pedunculated polyp like growth of conjunctiva, particularly from agricultural field with history of trauma, a retained conjunctival wooden foreign body should be ruled out first [10].

In conclusion, we would like to emphasize that with meticulous ocular examination and good clinical acumen we can avoid vision threatening complications because of retained foreign bodies and eye care professionals should keep in mind a retained foreign body as a differential diagnosis when dealing with inflamed conjunctival growths.

CONSENT

A written informed consent taken from the patient.

ETHICAL APPROVAL

It is not applicable.

ACKNOWLEDGEMENTS

Sincere thanks to Dr. V.V.L Narasimha Rao MS,. Our Professor and Supt. Govt. Regional Eye Hospital. Visakhapatnam AP.

COMPETING INTERESTS

Authors have declared that no competing interests exist.

REFERENCES

1.   Parsons Diseases of the Eye. 20th Edition; 2007.
2.   Insect wing tarsal foreign body causing conjunctival granuloma and marginal keratitis kalpana babu and rashmi eymaralihalli. Indian Journal of ophthalmology. 2009;57(6):473-474.
3.   Mke ST, Lui YH, KWli K. Case Report. Synthetic fibre granuloma of the conjunctiva. Hong Kong Med. Journal. 2015;21:77-9,
4.   Morsette et al. Periorbital foreign body – A case report. Journal of Medical case Report. 2012;6:9.
5.   Sheeja S, John Thaj A, Rehman Deep John, Renu S Raju. Missed diagnosis of a wooden intraorbital foreign body. Indian Journal of Ophthalmology. 2008;56(4):322-324.
6.   DonLiu, Sambal, Shail, KFUF. A retained orbital wooden foreign body. A surgical technique and Rationale. Ophthalmology. 2002;109(2). (Science Direct).

7.   Ishan Yadav, Rajendra P Maurya, Prashant Bhushan. Unrecognised large wooden intraorbital foreign body. Indian Journal of Clinical and Experimental Ophthalmology. 2015;1(1):50-55.

8.   Sagili Chandrasekhar Reddy. Retained wooden foreign body in the Orbit. International Journal of Ophthalmology. 2013;6(2):255-258.

9.   VanThong, James F, Mcguchin Jr, Eleanor M Smrgel. Intraorbital wooden foreign body; CT and MR appearance. American Journal of Neuroradiology. 1996;17:134-136.

10. Diagnosis and Management of a Wooden Orbital foreign Body-A case Report John A. Macrae. British Journal of Ophthalmology. 1979;63:848-851.

Cytomegalovirus Retinitis: Current State in People with HIV-AIDS in Peru

Bety Yáñez[1*]

[1]*Department of Ophthalmology, Hospital Nacional Dos de Mayo, Lima, Peru.*

Author's contribution

The sole author designed, analyzed and interpreted and prepared the manuscript.

<u>Editor(s):</u>
(1) Li Wang, Department of Ophthalmology, Cullen Eye Institute, Baylor College of Medicine, USA.
<u>Reviewers:</u>
(1) Anonymous, China.
(2) Francisco Jesús Sepúlveda Cañamar, Instituto Mexicano Seguro Social, México.
(3) Anonymous, Oakland University William Beaumont School of Medicine, USA.

ABSTRACT

Purpose: To describe the incidence and progression of cytomegalovirus retinitis (CMVR) in public hospital patients from Peru.
Study Design: Prospective study conducted in HIV-AIDS diagnosed patients.
Place and Duration of Study: Department of Ophthalmology and Department of Tropical Medicine, Hospital Nacional Dos de Mayo, from 2004 to 2013.
Methodology: Descriptive statistics were obtained for age, gender, associated disease, CMVR location and ganciclovir treatment. Data were analyzed by the Pearson Chi. Square test, Mann-Whitney test, and the two-tailed exact Fischer's Exact test. SPSS version 20.0 for Windows software program was used
Results: 2627 patients were evaluated, 75 had CMVR diagnosis. Active CMVR was found in 68 eyes (90.7%). Median age at diagnosis of CMVR was 37 years (IQR 30-41 years). Median CD4 level of 25 cells/µL (IQR 12.2-57.7 cells/µL), viral load > 1000,000 in 39 (52%) patients. Median mortality rate was 7.1 deaths per 1000 PY and mean survival time from HIV diagnosis to death was 29,5 months (95% 8,7-43,0 months) and from CMVR diagnosis, 6,2 months (95% IC 2,0-8,0 months). Duration since HIV diagnosis to CMVR onset was 12 months (IQR 3-48 months). Tuberculosis (TB) was present in 23 (30.7%) patients. Incidence rate of HIV patients with CMVR was 28.2 cases per 1000 PY. 51 patients received ganciclovir: endovenous 34 (91.17%), intravitreal 6 (26.5%) and orally 4 (11.8%).

Corresponding author: E-mail: byanez@hotmail.com

Conclusion: CMVR has a high prevalence in young people with an elevated value of HIV-TB co-infection (30.7%). CMVR diagnosis was a predictor for early mortality, including highly active antiretroviral therapy (ART).

Keywords: Cytomegalovirus retinitis; HIV; AIDS; blindness.

1. INTRODUCTION

There are 65,000 persons living in Peru with Human Immune Virus (HIV) – Acquired Immunodeficiency Syndrome (AIDS) infection. It is a concentrated epidemic, with a 0.23% of prevalence in general population and 12.4% in men with have sex with men [1].

In 2004 highly active antiretroviral therapy (ART) is initiated by Health Minister in hospitals and health centers. During 2011, 92.7% of the people that needed to receive ART and had access to the health system were receiving it. Between 2005 and 2011 the number of AIDS-related deaths, had been reduced by 55% [1,2].

HIV- AIDS patients with a CD4 count below of 50 cells / mL are more likely to have opportunistic infections that will cause death or disabilities that affect their quality of life in ART era [3].

Cytomegalovirus retinitis (CMVR) is a common opportunistic disease among HIV - AIDS patients, this infection contributes to mortality [4]. Before ART era, it was responsible of 90% HIV-related blindness in developed countries. Immune recovery produced by ART has resulted in an approximate 80% reduction in the incidence of CMV retinitis [5,6].

In developing countries, CMVR in AIDS patients is a neglected disease with no strategy for management and its complications. Their lower prevalence compared to the developed countries is explained by the fact that generally most lower-income patients living in Africa, Asia and Latin America die before the diagnosis [7]. Between 5% and 25% of all HIV-infected patients in the developing world can be expected to develop blindness at some time during their illness [8].

To define a strategy for CMVR diagnosis and treatment in our countries, is important know the epidemiological data. This study describes the incidence and progression of CMVR in public hospital patients from Peru.

2. METHODOLOGY

This prospective study was conducted in HIV-AIDS diagnosed patients treated at Hospital Nacional Dos de Mayo, a tertiary care hospital in Lima, Peru between April 2004 and December 2013. Institutional Ethics Committee approval was obtained before for this prospective study and consent forms were not required.

Patients were referred from Tropical Medicine Department for ophthalmological evaluation before starting ART (supported by the Global Fund). Demographic, HIV infection history, CD4 T cell counts, and plasma HIV viral load, associated diseases, characteristics and treatment of the CMVR data were obtained.

Dilated indirect fundoscopy was performed by an experimented ophthalmologist at the beginning and at 2-3 weekly intervals until CMVR was inactive. The diagnosis and site of CMVR was based on clinical features previously described [9]. Patients were treated with ganciclovir (endovenous, oral and/or intravitreal). Endovenous ganciclovir was given for two weeks at 7.5 to 15 mg/kg/day followed by maintenance therapy of 5 mg/kg/day. Intravitreal ganciclovir induction dose was 1000 µgr/0.1 ml twice weekly for the first week and maintenance dose one weekly to see inactivity of the disease. Oral ganciclovir was given for maintenance therapy at 1 g three times a day. An informed consent was obtained from all patients for each eye treated.

Descriptive statistics were obtained for age, gender, associated disease, CMVR location and ganciclovir treatment. Comparisons were done for survivors and deceased patients. Potential shorter survival time at CMVR diagnosis predictors were identified by extended Cox regression models. Data were analyzed by the Pearson Chi. Square test, Mann-Whitney test and when one of the numbers was less than 5, by the two-tailed exact Fischer's exact test. SPSS version 20.0 for Windows software program was used.

3. RESULTS

At the time the study was performed 2659 patients were diagnosed with HIV-AIDS. 2627 had ophthalmological examination and cytomegalovirus retinitis was found in 75 cases. In 26 patients damage was bilateral. CMVR was active in 68 eyes (90.7%). In Table 1 is shown that the median age at diagnosis of CMVR was 37 years (IQR 30-41 years). Males were 61 (81.3%). Median CD4 level of 25 cells/μL (IQR 12.2-57.7 cells/μL), viral load >1000,000 in 39 (52%) patients. Incidence rate of HIV patients with CMVR was 28.2 cases per 1000 PY. The duration since HIV diagnosis to CMVR onset was 12 months (IQR 3-48 months).

As indicated in Table 2, Tuberculosis (TB) was present in 23 (30.7%) patients. The most affected area in the retina was zone 1 in (55.4%) eyes. 51 patients received ganciclovir: endovenous 34 (91.17%), intravitreal 6 (26.5%) and orally 4 (11.8%). Inactivity of CMVR was observed at four weeks in 17 eyes with endovenous ganciclovir, three of them also received the drug via intravitreal. 46 patients had a minimum follow up of three months, with the longest observed follow-up of 9 years. CMVR was reactivated in 22 eyes (14.6%) of 16 patients. Nine cases of this group had CD4 counts <50 cells. Seven eyes (4.6%) showed immune reaction syndrome (vitreitis and macular edema).

Comparing deceased and survivors patients, there was no difference in demographic and clinical characteristics as is observed in Table 3.

Median mortality rate was 7.1 deaths per 1000 PY and mean survival time from HIV diagnosis to death was 29,5 months (95% 8,7-43,0 months) and from CMVR diagnosis, 6,2 months (95% IC 2,0-8,0 months). In the multivariate analysis was found that age at diagnosis of CMVR is not related to the patient's death as is shown in Table 4. The cumulative curve for survival of patients with CMVR is shown in Fig. 1.

4. DISCUSSION

Since 1983 to January 2014, a total of 52490 HIV and 31157 AIDS cases in Peru had been reported [1]. ART began in 2004 in public medical centers provided by Global Fund to Fight AIDS, Tuberculosis and Malaria. During 2011, 92.7% of the people that needed to receive ART and had access to the health system were receiving it. 62.3% of HIV cases and 72.2% of AIDS cases reported in 1983-2012, originate in Lima and Callao, urban regions inhabiting a third of the population of the whole country [1,2].

The prevalence of CMVR in HIV-AIDS patients in developing countries is generally lower than in industrialized countries explained this on the short survival time of this patients. Our results showed an overall incidence rate of CMVR of 28.2 cases per 1000 P Y, similar values are observed in Togo a country in sub-Saharan Africa (21.4%) [10]. It is remarkable that the highest value 62.4 cases per 1000 P Y was obtained in 2004 before starting ART.

The studied patients comprised young adults with a median age at diagnosis of CMVR of 37 years (IQR 30-41 years). Lowest levels of CD4 in most of the cases explain the highest incidence of CMVR compared with other reports [11,12]. The patients had severe immunosupression because a high percentage of them, requested medical care at an advanced stage of their disease. Factors preventing the prompt care of these patients were low socioeconomic and educational levels, plus stigma and discrimination in health centers similar to observed in other developing countries [1,8,11,13]. The beginning of CMVR was at a median of 12 months after HIV diagnosis (IQR 3-48 months) shorter than described in the literature (18 and 26 months) [11,14].

Mean onset of ART was two years after HIV diagnosis. This therapy significantly decreased CMVR incidence in this group of patients. While ART is free, other diagnostic tests must be paid by the patient to access to this program and receive therapy. Perhaps, this is one of the main reasons for delay in receiving treatment.

Median mortality rate was 7.1 deaths per 1000 PY and mean survival time from CMVR diagnosis was 6.2 months (95%, 2,0-8,0 months). The fact that the mortality rate in our study was lower than that found by Balo in Togo [10] and Tun in Myanmar [13], it can be explained that approximately one third of patients did not have follow-up. Survival time from CMVR was 6 months, early similar mortality, as described in previous studies in developing countries mentioned above. Sadly, it is observed that the, HIV epidemic continues to have a greater impact in terms of mortality in young population of our country, occupying the eighth leading cause of death in young (18-29 years old) [1].

Table 1. Demographic characteristics of HIV patients with cytomegalovirus retinitis in Lima –Peru, 2004 to 2013

Characteristic	Years										Total
	2004	2005	2006	2007	2008	2009	2010	2011	2012	2013	
CMV Retinitis, n (%)											
Male	16 (26.2)	9 (14.8)	6 (9.8)	3 (4.9)	5 (8.2)	4 (6.6)	5 (8.2)	2 (3.3)	7 (11.5)	4 (6.6)	61 (81.3)
Female	7 (50.0)	0	0	2 (14.3)	1 (7.1)	0	0	2 (14.3)	2 (14.3)	0	14 (18.7)
Total	23 (30.7)	9 (12.0)	6 (8.0)	5 (6.7)	6 (8.0)	4 (5.3)	5 (6.7)	4 (5.3)	9 (12.0)	4 (5.3)	75 (100.0)
Cumulative HIV cases, n	369	295	298	264	262	239	235	263	221	213	2659
Incidence (per 1000 PY)	62.3	30.5	20.1	18.9	22.9	16.7	21.2	15.2	40.7	18.7	28.2
Age (years), median [IQR]											
At HIV diagnosis	34.0 [27.0 – 40.0]	33.0 [30.5 – 44.0]	31.5 [25.0 – 35.5]	29.0 [23.0 – 34.0]	44.0 [31.2 – 60.0]	32.0 [28.2 – 45.5]	34.0 [25.5 – 40.0]	30.5 [29.0 – 33.5]	34.0 [25.0 – 43.0]	38.0 [32.5 – 45.0]	34.0 [28.0 – 39.0]
At CMVR diagnosis	38.0 [30.0 – 42.0]	37.0 [32.5 – 48.0]	33.0 [26.7 – 37.0]	29.0 [29.0 – 34.5]	44.5 [31.5 – 60.0]	36.5 [29.7 – 47.0]	40.0 [26.5 – 41.5]	33.0 [31.2 – 37.7]	36.0 [25.0 – 43.5]	44.0 [39.5 – 50.0]	37.0 [30.0 – 41.0]
At HAART initiation	38.5 [30.0 – 44.2]	35.0 [35.0 – 44.0]	34.0 [27.0 – 36.5]	29.0 [29.0 – 34.0]	44.5 [31.5 – 60.0]	36.0 [29.0 – 36.0]	40.0 [28.5 – 42.5]	33.0 [31.2 – 37.7]	35.0 [26.0 – 48.0]	38.0 [38.0 – 45.0]	36.0 [30.0 – 41.0]
CD4 count (cells/µL) Median [IQR]											
At CMVR diagnosis	20.0 [2.0 – 50.0]	25.0 [10.0 – 45.0]	43.5 [11.7 – 236.5]	26.0 [5.0 – 26.0]	25.0 [17.5 – 93.5]	286.5 [6.0 – 286.5]	23.0 [9.5 – 30.5]	8.0 [4.7 – 123.0]	57.0 [25.0 – 79.0]	333.0 [35.0 – 333.0]	25.0 [12.2 – 57.7]
Duration (months), median [IQR]											
HIV diagnosis to CMVR	24.0 [12.0 – 60.0]	48.0 [15.0 – 48.0]	15.0 [1.0 – 46.5]	8.5 [4.2 – 111.0]	4.5 [1.0 – 8.2]	25.5 [1.5 – 68.2]	24.0 [4.5 – 54.0]	12.5 [1.0 – 96.0]	1.0 [1.0 – 6.5]	25.5 [2.2 – 188.2]	12.0 [3.0 – 48.0]

Table 2. Clinical characteristics of HIV patients with cytomegalovirus retinitis in Lima –Peru, 2004 to 2013

Characteristic	2004	2005	2006	2007	2008	2009	2010	2011	2012	2013	Total
Associated disease, n (%)											
Tuberculosis	7 (30.4)	4 (44.4)	1 (16.7)	2(40.0)	0	2 (50.0)	0	1 (25.0)	3 (33.3)	3 (75.0)	23 (30.7)
Toxoplasmosis	0	0	0	0	0	0	0	1 (25.0)	1 (11.1)	0	2 (2.7)
Syphilis	0	0	0	0	2 (33.3)	2 (50.0)	0	0	0	0	4 (5.3)
Kaposis's Sarcoma	2 (8.7)	0	0	0	0	0	1 (20.0)	0	0	0	3 (4.0)
Non Hodgkin Lymphoma	0	0	0	0	0	0	0	0	2 (22.2)	0	2 (2.7)
CMVR location, n (%)											
Zone 1	15 (65.4)	3 (33.3)	3 (50.0)	3(60.0)	0	2 (50.0)	3(60.0)	1 (25.0)	3 (33.3)	2 (50.0)	35 (46.7)
Zone 2	2 (8.6)	0	1 (16.7)	0	3 (50.0)	1 (25.0)	2 (40.0)	3 (75.0)	5 (55.6)	2 (50.0)	19 (25.3)
Zone 3	6 (26.0)	6 (66.7)	2 (33.3)	2 (40.0)	3 (50.0)	1 (25.0)	0	0	1 (11.1)	0	21 (28-0)
Ganciclovir treatment, n (%)											
Endovenous	9 (39.1)	3 (33.3)	1 (16.7)	4 (80.0)	2 (33.3)	2 (50.0)	3 (60.0)	3 (75.0)	5 (55.6)	2 (50.0)	34 (45.4)
Intravitreal	3 (13.0)	0	2 (33.3)	0	0	1 (25.0)	0	0	0	0	6 (8.0)
Endovenous - intravitreal	1 (4.3)	0	3 (50.0)	0	2 (33.3)	1 (25.0)	2 (40.0)	1 (25.0)	4 (44.4)	1 (25.0)	15 (20.0)
Endovenous - oral	6 (26.1)	0	0	0	0	0	0	0	0	0	6 (8.0)
No report	4 (17.4)	6 (66.7)	0	1 (20.0)	2 (33.3)	0	0	0	0	1 (25.0)	14 (18.6)

Table 3. Characteristics of deceased and survivors patients with CMV retinitis, Peru 2004 to 2013

Characteristic	Deceased	Survivors	P value
CMVR, n (%)			0.09 [‡]
Male	13 (68.4)	48 (85.7)	
Female	6 (31.6)	8 (14.3)	
Age, median [IQR]			
At HIV diagnosis	29 [27.0 8.0]	34.5 [29.0–40.7]	0.027 [†]
At CMVR diagnosis	31 [29.0 8.0]	37.5 [30.2–46.2]	0.026 [†]
At HAART initiation	38 [30.0 9.5]	35.5 [30.0–43.0]	0.65 [†]
CD4 cells/μL, median [IQR]			
At CMVR diagnosis	17 [8.0–08.0]	26 [14.0–58.5]	0.63 [†]
Duration (months), Median [IQR]			
HIV diagnosis to CMVR	10 [2.0–48.0]	12 [3.0–48.0]	0.78 [†]
Associated disease, n (%)			0.52 [*]
TB	6 (31.6)	17 (30.4)	
Toxoplasmosis	1 (5.3)	1 (1.8)	
Syphilis	0	4 (7.1)	
Kaposi Syndrome	1 (5.3)	2 (3.6)	
Non Hodgkin Lymphoma	0	2 (3.6)	
No report	10 (52.6)	24 (42.9)	
ART, n (%)			0.11 [‡]
No	10 (52.6)	18 (32.1)	
Yes	9 (47.4)	38 (67.9)	
Ganciclovir treatment, n (%)			0.34 [*]
Endovenous	10 (52.6)	24 (42.9)	
Intravitreal	3 (15.8)	3 (5.4)	
Endovenous - intravitreal	2 (10.5)	13 (23.2)	
Endovenous - oral	2 (10.5)	4 (7.1)	
None	2 (10.5)	12 (21.4)	
CMVR location, n (%)			0.74 [*]
Zone 1	15 (78.9)	46(82.1)	
Zone 2	0(0.0)	2 (3.6)	
Zone 3	4(21.1)	8 (14.3)	

*Fisher's Exact test
† Mann-Whitney test
‡ Pearson Chi-Square test

Table 4. Hazard ratios for time-to-death after HIV diagnosis in patients with CMV retinitis in Peru, 2004 to 2013

Age	n	Unadjusted HR (95% C.I)*	P value	Adjusted HR (95% C.I)*	P value
At HIV diagnosis	75	0.94 (0.89 – 0.99)	0.031	0.98 (0.85 – 1.13)	0.82
At CMVR diagnosis	75	0.94 (0.89 – 0.99)	0.026	0.95 (0.83 – 1.09)	0.51

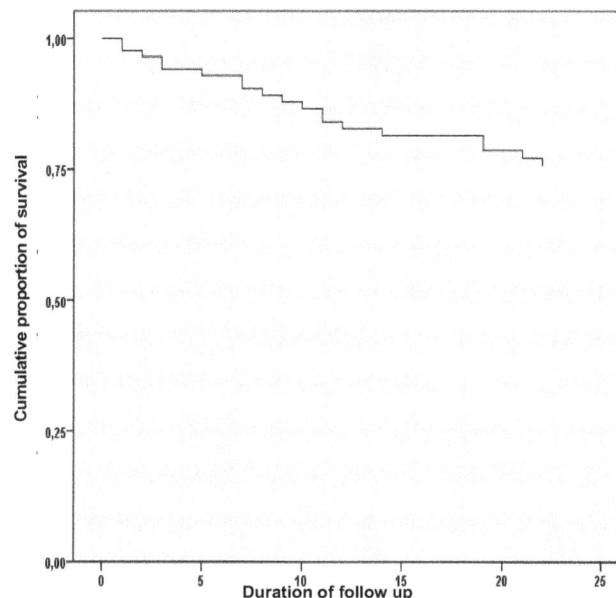

Fig. 1. Shows the Kaplan-Meier curve for survival

Peru is the second country with the most cases of patients with TB in Latin America, and has higher TB prevalence in HIV-AIDS patients. In this study, TB the most common associated disease was diagnosed in 23 patients (30.7%). HIV-TB co-infection is present in many countries of Latin America, and has an estimated prevalence of 25% [7]. National reports of 2013 showed that HIV-TB co-infection represents a serious public health problem in our country and only 42,4% of patients were treated [1,2].

In 55.4% of eyes, retinitis was localized in zone 1, an important retinal area which is associated with a high risk of vision loss. The management of CMVR consisted in intravenous initial therapy (induction therapy) and locally administered intravitreal ganciclovir as is reported previously [15,16]. Retinitis reactivation (10.6% of eyes) was observed generally after the first month. It is explained by many comorbidities in the patients, very low levels of CD4 and none or inadequate treatment with ganciclovir by the difficulty of accessing this medicine. At the beginning of the study, donated ganciclovir tablets were obtained

and 6 patients received in the maintenance therapy of CMVR for few months. It should be noted as a limitation of the study have not recorded the side effects of systemic treatment with intravenous ganciclovir as neutropenia, thrombocytopenia, rash, nephrotoxicity, and gastrointestinal symptom whose incidence is reduced with oral treatment.

CMVR is a neglected disease, largely undiagnosed and untreated. Workable diagnostic and therapeutic strategies have not yet been defined, and CMV is absent from current and pending World Health Organization (WHO) guidelines for the management of HIV in resource-limited settings [17]. Clinical risk factors recognized as predictors for CMVR, may be useful to clinicians and health policy experts in developing guidelines for screening, examination frequency targeted prophylaxis for CMVR in patients with AIDS [18].

Future care by Health Ministries in developing countries and WHO worldwide, will prevent that many HIV - AIDS young people be permanently blind by undiagnosed or poorly treated CMVR.

4. CONCLUSION

Results showed that cytomegalovirus retinitis has a high prevalence in young people with an elevated value of HIV-TB co-infection (30.7%). CMVR diagnosis was a predictor for early mortality, despite receiving ART.

CONSENT

It is not applicable.

ETHICAL APPROVAL

Institutional Ethics Committee approval was obtained.

ACKNOWLEDGEMENTS

The author wishes to acknowledge the assistance provided by Norma Pletikosic Silva in revising the text.

COMPETING INTERESTS

Author has declared that no competing interests exist.

REFERENCES

1. Informe Nacional sobre los progresos realizados en el País-Perú. Período enero 2012 – diciembre 2013. Accessed:15 December 2014. Available:http://www.unaids.org/sites/defau lt/files/country/documents//PER_narrative_ report_2014.pdf / (Spanish)
2. Reyes M, Pun M. Análisis de la situación epidemiológica del VIH/SIDA en el Perú, 2013. Ministerio de Salud de Salud. Dirección Dirección General de Epidemiología, 2013. Accessed:15 December 2014. Available:http://www.unaids.org/sites/defau lt/files/country/documents//PER_narrative_ report_2014.pdf / (Spanish)
3. Jabs DA. AIDS and ophthalmology. Arch Ophthalmol. 2008,126(8):1143–1146.
4. Deayton JR, Sabin CA, Johnson MA, Emery VC, Wilson P, Griffiths PD. Importance of cytomegalovirus viraemia in risk of disease progression and death in HIV-infected patients receiving highly active antiretroviral therapy. Lancet. 2004;363(9427):2116-2221.
5. Thorne JE, Jabs DA, Kempen JH, Holbrook JT, Nichols C, Meinert CL. Studies of Ocular Complications of AIDS Research Group. Incidence of and risk factors for visual acuity loss among patients with AIDS and cytomegalovirus retinitis in the era of highly active antiretroviral therapy. Ophthalmology. 2006;113(8):1432–1440.
6. Jabs DA. Cytomegalovirus retinitis and the acquired immunodeficiency syndrome – bench to bedside: LXVII Edward Jackson Memorial Lecture. Am J Ophthalmol. 2011;151(2):198–216.
7. Gao J, Zheng P, Fu H. Prevalence of TB/HIV co-infection in countries except China: A systematic review and meta-analysis. PLoS One. 2013;8(5):e64915.
8. Kestelyn PG, Cunningham ET Jr. HIV/AIDS and blindness. Bull World Health Organ. 2001;79(3):208–213.
9. Holland GN, Buhles WC Jr, Mastre B, Kaplan HJ. A controlled retrospective study of ganciclovir treatment for cytomegalovirus retinopathy. Use of a standardized system for the assessment of disease outcome. UCLA CMV Retinophathy. Study Group. Arch Ophthalmol. 1989;107(12):1759-1766.
10. Balo KP, Amoussou YP, Bechetoille A, Mihluedo H, Djagnikpo PA, Akpandja SM, Banla MJ. Cytomegalovirus retinitis and ocular complications in AIDS patients in Togo. J Fr Ophthalmol. 1999;22(10): 1042–1046.
11. Teoh S C, Wang PX, Won EPY. The epidemiology and incidence of cytomegalovirus retinitis in the HIV population in Singapore over 6 years. Invest Ophthalmol Vis Sci. 2012;53(12):7546–7552.
12. Pertel P, Hirschtick R, Phair J, Chmiel J, Poggensee L, Murphy R. Risk of developing cytomegalovirus retinitis in persons infected with the human immunodeficiency virus. J Acquir Immune Defic Synd. 1992;5(11):1069-1074.
13. Tun N, London N, Kyaw Kyaw M, Smithuis F, Ford N, Margolis T, Drew WL, Lewallen S, Heiden D. CMV retinitis screening and treatment in a resource-poor setting: Three-year experience from a primary care HIV/AIDS programme in Myanmar. Journal of the International AIDS Society. 2011;14:41.

14. Pauriah M, Ong EL. Retrospective study of CMV retinitis in patients with AIDS. Clin Microbiol Infect. 2000;6(1):14–18.

15. Kempen JH, Jabs DA, Wilson LA, Dunn JP, West SK, Tonascia J. Mortality risk for patients with cytomegalovirus retinitis and acquired immunodeficiency syndrome. Clin Infect Dis. 2003;37(10):1365-1373.

16. Jabs DA, Ahuja A, Van Natta M, Dunn JP, Yeh S. Studies of the ocular complications of AIDS research group. Comparison of treatment regimens for cytomegalovirus retinitis in patients with AIDS in the era of highly active antiretroviral therapy. Ophthalmology. 2013;120(6):1262-1270.

17. Heiden D, Ford N, Wilson D, Rodriguez WR, Margolis T, Janssens B, Bedelu M, Tun N, Goemaere E, Saranchuk P, Sabapathy K, Smithuis F, Luvirika E, Drew WL. Cytomegalovirus retinitis: The neglected disease of the AIDS pandemic. PLoS Med. 2007;4(12):e334.

18. Hodge WG, Boivin JF, Shapiro SH, Lalonde RG, Shah KC, Murphy BD, Dionne MA, Goela A. Clinical risk factors for cytomegalovirus retinitis in patients with AIDS. Ophthalmology. 2004;111(7):1326-1333.

Diplopia and Strabismus in Diabetics (Type II) and Non-diabetics in Yazd, Iran

Mitra Dehghan Harati[1], Mohammad Reza Besharati[2*], Elahe Abbasi Shavazi[1], Mohammad Afkhami Ardekani[3], Samira Salimpur[4] and Sajjad Besharati[5]

[1]*Geriatric Ophthalmology Research Center, Shahid Sadoughi University of Medical Sciences, Yazd, Iran.*
[2]*Department of Ophthalmology, Geriatric Ophthalmology Research Center, Shahid Sadoughi University of Medical Sciences, Yazd, Iran.*
[3]*Department of Endocrinology, Diabetes Research Center, Shahid Sadoughi University of Medical Sciences, Yazd, Iran.*
[4]*Department of Ophthalmology, Shahid Sadoughi University of Medical Sciences, Yazd, Iran.*
[5]*Shahid Beheshti University of Medical Sciences, Tehran, Iran.*

Authors' contributions

This work was carried out in collaboration between all authors. Author MRB designed the study, Author MDH wrote the protocol, and wrote the first draft of the manuscript, and collected the data and revised. Author EAS managed the literature searches, and revised. Author MAA did expert consultation. Author SS collaborated in collecting data, and author SB collaborated in revising. All authors read and approved the final manuscript.

Editor(s):
(1) Tatsuya Mimura, Department of Ophthalmology, Tokyo Women's Medical University Medical Center East, Japan.
(2) Kota V Ramana, Department of Biochemistry & Molecular Biology, University of Texas Medical Branch, USA.
Reviewers:
(1) Jose Francisco de Sales Chagas, Department of Surgery. School of Medicine. Catholic University Campinas, Brazil.
(2) Anonymous, Northwestern University, USA.
(3) Anonymous, University of Incarnate Word, USA.
(4) Fernanda Teixeira Krieger, Doutora em Oftalmologia pela Faculdade de Medicina de Ribeirão Preto da Universidade de São Paulo - USP-Ribeirão Preto (SP) – Brazil.

ABSTRACT

Purpose: To describe the frequency of diplopia and strabismus in diabetics (Type II) and non-diabetics in Yazd, Iran.
Methods: This is a cross-sectional study on 3000 patients including 1500 diabetics (type II) and 1500 non-diabetics in Yazd from 2011 to 2012.Based on aims, a questionnaire was designed and data including, demographic data, duration of diabetes, presence of diplopia or strabismus,

*Corresponding author: E-mail: besharaty@gmail.com

duration of them, and involved cranial nerves were gathered and documented. Data were analyzed by SPSS (ver. 16) using descriptive statistics, chi-square, fisher and T tests.

Results: Diplopia existed in 6(0.4%) diabetic and 13(0.9%) non-diabetic patients, without statistically significant difference (p-value=0.107). Strabismus existed in 6(0.4%) diabetic and 10(0.7%) non-diabetic patients, without statistically significant difference (p-value=0.316).Mean duration of diabetes was 11±7.42 years. There was no statistical difference between the two groups in terms of gender. Sixth nerve palsies were accounted for the majority of patients with strabismus in the two groups.

Conclusion: There was no statistically significant difference in frequency of diplopia and strabismus between diabetics and non-diabetics.

Keywords: Diplopia; strabismus; diabetics; non-diabetics.

1. INTRODUCTION

The ability to maintain visual axis alignment depends on coordination of eye movements. Diabetes mellitus (DM) is a rare benign cause of cranial neuropathy. Extra-ocular motility disorders may occur in diabetic patients, secondary to diabetic neuropathy, involving third, fourth, or sixth cranial nerves [1]. Many factors cause disruption of alignment and lead to diplopia or eye deviation. Cranial nerve palsy is one of them that may be precipitated by diabetes [2]. Diabetic mono-neuropathy appears to be a serious problem from a diagnostic and therapeutic point of view. Cranial neuropathies in diabetic patients are extremely rare and occur in older individuals with long duration of diabetes [3-5]. Ophthalmoplegia is usually seen in patients with mild and long term diabetes, so it associates with complications such as retinopathy, neuropathy and lens opacity [6].

Strabismus is misalignment of eyes in any direction [7]. Paralysis strabismus is a diagnostic and therapeutic challenge in ophthalmology. Isolated sixth nerve palsy is usually associated with diabetes, hypertension and atherosclerosis [8].

Different incidences of cranial nerve palsies in diabetic patients have been reported. Patients with diabetes have a 10-fold increase in the incidence of cranial nerve palsy, with an incidence of 1% among diabetics compared with an incidence of 0.1% for the non-diabetic population [4]. In the present study, we have reported the relative frequency of diplopia and strabismus in diabetics (Type II) and non-diabetics in Yazd, Iran.

2. MATERIALS AND METHODS

In this cross-sectional study, we studied 3000 patients including 1500 diabetics (type II) referred to Yazd diabetes center and 1500 non-diabetics from ophthalmology clinic of Shahid Sadughi hospital, Yazd, from 2011 to 2012.

Based on aims, a questionnaire designed and data including, demographic data, duration of diabetes, presence of diplopia or strabismus and duration of them, and involved cranial nerves were gathered and documented. Inclusion criteria were admitted non-diabetic patients in ophthalmology clinic of Shahid Sadughi hospital, Yazd, for any reason and type II diabetic patients referred to diabetes center for any reason. Patients with congenital strabismus were excluded. The questionnaire was completed by a general practitioner. Primary status of patients was detected and suspicious cases were referred to ophthalmologist for orthoptic evaluation.

Collected data were analyzed by SPSS (version 16) based on aims, using descriptive statistics, chi-square, fisher and T tests. Statistically significance level was set at 0.05.

3. RESULTS

In this study, 3000 patients including 1500 diabetics [639(42.6%) males and 861(57.4%) females] and 1500 non-diabetics [628(41.9%) males and 872(58.1%) females] were selected. There was no statistical difference between the two groups in terms of gender (p-value=0.684). Mean duration of diabetes was 11±7.42 years. Mean age in diabetic and non-diabetic groups was 61.04±10.84 and 36.32±12.63 respectively, with statistical difference (p-value<0.001). Overall, the mean age of patients with and without diplopia was 45±13.11 and 48.70±17.09 respectively, without statistically differences (p-value= 0.346). Also, the mean age of patients with and without strabismus was 46.5±11.72 and 48.69±17.09 respectively, without statistically differences (p value= 0.608). The mean age of diabetic and non-diabetic patients with diplopia was 51±13.26 and 42.23±12.58 respectively, without statistically differences (p-value= 0.18). Also, the mean age of diabetic and non-diabetic patients with strabismus was 51±13.26 and 43.8±10.47 respectively, without statistically differences (p-value= 0.24). Therefore, we ignored the role of age in frequency of diplopia and strabismus in the two groups.

As indicated in Table 1, diplopia existed in 6(0.4%) diabetic patients and 13(0.9%) non-diabetics. The difference between the two groups was not statistically significant (p-value=0.107). Also, strabismus existed in 6(0.4%) diabetic patients and 10(0.7%) non-diabetics without statistically significant difference (p-value=0.316). Table 2 shows the mean age of patients with and without diplopia and strabismus in diabetic and non- diabetic groups. As indicated in Table 2, mean age in diabetic patients with diplopia was 51±13.26 while in diabetic patients without diplopia was 61.08±10.82 which shows statistically significant difference between the two groups (P-value=0.023). Mean age in diabetic patients with strabismus was 51±13.26 while in diabetic patients without strabismus was 61.08±10.82 which shows statistically significant difference between the two groups (P-value=0.023).

Mean age in non-diabetic patients with diplopia was 42.23±12.58 and in non-diabetic group without diplopia was 36.27±12.62; the difference between the two groups was not statistically significant (P-value=0.09).

Mean age in nan-diabetic patients with strabismus was 43.8±10.47and in nan-diabetic patients without strabismus was 36.27±12.63and the difference between the two groups was not statistically significant (P-value=0.06). We conclude from Table 2 that effect of diabetes on cranial nerve palsy is stronger than age. So statistical difference in the mean age between two groups don't have strong effect on result of our study.

Paralysis was the cause of strabismus in 6 diabetic patients and 7 non-diabetic patients. Sixth nerve palsy was accounted for the majority of patients with strabismus in the two groups, with 5 and 7 cases in diabetics and non-diabetics respectively.

As the frequency of diplopia and strabismus in all patients in terms of gender is shown in Table 3, the difference between the two groups was not statistically significant. Overall, 9 patients (3 diabetics and 6 non-diabetics) had systemic disease comorbidity such as hypertension (4 patients), hyperlipidemia (2 patients), thyroid disease (1 patient), hypertension and thyroid disease (1 patient), hyperlipidemia and thyroid disease (1 patient).

4. DISCUSSION

Approximately 1-14% of diabetics have ocular motor nerves palsy during the course of the disease [9,10]. Despite being a rare entity in diabetes mellitus, ophthalmoplegia is associated with great anxiety for patients, and often appears to be a serious problem from a diagnostic and therapeutic point of view [5].

Table 1. Frequency of diplopia and strabismus in diabetic and non-diabetic group

Cases / Groups	With diplopia	Without diplopia	P value	With strabismus	Without strabismus	P value
Diabetics	6(0.4%)	1494(99.6%)	0.107	6(0.4%)	1494(99.6%)	0.316
Non-diabetics	13(0.9%)	1487(99.1%)		10(0.7%)	1490(99.3%)	
Total	19(0.6%)	2981(99.4%)		16(0.5%)	2984(99.5%)	

Chi-square test

Table 2. The mean age of different groups

* / Groups	With diplopia	Without diplopia	P-value	With strabismus	Without strabismus	P-value
Diabetics	51±13.26	61.08±10.82	0.023	51±13.26	61.08±10.82	0.023
Non-diabetics	42.23±12.58	36.27±12.62	0.09	43.8±10.47	36.27±12.63	0.06

*T test; *Mean age±SD*

Table 3. The frequency of diplopia and strabismus in all patients based on gender

Gender / Patients	Male	Female	p-value
With diplopia	8(0.6%)	11(0.6%)	0.991
Without diplopia	1259(99.4%)	1722(99.4%)	
With strabismus	7(0.6%)	9(0.5%)	0.902
Without strabismus	1260(99.4%)	1724(99.5%)	

Chi-Square test

In the present study, we reported diplopia in 0.4% diabetic patients and in 0.9% non-diabetics. Also strabismus existed in 0.4% diabetic patients and in 0.7% non-diabetics without any statistically significant difference.

Large randomized clinical trials on individuals with type 1 or type 2 DM have conclusively demonstrated that reduction in chronic hyperglycemia prevents or delays microvascular complications. Genetic and other unknown factors may affect the development of complications. For example, despite long-standing DM, some individuals never develop nephropathy or retinopathy [9]. Blood sugar might be controlled in patients referred to diabetes centers so that incidence of complications such as diplopia and strabismus would be lower than expected. Moreover, among diabetic patients with diplopia and strabismus, 2 cases had hypertension and 1 case had hypertension and hyperlipidemia. Among non-diabetic patients with diplopia and strabismus, 4 cases had hypertension, 2cases had hyperlipidemia and 2 cases had thyroid disease that may be as a disturbing factor on development of cranial nerves palsy. Also, overlapping between causes of cranial nerve palsy in both groups could cause no statistically significant difference between the two groups.

The frequency of diplopia and strabismus (cranial nerve palsy) in diabetic patients in our study was 0.4%. According to Greco's study, 0.75% of 8150 diabetic patients had cranial nerve palsy during 12 years6. Also, based on another study by Greco [5], 0.4% of 6765 diabetic patients had ophthalmoplegia that is consistent with our results. In Chebel study, 16 patients with DM were associated with ocular motor nerves palsy. All of those complaining of acute diplopia with headaches were recorded and there was a female predominance with mean age of 67±13.9 years. A long history of DM was observed in all patients, with mean duration of 16±5.8 years (ranging from 5-27 years) [10].Mean duration of diabetes in our study was 11±7.42 years too.

Other vascular risk factors or chronic diseases in Chebel reports were arterial hypertension in 9 patients and hyperlipidemia in 4 cases, which was more than vascular risk factors in our report.

In our study, all diabetic patients with diplopia had strabismus. In Greco study5, all patients were presented with clinical signs of affected cranial ocular nerves including double vision, loss of or impaired motility of the eyeball, and deviation of the eyeball. The frequency of strabismus in other studies is near to non-diabetics in our survey [11].

Paralysis of the sixth cranial nerve is identified as the most common type in some literature [12-14], while the third cranial nerve was the most affected in some others [5,10,15,16]. In our patients, the sixth nerve was the most frequently involved which versus Greco reports. No palsy of the fourth nerve was reported in the same period as others; this finding confirms that the trochlear nerve is the least involved in diabetic ophthalmoplegia [5].

5. CONCLUSION

According to this study, no statistically significant difference was seen in frequency of diplopia and strabismus between diabetic and non-diabetic groups.

CONSENT

Not applicable.

ETHICAL APPROVAL

Local Ethics Committee approval was obtained for this retrospective study and consent forms were not required.

COMPETING INTERESTS

Authors have declared that no competing interests exist.

REFERENCES

1. Urso DL, Formaro L, Scattarella L, Curia A, Passavanti G. Sixth cranial nerve palsy associated with diabetes. Recenti Prog Med. 2011;102(1):20-22.
2. Acaroglu G, Akinci A, Zilelioglu O. Retinopathy in patients with diabetic ophthalmoplegia. Ophthalmoplegia. 2008;222(4):225-228.
3. Boulton AJM, Arezzo JC, Lamik RA, Sosenko JM. Diabetic somatic neuropathies. Diabetes Care. 2004;27:1458–1486.
4. Watanabe K, Hagura R, Akanuma Y, Takasu T, Kajinuma H, Kuzuya N, Irie M. Characteristics of cranial nerve palsies in diabetic patients. Diabetes Res Clin Pract. 1990;10:19–27.
5. Greco D, Gambina F, Maggio F. Ophthalmoplegia in diabetes mellitus. Acta Diabetol. 2009;46(1):23-26.
6. Greco D, Gambina F, Pisciotta M, Abrignani M, Maggio F. Clinical characteristics and associated comorbidities in diabetic patients with cranial nerve palsies. J Endocrinol Invest. 2012;35(2):146-149.
7. Falahati J, Jadidi R. Exodeviation prevalence in patients referring with headache or asthenopia to the ophthalmology clinic of Amir Kabir Hospital of Arak in 2006. Arak University of Medical Sciences Journal. 2010;13(1):113-118.
8. Zafer K, Yahya C, Mcem U, Kazim U, Meryem K, Sait A. Isolated bilateral sixth nerve palsy secondary to metastatic carcinoma: a case report with a review of the literature. Clini Neurology and Neurosurgery. 2003;106(1):51-55.
9. El Mansouri Y, Zaghloul K, Amraoni A. Oculomotor paralysis in the course of diabetes. JFr Ophthalmol. 2000;23(1):14-18.
10. Chebel S, Bouatay AB, Ammar M, Ben-Yahia S, Khairallah M, Ayed MF. Diabetes mellitus-associated ocular motor nerve palsies. Neurosciences. 2009;14(4):386-8.
11. Ojaghi H, Masoumi R, Chegini AR. Level of visual disorders in clients referred to medical exemption commission of Alavi hospital in Ardabil. Iranian Journal of Military Medicine. 2011;12(4):235-240.
12. Rush JA, Younge BR. Paralysis of cranial nerves III, IV, and VI: cause and prognosis in 1000 cases. Arch Ophthalmol. 1981;99:76–79.
13. Lazzaroni F, Laffi GL, Galuppi V, Scorolli L. Paralysis of oculomotor nerves in diabetes mellitus. A retrospective study of44 cases. Rev Neurol Paris. 1993;149:571–573.
14. Tiffin PA, MacEwen CJ, Craig EA, Clayton G. Acquired palsy of the oculomotor, trochlear and abducens nerves. Eye. 1996;10:377–384.
15. Berlit P. Isolated and combined pareses of cranial nerves III, IV, and VI. A retrospective study of 412 patients. J Neurol Sci. 1991;103:10–15.
16. Dominguez D, Gomensoro J, Temesio P, Rodriguez-Barrios R. Diabetic ophthalmoplegia. Acta Diabet Lat. 1974;11:198–205.

4

Rasayana Pills in Cataract- An Integration of Ancient Knowledge and Scientific Evidences

Amandeep Kaur[1], Vikas Gupta[1], Ajay Francis Christopher[1] and Parveen Bansal[1*]

[1]*Division of Herbal Drug Technology, University Centre of Excellence in Research, Baba Farid University of Health Sciences, Faridkot, India.*

Authors' contributions

This work was carried out in collaboration between all authors. Authors AK and PB designed the study, wrote the protocol, and wrote the first draft of the manuscript. Authors VG, AFC and PB managed the literature searches. All authors read and approved the final manuscript.

Editor(s):
(1) Li Wang, Department of Ophthalmology, Cullen Eye Institute, Baylor College of Medicine, USA.
Reviewers:
(1) Sagili Chandarsekhara Reddy, University of Malaysia, Kuala Lumpur, Malaysia.
(2) Anonymous, Mansoura University, Egypt.

ABSTRACT

Introduction: Cataract is a principal cause of blindness in the world. Surgery, the major prevailing therapeutic approach for cataract is laced with various complications that include iris prolapse, raised intraocular pressure, infection, cystoid macular oedema and posterior capsular opacification. So world is looking towards more robust and natural ways to prevent cataract.

Aim: *Rasayana* therapy (specially *Caksusya Rasayana*) have been known to play an important role in prevention and cure of eye disorders. This manuscript intends to highlight hypothesis along with the scientific evidences in favour of role of *Rasayanas* in prevention and cure of cataract

Methodology: Extensive internet search and literature search related to Ayurvedic texts on *Rasayana* was conducted. Local Ayurveda experts were contacted to know about commonly used *Rasayana* preparations in cataract. Based on that, *Rasayana* components of these single preparations/polyherbal preparations were searched for their antioxidant, aldose reductase inhibitor and antiglycating activity.

Results: Metadata analysis and perusal of ancient texts on Ayurveda and scientific studies on the evidences in favour of some *Rasayanas* and some specific *Caksusya Rasayana* show ability of *Rasayana* to act as anticataract agents by acting through one or the other molecular mechanism. It is also important to note that some of these *Rasayanas* like *Yashthimadhu, Shunthi, Haridra,*

Corresponding author: E-mail: bansal66@yahoo.com, aman11091991@gmail.com

Amalaki, Tulsi, Pippali and *Triphala Rasayana* are very common component of daily kitchen use and can be a better therapy for patient compliance.

Conclusion: From the metadata analysis it may be concluded that most of the *Rasayanas* possess antioxidant, antiglycating and aldose reductase inhibitory activity, either singly or simultaneously and thus they can prevent or revert changes responsible for cataract pathogenesis. So it is pertinent to mention here that use of *Rasayana* therapy have the potentials to work against the development of cataract and should be explored for scientific evidences for mechanism of action.

Keywords: Antioxidants; cataract; free radicals; Caksusya Rasayana.

1. INTRODUCTION

Cataract, a principal cause of blindness in the world is characterized by the clouding of the eye's natural lens, due to aggregation of proteins in the lens resulting in clouding of the lens and formation of cataract. According to most recent estimates by World Health Organization (WHO), 47.8% of global blindness is due to cataract whereas in India cataract is the principal cause of blindness accounting for 77.5% of blindness [1]. India is one of the signatories in a program "Vision 2020" for elimination of avoidable blindness that can occur due to numerous reasons like aging, infection in new born babies, injury or poor development prior to birth or during childhood or due to complications of various diseases like diabetes or on exposure to toxic substances like UV radiations and various drugs such as corticosteroids or diuretics. There is strong scientific evidence that free radicals and the oxidative stress play an important role in the pathogenesis of cataract [2].

In the early stages of the disease, optimal refractive management and advice on glare reduction can reduce the impact of cataract formation. Surgery is considered when these measures are no longer adequate for the patient's visual needs. The major therapeutic step that can be taken to cure cataract is surgery, but it has its own limitations. Significant intraoperative complications of phacoemulsifaction in experienced hands are rare. Early post-operative complications (iris prolapse, raised IOP and infection) and most common late complications are Cystoid Macular Oedema (CMO) and Posterior Capsular Opacification (PCO) [3]. So there is an urgent need of more robust and natural ways to prevent cataract. One of the important factors that can play a role in prevention of any and many diseases is the diet of people.

Rasayana chikitsa or rejuvenation (making young again) therapy is one of the traditional anti-cataract strategies in Ayurveda. However complete prevention or cure of cataract is possible only if anti-cataract therapy is applied before a critical age. *Rasayana* is one of the eight branches of Ayurveda and are special herbs, fruits or any other form of medication that destroys the old age and disease through the conservation, transformation, and revitalization of energy. To live long and healthy life is the desire of every person, so the main aim of Ayurvedic rejuvenation therapy or *Rasayana* therapy is to restore spirit and attain longevity. It is also known to reverse the disease process and prevent re-occurrence. *Rasayana* therapy is used as a preventive therapy which replenishes the vital fluids of our body, thus keeping us away from diseases [4]. It is one of the important traditional therapies that implies *Caksusya Rasayana* for treatment and prevention of eye disorders. Further the 'caksusya–rasayana' (preservation and promotion of ocular heath) approach of Ayurveda certainly provide safe and clinically effective ophthalmic drugs having diversified effects may be judiciously used to tackle intractable problems of the eye. This manuscript intends to highlight hypothesis along with the scientific evidences in favour of role of commonly used *Rasayanas* that are inadvertently used in kitchen and other *Rasayanas* in prevention and cure of cataract.

2. MATERIALS

Extensive internet search and literature search related to Ayurvedic texts on *Rasayana* was conducted. Pathogenesis of cataract and role of *Rasayana* in various disorders was also reviewed. Local Ayurveda experts were contacted to know about commonly used *Rasayana* preparations in cataract. Based on that, *Rasayana* components of these single preparations/polyherbal preparations were searched for their antioxidant, aldose reductase inhibitor and antiglycating activity.

2.1 Pathogenesis of Cataract

A cataract is a cloudy or opaque area in the lens of the eye that ultimately results in the loss of vision in people over the age of 40 years. The pathways involved in the pathogenesis of cataract are oxidative stress, non-enzymatic glycation and polyol pathway [2,5,6].

2.1.1 Oxidative stress

Oxidative stress is the main cause involved in formation of cataract. On exposure to Reactive Oxygen Species (ROS) like peroxide, superoxide and hydroxyl radicals, UV radiations, smoking and other environment factors, the proteins of the eye lens undergo aggregation and post translational modifications [2]. Hydrogen peroxide (H_2O_2), which is derived from sources both inside and outside the lens, has been considered as the major oxidant in the pathogenesis of cataract. The healthy eye lens contains antioxidants like glutathione, ascorbate and catalase that protect lens proteins against ROS. Glutathione is one of the most important antioxidant found in eye lens. Reduced glutathione (GSH) reacts with ROS and is converted to its oxidized form (GSSG). GSH is restored through the action of the enzyme glutathione reductase (GR). H_2O_2 is eliminated by GSH, or through the action of the enzymes glutathione peroxidase and catalase. Although there is a protective mechanism in the eye lens, yet there is development of oxidative stress. It can occur when there is an imbalance between the production of Reactive Oxygen Species (ROS) and the cellular antioxidant defence mechanisms (protective mechanism). At the same time with increasing age, the activity of these defence mechanisms decreases resulting in protein aggregation and ultimately lens opacification and cataract.

2.1.2 Non-enzymatic glycation

In hyperglycaemic conditions, the increased glucose levels in the aqueous humour may get attached to the lens proteins without the help of enzymes. This process is called non-enzymatic glycation, which leads to the formation of ketoamines termed as Amadori Products and further on oxidation gives rise to Advanced Glycation End products (AGEs) [5]. Accumulation of AGEs results in the generation of free radicals like superoxide radicals (O_2^-) and hydrogen peroxides (H_2O_2), which are involved in development of cataract.

2.1.3 Polyol pathway

In diabetes, there is high concentration of glucose in the aqueous humour, which is passively transported into the lens. The enzyme Aldose Reductase (AR) catalyzes the conversion of glucose to sorbitol through the polyol pathway and it results in intracellular accumulation of sorbitol which further leads to osmotic changes resulting in degeneration of hydropic lens fibers, electrolyte imbalance and formation of cataracts [6].

2.2 Role of *Rasayana* in cataract

2.2.1 Definition of Rasayana [7]

The excerpts from Ayurveda demonstrate that with the application of *Rasayana* treatment, one attains longevity, memory, intelligence, freedom from disorders, youthful age, excellence of luster, complexion and voice, oratory, optimum strength of physique and sense organs, respectability and brilliance. It means the attaining the excellent *Rasa* etc.

2.2.2 Rasayana benefits as per Ayurveda [8]

The excerpts narrate that as was the nectar to the gods and ambrosia for the serpents, so was the *Rasayana* for the great *sages* in early times. The persons using *Rasayana* treatment in early ages lived very long life unaffected by old age, debility, illness and untimely death. One who uses the *Rasayana* treatment methodically attains not only long life but also the auspicious status enjoyed by the godly sages.

दीर्घमायुः स्मृतिं मेधामारोग्यं तरुणं वयः । प्रभावर्णस्वरौदार्यं देहेन्द्रियबलं परम् ॥ ७ ॥

वाक्सिद्धिं प्रणतिं कान्तिं लभते ना रसायनात् । लाभोपायो हि शस्तानां रसादीनां रसायनम् ॥ ८ ॥

dīrghamāyuḥ smṛtiṁ mēdhāmārōgyaṁ taruṇaṁ vayaḥ|
prabhāvaṇasvaraudāryaṁ dēhēndriyabalaṁ param||7||
vāksiddhiṁ praṇatiṁ kāntiṁ labhatēnā rasāyanāt|
lābhōpāyō hi śastānāṁ rasādīnāṁ rasāyanam||8||

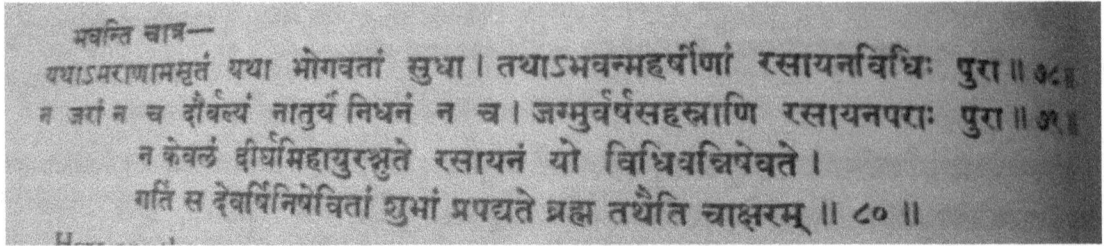

yathamranaamamritam yatha bhogvatam sudha!
Tathabhavnamharsheenam rasayanavidhi pura!!
Na jaram na ch daurbalyam naaturyam nidhanm na ch!
Jagmurvarshashasatraane rasaayanapraa pura!!
Na kewalam deeraghmehayurshrunte rasayanam yo vidhivatreshevate!
Gatim sa devarsheeneshevitam shubham prapdhhate brahma tatheti chaaksharm!!

2.2.3 Theory and concept of *Rasayana*

In terms of Ayurveda, the physical structure consists of 7 *dhatus* i.e. *Rasa* (nutrition part of blood), *Rakta* (Blood cells), *Mamsa* (Muscles and Soft tissue), *Medha* (Lipids), *Asthi* (Bones and Cartilages), *Majja* (Marrow) and *Sukra* (Vital fluid). The word *Rasayana* consists of term *'rasa'* which means nutrition part of blood and *'ayana'* which means circulation and promotion or path. In other words *Rasayana* means nutrition and its transportation in the body. The main concept of *Rasayana* therapy is that according to Ayurveda, the health of all *dhatus* (tissues) of the body is influenced by the qualities of *'Rasa dhatu'*. So any medication, which improves the quality of *'Rasa'(Rasayana)* should strengthen the quality of all *dhatus* of the body and when the quality of all *dhatus* enhances or strengthens, it results in longevity, strong immune system to fight against diseases, development of body and youthfulness [9]. This therapy is normally recommended after 45 yrs of age, in both male and female. The *Rasayana* measures and remedies produce their effect at the level of *Rasa* by directly acting as a nutrient by promoting nutrient value of plasma, at the level of *Agni* by promoting biofire system responsible for digestion and metabolism or at the level of *Srotas* by promoting microcirculation and tissue perfusion. Other than the above mentioned modes of action, most of the *Rasayanas* exhibit specific action on various organs and tissues and thus they are used for specific indications like *Medhya Rasayana* as brain tonic, *Hrdya Rasayana* as cardiotonic, *Twacya Rasayana* as skin tonic, *Kesya Rasayana* as hair tonic, *Caksusya Rasayana* as eye tonic etc.

2.2.4 Mechanism of action of *Rasayana*

It has been studied that generation of free radicals and oxidative stress are involved in pathogenesis of cataract. Free radicals (electrically charged molecules) attack lens cells, cross through cell membranes to react with the nucleic acids, proteins, and enzymes present in the lens. This attack by free radicals is known as oxidative stress, causing cells to lose their structure, function and ultimately destroy them. Free radicals are continuously produced by our body's use of oxygen such as in respiration and some cell-mediated immune functions. They are also generated on an exposure to toxic substances, environmental pollutants, smoke, automobile exhaust, radiations etc. Normally, a balance exists between the amount of free radicals generated in the body and the antioxidant defence systems, which scavenge free radicals, preventing them to cause hazardous effects in the eye lens. However with age, there is decrease in the activity of antioxidant defence systems leading to oxidative stress and subsequent disease development.

Rasayanas are rejuvenating agents, nutritional supplements and possess strong antioxidant activity. They exhibit antagonistic actions on the oxidative stressors and thus prevent formation of different free radicals. They have been found to be a rich source of antioxidants [10]. It has been reported that antioxidant activity of any *'Rasayana'* is 1000 times more potent than ascorbic acid, α-tocopherol and probucol [11]. *Rasayanas* act as preventive antioxidants, attempt to stop formation of ROS [12], scavenge free radicals [13], repair and reconstitute through repair enzymes [14].

2.2.5 *Rasayanas* beneficial role in cataract

It is evident from literature that formation of free radicals plays important role in development of cataract [2]. Therefore, antioxidants are used as a preventive measure in cataract. As it has been discussed earlier that *Rasayanas* has potent antioxidant activity, so it can prove beneficial in cataract. Different *Rasayanas* which exhibit anticataract activity has been enlisted in Fig. 1.

2.2.6 Potential *Rasayanas* in Ayurveda for cataract

2.2.6.1 Amalaki Rasayana

Amalaki Rasayana is herbal formulation mentioned in Ayurveda to prevent cataract. It is extensively used in making Ayurvedic medicines because of its miraculous actions. According to Ayurveda regular usage of *Amla* will make you live more than 100 years like a youth. It is supposed to rejuvenate all the organ systems of the body, provide strength and wellness. It keeps us away from all the diseases by boosting our immune system. *Emblica officinalis* as the main ingredient that is rich source of vitamin C; so, it

possesses antioxidant as well as free radical scavenging activity to minimize free radical induced damage in cataract. Regular use of *Amalaki Rasayana* makes eyes healthy. Various studies confirm the total phenolic and tannin content, free radical scavenging activity, superoxide radical scavenging activity and reducing power [15] of *Emblica officinalis*. It is also known to possess aldose reductase inhibitory activity [16].

2.2.6.2 Ashwagandha Rasayana

Dried roots of *Withania somnifera*, commonly known as "Indian Winter cherry" or "Indian Ginseng". The name *Ashwagandha* is from the Sanskrit language and is a combination of the word *Ashva*, meaning horse, and *gandha*, meaning smell. The root has a strong aroma that is described as "horse-like."

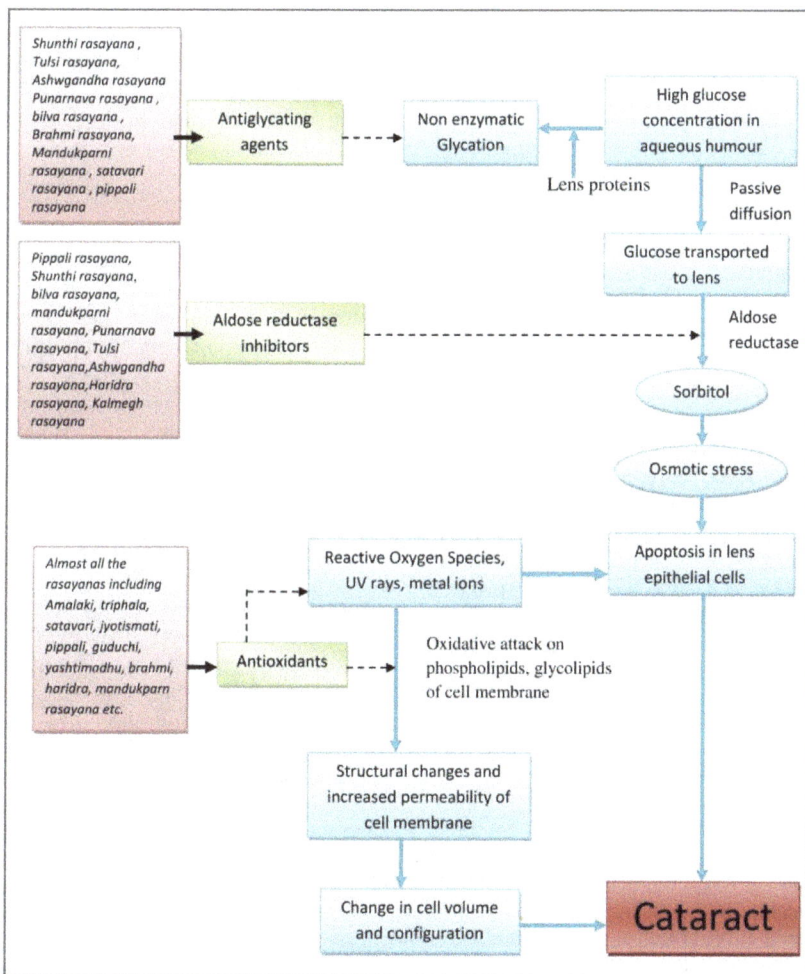

Fig. 1. Diagrammatic representation of mechanism of action of various *Rasayanas*

It is one of the most important herb of Ayurveda (the traditional system of medicine in India) used for millennia as a *Rasayana* for its wide ranging health benefits. *Ashwagandha* is commonly available as a *churna*, a fine sieved powder that can be mixed with water, *ghee* (clarified butter) or honey. A herbal formulation containing *Ashwagandha* has also shown an anti-oxidant activity which is having natural antioxidant, self replicating and sustained action. The studies reveal that it acts as antioxidant [17], antiglycating agent [18] and aldose reductase inhibitor [19]. It contains withanolides, piperidine and pyrrolidine alkaloids, flavonol glycosides and phenolic acids.

2.2.6.3 Bilva Rasayana

Also known as the "Wood Apple", *Aegle marmelos* or Bael, is a species native to India. *Bilva* tree is considered to be sacred to the Hindus. A famous drink known as *sharbet* (Syrup) is made from the bael fruit and it has been known for its medicinal values since 2000 BC. It contains protein, beta-carotene, vitamins, thiamine, riboflavin and vitamin C, aegelin [20], lupeol [21], cineol [22], citral [23], citronellal [24], cuminaldehyde [25], eugenol [26], marmesinin [27] as the chief constituents. Studies confirm that it is an antioxidant [28], antiglycating agent [29] as well as inhibitor of aldose reductase [30]. So, it plays significant role in prevention of cataract.

2.2.6.4 Brahmi Rasayana

It is known as *Jalanimba* or *Bacopa monniera*. The name *Brahmi* is derived from the word "Brahma", the mythical "creator" in the Hindu pantheon. This extracted oil is very beneficial and can be used to treat a number of different ailments in Ayurveda as well as Japanese traditional medicine. *Bacopa monniera* contains luteolin, apigenin, quercetin, hersaponin alkaloid viz herpestine [31-33]. It is responsible for antioxidant activity [34].

2.2.6.5 Guduchi Rasayana

Also known as *Tinospora cordifolia*, or Amrita, is an immune system boosting herb that can potently reduce the symptoms of allergic rhinitis. It is a promising anti-cancer herb and may provide benefits for people with diabetes. Alcoholic root extract has antioxidant defence mechanism in alloxan induced diabetic rats. The herb has strong free radical scavenging

properties against reactive oxygen and nitrogen species as revealed by electron paramagnetic resonance spectroscopy. *Guduchi* is also a powerful *Rasayana*(longevity enhancer) even by itself, but especially when combined with complementary herbs. It contains alkaloids-berberine, palmatine, tembetarine, magnoflorine [35-39], sesquiterpenoid-tinocordifolin [40]. *Guduchi* have tendency to act as antioxidant [41] and inhibit aldose reductase [42].

2.2.6.6 Haridra Rasayana

Haldi(*Curcuma longa*) is commonly used spice in most of kitchens in India and abroad. Curcumin is an important active component of *haldi*. *Haridra's* ability to reduce oxidative stress makes it helpful in the management of conditions such as leukoplakia, diabetes mellitus, chronic eye disease and tissue injury. *Haridra* inhibits aldose reductase enzyme [19]. Also it is an antioxidant [43], antiglycating agent as it exhibited significant inhibitory activity against AGEs formation [44]. It is potent antioxidant that can neutralize free radicals due to its chemical structure and it also boosts the activity of the body's own antioxidant enzymes.

2.2.6.7 Jyotismati Rasayana

Popularly being described as *Jyotishmati*, this plant has an important role in enhancing cognitive function and the natural luminosity (*jyoti*) of the mind (*mati*), commonly known as *Malkangni, Jyotishmati*, Intellect Tree, Black oil, Bitter sweet, is an important Indian medicinal plant (*Celastrus paniculata*,) belonging to family Celastraceae. The phytochemical profile of *Jyotismati* shows the presence of terpenoids, flavonoids, glycosides and saponins. Petroleum ether extracts of *Celastrus paniculatus* seeds exhibited significant role in medicinal chemistry for formulation of life saving drugs. *Jyotismati* oil is used in formulation of Ayurvedic eye drops for the treatment for cataract. The strong antioxidant activity of this plant has been evaluated by phytochemical examination [45].

2.2.6.8 Mandukparni Rasayana

Also known as Gotu kola, Indian Pennywort, Jal Brahmi and has been used since ancient times as a medicinal herb. *Centella asiatica*, almost whole plant is of great importance. A study revealed that it contains alkaloids, flavonoids, phenols and tannins [46]. It possesses antioxidant [47], aldose reductase inhibitory activity [48] as well as antiglycating activity [49].

2.2.6.9 Pippali Rasayana

It is known as *Piper longum* or long pepper. It is having slender, aromatic, perennial climber, with woody roots and numerous wide ovate, cordate leaves. The active constituents responsible for the desired activity are α-terpineol, 1, 8-cineol, citral, α-pinene, piperolnol, vitamin A, C, E, K and β-carotene [50]. *Pippali* is a centre of attraction as sources of effective antioxidants Vitamins A, Vitamin E, Vitamin K are the major vitamins found in the *Pippali*. So it has the potential to prevent cataract. It is evident from the study that *Pippali* proteins act as antioxidants by inhibiting lipid peroxidation and by scavenging free radicals [51]. A study has been conducted to detect aldose reductase inhibitory activity of *Piper longum* [52].

2.2.6.10 Punarnava Rasayana

It is rightly called *Punarnava (Boerhavia diffusa)* as it brings back lost vigour and vitality. This is a miracle herb with wonderful health benefits and medicinal uses. Regular consumption of *Punarnava* root decoction or the dried root powder mixed with honey daily has been recommended for all the disorders of the eyes like night blindness, glaucoma, gradually reducing vision, cataract and persistent irritation in the eyes. It contains sitosterol, esters of sitosterol, punarnavine, boerhaavia acid, boeravinone, palmitic acid and other flavonoids and phenols responsible for antioxidant activity [53]. The fresh juice of its roots instilled into eyes, mitigates the ailments of the eyes like night blindness and conjunctivitis.

2.2.6.11 Satavari Rasayana

It is a very well known *Rasayana* that contains parts of *Asparagus racemosus,* belonging to family Asparagaceae. *Satavari* means "who possesses a hundred husbands or acceptable to many". In Ayurveda, this amazing herb is known as the "Queen of herbs", because it promotes love and devotion. The health benefits of *Satavari* are inumerable and include fertility, relief from pre-menstrual syndrome, cancer, diabetes, hangover, cataract, rheumatism, tuberculosis, depression, neurodegenerative diseases, and convulsions. It also reduces urinary tract infections and blood cholesterol. Asparagus is a source of vitamin A, which is essential for good vision. Due to the presence of antioxidants, it helps in defending the retina from the damage caused by the oxygen-free radicals.

The presence of the amino acid glutathione in asparagus also helps in reducing the risk of eye ailments such as cataracts and night blindness. Apart from this, it contains polycyclic alkaloid- Aspargamine A, pyrrolizidine alkaloid [54,55], isoflavones known as 8-methoxy- 5, 6, 4-trihydroxy isoflavone-7-0-beta-D-glucopyranoside [56], polysacharides [57], flavanoids- quercitin, rutin and hyperoside are present in flower and fruits [58]. The antioxidant, antiglycating activity and aldose reductase inhibitory activity of *Satavari* has been studied [59].

2.2.6.12 Shunthi Rasayana

Shunthi or *sonth* as is popularly called is dried form of ginger, botanically called *Zingiber officinale*. Shunthi/sonth is prepared after drying ginger by processing it through lime water. *Shunthi/sonth* is one of the constituent of commonly used *Trikatu* powder. It is beneficial in prevention of eye disorders. *Zingiber officinale* contains gingerol which is very effective agent for anticipation of ultra violet B (UVB)-induced reactive oxygen species production [60] and also it contains 2-(4-hydroxy-3-methoxyphenyl) ethanol responsible for aldose reductase inhibitory activity [61]. It is also revealed that *Shunthi* possesses antiglycating activity [62].

2.2.6.13 Triphala Rasayana

Triphala is listed in Ayurveda system of medicine and also referenced in traditional Indian texts *Charaka samhita* and *Sushruta samhita*. It is an important medicine of *Rasayana* group and is believed to promote health, immunity and longevity. As per ancient experiences, Indian people are saying that "One Doesn't need to have a mother to take care of you, as long as you take *Triphala* every day." The word *Triphala* means "three fruits." *Triphala* is a very famous and traditional herbal combination used extensively by Ayurvedic healers. This formulaton mainly contains equal parts three herbs, i.e. *Terminalia belerica* (*Vibheetaki*), *Terminalia chebula* (*Haritaki*) & *Emblica officinalis* (*Amla*). Although *Triphala* is most commonly used to cleanse and tone the digestive tract, it is in reality an Ayurvedic *Rasayana*-a rejuvenative herbal blend that delivers benefits to the physiology as a whole. On its phytochemical analysis, it was depicted that *Triphala* contains alkaloidal content, tannins and phenolic compounds, flavonoids, saponins and anthraquinon glycosides [63]. This polyherbal formulation is rich in antioxidant and free radical scavengers thus prevent lipid peroxidation [64]. Consumption of *Maha Triphala Ghrit* along with milk has been indicated in cataract prevention.

2.2.6.14 Tulsi Rasayana

Holi basil *(Ocimum sanctum)* popularly known in India as *'Tulsi'* is worshipped every morning by most Hindus. It is perhaps the most sacred plant in India and is referred to in Ayurveda for its healing and life giving properties. Basil juice is an effective remedy for eye disorders and night-blindness caused by deficiency of vitamin A. Vitamin C, Vitamin A, ursolic acid and the essential oils in *Tulsi*, are excellent anti oxidants and protects the body from nearly all the damages caused by the free radicals. Eyewash with water soaked with few leaves of *Tulsi* soothes eyes and reduces stress. A regular consumption can protect from all the damages done by the free radicals, such as cataract, macular degeneration, glaucoma, vision defects, opthalmia etc. *Tulsi* is a good antioxidant [65], antiglycating agent [66] and aldose reductase inhibitor [19,67] and ultimately beneficial in prevention of cataractogenesis.

2.2.6.15 Yashtimadhu Rasayana

Yashtimadhu is also commonly known as Liquorice *(Glycyrhizza glabra)* renowned for its roots. It contains Semilicoisoflavone B (aldose reductase inhibitor), other than this it contains flavonoids responsible for antioxidant [68], aldose reductase inhibitory and antiglycating activity [69]. It is recommended as *Caksusya Rasayana,* washing eyes with *Yashtimadhu* soaked water has been recommended for preventing eye disorders including cataract.

3. RESULTS AND DISCUSSION

From Table 1, it is very much clear that the *Rasayanas* possess anticataract activity and demonstrate the same through established mechanism. It has been found that these *Rasayanas* act through their antioxidant, antiglycating and aldose reductase inhibitor activity. Metadata analysis and perusal of ancient texts on ayurveda and scientific studies on the evidences in favour of some Rasayanas and some specific Caksusya Rasayana show ability of Rasayana to act as anticataract agents by acting through one or the other molecular mechanism. It is also important to

Table 1. *Rasayanas* having anti-cataract activity

S. no.	*Rasayana*	Main composition	Mechanism of action
1.	Amalaki Rasayana	Fruits of *Emblica officinalis*	Antioxidant, AR inhibitor
2.	Ashwgandha Rasayana	*Withania somnifera*	Antioxidant, AR inhibitor, antiglycating agent
3.	Bilva Rasayana	*Aegle marmelos*	Antioxidant, AR inhibitor, antiglycating agent
4.	Brahmi Rasayana	*Bacopa monniera*	Antioxidant
5.	Guduchi Rasayana	*Tinospora cordifolia*	Antioxidant, AR inhibitor
6.	Haridra Rasayana	*Curcuma longa*	Antioxidant, AR inhibitor, antiglycating agent
7.	Jyotismati Rasayana	*Celastrus paniculatus*	Antioxidant
8.	Mandukparni Rasayana	*Centella asiatica*	Antioxidant, AR inhibitor, antiglycating agent
9.	Pippali Rasayana	*Piper longum*	Antioxidant, AR inhibitor
10.	Punarnava Rasayana	*Boerhaavia diffusa*	Antioxidant
11.	Satavari Rasayana	*Asparagus racemosus*	Antioxidant, antiglycating agent, AR inhibitor
12.	Shunthi Rasayana	*Zingiber officinale*	Antioxidant, AR inhibitor, antiglycating agent
13.	Triphala Rasayana	fruits of *Terminalia belerica, Terminalia chebula & Emblica officinalis*	Antioxidant
14.	Tulsi Rasayana	*Ocimum sanctum*	Antioxidant, AR inhibitor, antiglycating agent
15.	Yashtimadhu Rasayana	*Glycyrhizza glabra*	Antioxidant, AR inhibitor, antiglycating agent.

AR- Aldose reductase

note that some of these *Rasayanas* like *Yashthimadhu, Shunthi, Haridra, Amalaki, Tulsi, Pippali* and *Triphala Rasayana* are very common component of daily kitchen use and can be a better therapy for patient compliance. As cataract is much more prevalent in diabetics and keeping in view all the molecular mechanisms through which these *Rasayanas* could exert anticataract activity, it can be suggested that diabetics should be suggested to use these *Rasayanas* to keep away from cataract.

4. CONCLUSION

Although there are significant advancements in modern medicine for curing the cataract, yet traditional medicine viz *Rasayana* therapy remains one of the important pillars of preventing and curing cataract. This manuscript catches up the eyes towards the scientific evidences in favour of some *Rasayanas* and some specific *Caksusya Rasayana* that have the ability to act as anticataract agents by acting through one or the other molecular mechanism. It is also important to note that some of these *Rasayanas* like *Yashthimadhu, Shunthi, Haridra, Amalaki, Tulsi, Pippali* and *Triphala Rasayana* are very common component of daily kitchen use. From the metadata analysis it may be concluded that most of the *Rasayanas* possess antioxidant, antiglycating and aldose reductase inhibitory activity, either singly or simultaneously and thus they can prevent or revert changes responsible for cataract pathogenesis. So it is pertinent to mention here that use of *Rasayana* therapy have the potentials to work against the development of cataract and should be explored for scientific evidences for mechanism of action.

CONSENT

It is not applicable.

ETHICAL APPROVAL

It is not applicable.

COMPETING INTERESTS

Authors have declared that no competing interests exist.

REFERENCES

1. John N, Rachel J, Vashist P, Murthy GV. Rapid assessment of avoidable blindness in India. PLoS One. 2008;3:e2867. DOI:10.1371/journal.pone.0002867

2. Ottonello S, Foroni C, Carta A, Petrucco S, Maraina M. Oxidative stress and age-related cataract. Ophthalmologica. 2000; 214:78-85.

3. Yorston D. Cataract complications. Community Eye Health Journal. 2008; 21(65):1-3.

4. Chulet R, Pradhan P. A review on rasayana. Phcog Rev. 2009;3(6):229-34.

5. Odjakova M, Popova E, Al Sharif M, Mironova R. Plant-derived agents with anti-glycation activity; 2012. Available:http://dx.doi.org/10.5772/48186

6. Pollreisz A, Schmidt-Erfurth U. Diabetic cataract—pathogenesis, epidemiology and treatment. Journal of Ophthalmo-logy. 2010; 2010:1-8.

7. Sharma PV. Charak Samhita, Section 6, Chapter 1, Qtr 1. Varanasi: Chaukhambha Orientalia. 1998;3-4, Shloka 7-8.

8. Sharma PV. Charak Samhita, 4th Edition, Section 6, Chapter 1, Qtr 1. Varanasi: Chaukhambha Orientalia. 1998;2, Shloka 78-80.

9. Panday KK. Comprehensive human physiology. Varanasi: Chowkhamba Karishnadas Academy; 2011.

10. Brahma S.K, Debnath PK. Therapeutic importance of rasayana drugs with special reference to their multi-dimensional actions. Aryavaidyan. 2003;16:160–3.

11. Sharma HM, Hanna AN, Kauffman EM, Newman HA. Inhibition of human low-density lipoprotein oxidation in vitro by Maharishi Ayurveda herbal mixtures. Pharmacol Biochem Behav. 1992; 43(4):1175–82.

12. Sies H, Murad F. Antioxidants in disease mechanisms and therapy. Advances in Pharmacology. New York: Academic Press; 1996.

13. Cadenas E, Packer L. Hand book of antioxidants. New York: Plenum Publishers; 1996.

14. Halliwell B, Aruoma OI. DNA and free radicals. Boca Raton Press: Minuteman press; 1993.

15. Samarakoon SMS, Chandola HM, Shukla VJ. Evaluation of antioxidant potential of amalakayas rasayana: A polyherbal ayurvedic formulation. International Journal of Ayurveda Research. 2011;2(1):23-8.

16. Suryanarayana P, Kumar PA, Saraswat M, Petrash JM, Reddy GB. Inhibition of aldose reductase by tannoid principles of *Emblica*

officinalis: implications for the prevention of sugar cataract. Mol Vis. 2004;10:148-54.

17. Shahriar M, Hossain I, Sharmin FA, Akhter S, Haque A, Bhuiyan MA. *In vitro* antioxidant and free radical scavenging activity of *Withania somnifera* Root. Iosr Journal of Pharmacy. 2013;3(2):38–47.

18. Babu VP, Gokulakrishnan A, Dhandayuthabani R, Ameethkhan D, Kumar CV, Ahamed MI. Protective effect of *Withania somnifera* (Solanaceae) on collagen glycation and cross-linking. Comp Biochem Physiol B Biochem Mol Biol. 2007;147(2):308-13.

19. Halder N, Joshi S, Gupta SK. Lens aldose reductase inhibiting potential of some indigenous plants. J Ethnopharmacol. 2003;86:113-6.

20. De Smet PA. The role of plant derived drugs and herbal medicines in healthcare. Drugs. 1997;54(6):801-40.

21. Shu YZ. Recent natural products based drug development: A Pharmaceutical industry perspective. J Nat Prod. 1998; 61(8):1053-71.

22. Biswas K, Chattopadhyay I, Banerjee RK, Bandyopadhyay U. Biological activities & medicinal properties of neem (*Azadirachta indica)*. Curr Sci. 2002;82(11):1336-45.

23. Chattopadhyay I, Biswas K, Bandyopadhyay U, Banerjee RK. Turmeric & curcumin: biological actions & medicinal applications. Curr Sci. 2004; 87:44-53.

24. Bandyopadhyay U, Biswas K, Chattopadhyay I, Ganguly CK, Chakraborty T, Battacharya K, et al. Gastroprotective effect of neem (*Azadirachta indica*) bark extract: Possible involvement of H+ K+ ATPase inhibition and scavenging of hydroxyl radical. Life Sci. 2002;71(24):2845-65.

25. Chattopadhyay I, Bandyopadhyay U, Banerjee RK. Mechanism of antiulcer effect of neem (*Azadirachta indica*) leaf extract: Effect on H+K+ATPase, oxidative damage and apoptosis. Inflammopharmacology. 2004;12(2):153-76.

26. Chattopadhyay I, Bandyopadhyay U, Biswas K, Maity P, Banerjee RK. Indomethacin inactivates gastric peroxidase to induce reactive oxygen mediated gastric mucosal injury & curcumin protect it by perventing peroxidase inactivation & scavenging reactive oxygen. Free Radical Biology & Medicine. 2006;40(8):1397-408.

27. Swarnakar S, Ganguly K, Kundu P, Banerjee A, Maity P, Sharma AV. Curcumin regulates expression & activity of matrix metalloproteinases 9 & 2 during prevention & healing of indomethacin induced gastric ulcer. J Biol Chem. 2005; 280(10):9409-15.

28. Upadhya S, Shanbhag KK, Suneetha G, Naidu BM, Upadhya S. A study of hypoglycemic and antioxidant activity of *Aegle marmelos* in alloxan induced diabetic rats. Indian J Physiol Pharmacol. 2004;48(4):476–80.

29. Panaskar SN, Joglekar MM, Taklikar SS, Haldavnekar VS, Arvindekar AU. *Aegle marmelos* correa leaf extract prevents secondary complications in streptozotocin-induced diabetic rats and demonstration of limonene as a potent antiglycating agent. Journal of Pharmacy and Pharmacology. 2013;65(6):884-94.

30. Sankeshi V, Kumar PA, Naik RR, Sridhar G, Kumar MP, Gopal VV, et al. Inhibition of aldose reductase by *Aegle marmelos* and its protective role in diabetic cataract. J Ethnopharmacol. 2013;149(1):215-21.

31. Bhandari P, Kumar N, Singh B, Kaul VK. Bacosterol glycoside, a new 13, 14-seco-steroid glycoside from *Bacopa monnieri*. Chem Pharm Bull. 2006;54(2):240-1.

32. Ghosh T, Maity TK, Singh J. Antihyperglycemic activity of bacosine, a triterpene from *Bacopa monnieri*, in alloxan-induced diabetic rats. Planta Med. 2011;77(8):804-8.

33. Bhandari P, Kumar N, Gupta AP, Singh B, Kaul VK. A rapid RP-HPTLC densitometry method for simultaneous determination of major flavonoids in important medicinal plants. J Sep Sci. 2007;30(13):2092-6.

34. Mathur A, Verma SK, Purohit R, Singh SK, Mathur D, Dua VK et al. Pharmacological investigation of *Bacopa monnieri* on the basis of antioxidant, antimicrobial and anti-inflammatory properties. Journal of Chemical and Pharmaceutical Research. 2010;2(6):191-8.

35. Kumar S, Verma NS, Pande D, Srivastava PS. In vitro regeneration and screening of berberine in *Tinospora cordifolia*. J Med Arom Plant Sci. 2000;22:61.

36. Bisset NG, Nwaiwu J. Quaternary alkaloids of *Tinospora* species. Planta Medica. 1983;48:275-9.

37. Pachaly P, Schneider C. Alkaloids from *Tinospora cordifolia* Miers. Arch Pharm. 1981;314:251-6.

38. Qudrat-I-Khuda M, Khaleque A, Ray N. *Tinospora cordifolia*. I. constituents of the plant fresh from the field. Sci Res. 1964; 1:177-83.

39. Padhya MA. Biosynthesis of isoquinoline alkaloid berberine in tissue cultures of *Tinospora cordifolia*. Indian Drugs. 1986; 24:47-8.

40. Maurya R, Handa SS. Tinocordifolin, a sesquiterpene from *Tinospora cordifolia*. Phytochemistry. 1998; 49:1343-6.

41. Premanath R, Lakshmidevi N. Studies on Anti-oxidant activity of *Tinospora cordifolia* (Miers.) leaves using in vitro models. Journal of American Science. 2010; 6(10):736−43.

42. Nadig PD, Revankar RR, Dethe SM, Narayanaswamy SB, Aliyar MA. Effect of *Tinospora cordifolia* on experimental diabetic neuropathy. Indian J Pharmacol. 2012;44:580−3.

43. Choi HY. Antioxidant activity of *Curcuma longa* L. novel foodstuff. Mol Cell Toxicol. 2009;5(3):237-42.

44. Gutiérrez RMP, Diaz SL, Reyes IC, Gonzalez AMN. Anti-glycation effect of spices and chilies uses in traditional mexican cuisine. Journal of Natural Products. 2010;3:95-102.

45. Verma A, Ahirwar AK. Phytochemical examination and evaluationof in-vitro antioxidant potential activity of *Celastrus paniculatus* seeds extract. International Journal of Scientific Research. 2014; 3(1):46−8.

46. Desai SS, Shruti K, Sana S, Sapna P, Zainab M, Swati H, et al. Phytochemical analysis, free radical scavening and antioxidant profiling using chromatographic techniques for *Centella asiatica*. International Journal of Biotechnology and Bioengineering Research. 2013;4(7):687-96.

47. Adtani P, Malathi N, Chamundeeswari D, Dinesh MG. In-vitro antioxidant activity of ethanolic extracts of *Centella asiatica* L., *Oregano vulgare* sub. sp hirtum and *Ocimum basilicum* L. via five model systems. Indian Journal of Research in Pharmacy and Biotechnology. 2014; 2(3):1230-6.

48. Matsuda T, Kuroyanagi M, Sugiyama S, Umehara K, Ueno A, Nishi K. Cell differentiation inducing diterpenes from *Andrographis paniculata* Nees. Chem Pharm Bull. 1994;42:1216–25.

49. Maramaldi G, Togni S, Franceschi F, Lati E. Anti-inflammaging and antiglycation activity of a novel botanical ingredient from african biodiversity (Centevita™). Clinical. Cosmetic and Investigational Dermatology. 2014;7:1-9.

50. Meghwal M, Goswami TK. Nutritional constituent of black pepper as medicinal molecules: A review. Open Access Scientific Reports. 2012;1(1). DOI:10.4172/scientificreports.129.

51. Dinesha R, Chikkanna D. Antioxidant activities of pippali (*Piper longum*) proteins. Indian Journal of Pharmaceutics and Drug Analysis. 2014;2(11):811–4.

52. Kumar S, Sharma S, Vasudeva N. Screening of antidiabetic and antihyper-lipidemic potential of oil from *Piper longum* and Piperine with their possible mechanism. Expert Opinion on Pharmaco-therapy. 2013;14(13):1723-36.

53. Bhardwaj R, Yadav A, Sharma R. Phytochemicals and antioxidant activity in *Boerhavia diffusa*. International Journal of Pharmacy and Pharmaceutical Sciences. 2014;6(1):344−8.

54. Sekine T, Fukasawa N, Kashiwagi Y, Ruangrungsi N, Murakoshi I. Structure of asparagamine A, a novel polycyclic alkaloid from *Asparagus racemosus*. Chemi Pharma Bull. 1994a;42(6):1360-2.

55. Sekine T, Ikegami F, Fukasawa N, Kashiwagi Y, Aizawa T, Fujii Y, et al. Structure and relative stereochemistry of a new polycyclic alkaloid, asparagamine A, showing anti-oxytocin activity, isolated from *Asparagus racemosus*. J Chem Soc Perkin Trans. 1995;1:391-3.

56. Saxena VK, Chourasia S. A new isoflavone from the roots of *Asparagus racemosus*. Fitoterapia. 2001;72(3):307-9.

57. Kamat JP, Boloor KK, Devasagayam TP, Venkatachalam SR. Antioxidant properties of *Asparagus racemosus* against damage induced by gamma-radiation in rat liver mitochondria. J Ethnopharmacol. 2000; 71(3):425-35.

58. Sharma SC. Constituents of the fruits of *Asparagus racemosus* Willd. Pharmazie. 1981; 36:709-710.

59. Vadivelan R, Dipanjan M, Umasankar P, Dhanabal SP, Satishkumar MN, Antony S, et al. Hypoglycemic, antioxidant and hypolipidemic activity of *Asparagus racemosus* on streptozotocin-induced

diabetic in rats. Advances in Applied Science Research. 2011;2(3):179-85.

60. Ghosh AK, Banerjee S, Mullick HI, Banerjee J. *Zingiber officinale*: A natural gold. International Journal of Pharma and Bio Sciences. 2011;2(1):283-94.

61. Li Y, Tran VH, Duke CC, Roufogalis BD. Preventive and protective properties of *Zingiber officinale* (Ginger) in diabetes mellitus, diabetic complications, and associated lipid and other metabolic disorders: A Brief Review. Evidence-Based Complementary and Alternative Medicine. 2012;2012:1-10.

62. Saraswat M, Suryanarayana P, Reddy PY, Patil MA, Balakrishna N, Reddy GB. Antiglycating potential of *Zingiber officinalis* and delay of diabetic cataract in rats. Molecular Vision. 2010;6:1525-37.

63. Varma RK, Manjusha R, Harisha CR, Shukla VJ. Pharmacognostical and physiochemical analysis of triphaladi yoga: An ayurvedic polyherbal formulation. Journal of Pharmaceutical and Scientific Innovation. 2012;1(6):9-12.

64. Shashildhara CS, Bharath Raj KC, Aswathanarayana BJ. A comparative study of anti cataract activity of triphala and its constituents. International Research Journal of Pharmacy. 2012;3(5):407–10.

65. Devi PU. Radioprotective, anticarcinogenic and antioxidant properties of Indian holy basil *Ocimum sanctum* (tulsai). Indian Journal of Experimental Biology. 2001; 39:185-90.

66. Kaewnarin K, Shank L, Niamsup H, Rakariyatham N. Inhibitory effects of lamiaceae plants on the formation of Advanced Glycation Endproducts (AGEs) in model proteins. Journal of Medical and Bioengineering. 2013;2(4):224-7.

67. Pavithra N, Sathish L, Kumar SM, Venkatarathanamma VA, Pushpalatha H, Bhanuprakash Reddy G, et al. In-vitro studies on α-Amylase, α-Glucosidase and aldose reductase inhibitors found in endophytic fungi isolated from *Ocimum sanctum*. Current Enzyme Inhibition. 2015; 11(2):129-36.

68. Chopraa GPKP, Saraf BD, Inam F, Deo SS. Antimicrobial and antioxidant activities of methanol extract roots of *Glycyrrhiza glabra* and HPLC analysis. International Journal of Pharmacy & Pharmaceutical Sciences. 2013;5(2):157-60.

69. Alqahtani A, Hamid K, Kam A, Wong KH, Abdelhak Z, Razmovski-Naumovski V, et al. The pentacyclic triterpenoids in herbal medicines and their pharmacological activities in diabetes and diabetic complications. Curr Med Chem. 2013; 20(7):908-31.

5

Evaluation of Structural Changes in the Retina of Patients with Schizophrenia

Mafalda Mota[1*], Peter Pêgo[1], Catarina Klut[2], Inês Coutinho[1], Cristina Santos[1], Graça Pires[1], Teresa Maia[2] and António Melo[1]

[1]Department of Ophthalmology, Hospital Professor Doutor Fernando Fonseca, Lisboa, Portugal.
[2]Departmentof Psychiatry, Hospital Professor Doutor Fernando Fonseca, Lisboa, Portugal.

Authors' contributions

This work was carried out in collaboration between all authors. Author MM designed the study, wrote the protocol and wrote the first draft of the manuscript. Author PP performed the statistical analysis. Author CK participated in the design of the study and recruited patients with schizophrenia. Authors IC, CS, GP and AM managed the analyses of the study. Author TM made the cognitive assessment of patients with schizophrenia. All authors reviewed and approved the research protocol and also the final manuscript.

Editor(s):
(1) Jimmy S. M. Lai, Department of Ophthalmology, The University of Hong Kong, Hong Kong and Honorary Consultant Ophthalmologist, Queen Mary Hospital, Hong Kong.
Reviewers:
(1) S. K. Prabhakar, Ophthalmology, JSS University, India.
(2) Gabor Nemeth, Department of Ophthalmology, University of Debrecen, Debrecen, Hungary.
(3) Anonymous, University of Eastern Finland, Finland.

ABSTRACT

Aim: To understand the potential of evaluating the thickness of the retinal nerve fiber layer (RNFL) and macular volume in patients with schizophrenia, using Optical Coherence Tomography (OCT), and its possible application to monitor this disorder.
Study Design and Participants: Cross-sectional study that included two groups, one with 20 patients diagnosed with schizophrenia and a control group with 20 healthy volunteers. Patients with schizophrenia were divided into two subgroups, one with less than 5 years of illness duration and the other with more than 5 years. Both groups underwent OCT. The study was conducted between April 2014 and July 2014, with the collaboration of the Ophthalmology and Psychiatry departments.
Results: Schizophrenic patients showed a significant decrease in all measurements of the macula, volume and thickness, when compared to the control group (p<0.05). No differences were found between groups regarding RNFL thickness, although there was a correlation between disease

---

Corresponding author: E-mail: mafaldamsbm@gmail.com

duration and decreased overall RNFL thickness (r=-0.338; p=0.033). Comparison between the group with schizophrenia for less than five years and the group with more than 5 years, revealed statistically significant differences in volume (p=0.021) and thickness (p=0.018) of the temporal outer ring of the macula.

Conclusion: Results suggest that there are differences in the retina in patients with schizophrenia. These data support the hypothesis of a neurodegenerative component of the disorder. OCT is a noninvasive exam that, although non-specific, can be useful either to diagnose or monitor disease progression.

Keywords: Schizophrenia; OCT; macula; RNFL.

1. INTRODUCTION

Schizophrenia is a complex clinical entity that affects around 24 million people worldwide [1]. It is a chronic mental disorder. It is mainly defined according to current classifications, as a function of the psychotic symptoms. However, this syndrome is also defined as a function of various other dimensions, including cognitive, emotional and volitional, all responsible for most of the functional impairment of these patients.

Schizophrenia has been intensely studied over the past century, remaining however poorly understood with regard to its etiology and pathophysiology. One of the lines of research has focused on the existence of changes in the central nervous system. Several neuro-imaging studies have shown structural changes, such as ventricular enlargement and reduced total brain volume, mainly due to loss of gray matter [2,3].These changes are already present at the first psychotic episode and even during the prodromal period, and tend to worsen with disease progression. Although available evidence suggests that the pathological process starts during neurodevelopment, the extension of the relative contribution of a neurodegenerative process is still unclear [4].

The effect of antipsychotics on the structure of the central nervous system is not consensual, and there are studies with positive and negative results regarding their ability to alter brain volume, and some studies even suggest a differential effect of typical and atypical antipsychotics. A recent meta-analysis concluded that there appears to be a longitudinal decrease in gray matter in patients with schizophrenia, which correlates with a higher cumulative exposure to antipsychotics, but this is not the only factor involved in this process [5].

It is increasingly important to find new noninvasive methods to study the brain and its function, so that the patient may be more comfortably monitored.

In this context, it is important to understand the potential of evaluating the thickness of the retinal nerve fiber layer (RNFL) by Optical Coherence Tomography (OCT) in patients with neurological and/or psychiatric disorders, such as schizophrenia. OCT allows to access non-myelinated cells *in vivo*, without the need for other more invasive and costly neuro-imaging studies neuro-imaging studies, with exposure to radiation.

OCT allows a non-invasive assessment and monitoring of various eye pathologies, such as glaucoma and retinal disorders. Its use has been increasingly extended to other areas of medicine, as a useful tool to access retinal ganglion cells. In other neurological disorders, such as Alzheimer's disease and Parkinson's disease, the relationship between the decrease in RNFL thickness and the atrophy of brain tissue has been studied, with positive and promising results. Therefore, the aim of this study was to ascertain if OCT can also be useful in schizophrenia, and if OCT measurements correlate with disease progression, so that, in the future, these patients have a non-invasive, harmless and convenient method for monitoring/staging.

Retina is thus a possible "window to the brain" that remains to be opened. This study provides a step further in discovering the potential of this neurological tissue for the evaluation of pathologies other than strictly ophthalmological.

The aim of this study is to understand the potential of evaluating the thickness of the retinal nerve fiber layer (RNFL) and macular volume and thickness in schizophrenic patients, using OCT and its possible application to monitor this pathology.

2. MATERIALS AND METHODS

Cross-sectional, observational study, conducted at Hospital Prof. Dr. Fernando da Fonseca (HFF), between April 2014 and July 2014.

The population sample consisted of 20 patients with the diagnosis of schizophrenia based on the criteria of the *International Classification of Diseases 10th Revision Procedure Classification System* (ICD 10), clinically stable, with regular follow-up in the Psychiatric Department of HFF.

Schizophrenic patients were divided into 2 groups, depending on the duration of illness. One group with less than 5 years duration of illness (10 patients) and one group with more than 5 years duration of illness (10 patients).

Patients were evaluated in Psychiatry consultation, taking into account: duration of illness; age of onset; therapy with typical or atypical antipsychotics; compliance to therapy - Scale "Medication Adherence Rating Scale" (MARS); and degree of positive or negative symptomatology, and general psychopathology - Scale "Positive and Negative Syndrome Scale" (PANSS). Cognitive functioning was also assessed using the following cognitive tests: "Standardized Cognitive Assessment Conde de Ferreira" (SCACF, Prof. Marques Teixeira), comprising: STROOPTest, Wisconsin Card Sorting Test, HVLT-R (Hopkins Verbal Learning Test - Revised), TMT (Trail Making Test) and WMS-III (Wechsler Memory Scale). In this evaluation results were provided as a function of different cognitive domains, such as attention and focus, learning and memory, executive function and processing speed.

The control group consisted of 20 gender- and age-matched healthy individuals.

Both groups were given a General Health Questionnaire, were generally assessed at an Ophthalmology consultation, and underwent OCT, with software to study the macula (volume and thickness) and the optical disc (RNFL thickness).

2.1 Inclusion Criteria

Men and women over 18 years of age, diagnosed with schizophrenia, based on the criteria of ICD 10, with the ability to provide informed consent. The research followed the tenets of the Declaration of Helsinki, and the protocol was approved by the HFF ethics committee.

2.2 Exclusion Criteria

All participants that, in the General Health Questionnaire, were found to have other degenerative or neurological diseases, general systemic diseases that could affect the eye, such as autoimmune or infectious diseases, and history of traumatic brain injury associated with loss of consciousness. During the evaluation in Psychiatry consultation, participants who presented episodes of acute decompensation, with current history of prominent addictive behaviors (alcohol or other illegal drugs), with personal history of macrostructural lesions of the central nervous system, and other relevant co-morbid psychiatric disorders, particularly mental retardation or dementia, were also excluded. Ophthalmological exclusion criteria were: refractive error ≥ -6.00 D; BCVA(best corrected visual acuity)< 8/10; intraocular pressure (IOP) ≥ 22 mmHg; opacification of transparent media of the eye; change of excavation/upper disc > 0.4; and pathology of the retinal posterior pole, such as diabetic retinopathy, hypertension or another.

2.3 Optical Coherence Tomography (OCT)

The OCT SPECTRALIS® (Heidelberg Engineering GmbH) was used for the study of the macula and optical disc. This device uses confocal laser scanning for image acquisition, through focus of the laser beam on the retina. Two different beams of light (infrared, IR) are used simultaneously, in order to obtain 3D volume scans. These beams are periodically deflected through oscillating mirrors, thus allowing a sequential scan of the retina. Being linked to a normative database, it is possible to compare thickness and volume of the various layers of the retina, by comparing the values obtained from an individual with the database of normal individuals. Thus, it is possible to obtain high resolution spatial images, with a scanning proximity of 11 μm. This device incorporates the active tracking system of eye movement (TruTrack) and fovea-disc alignment technology (FoDi), allowing to capture two images in the exact same position, compensating for the eye and head movement of the patient.

Macula assessments were conducted using the macular assessment protocol *"fastHR"*, and the 9 sectors defined by the *"Early Treatment Diabetic Retinopathy Study* (ETDRS) were obtained, having been evaluated 3 circles of 1, 3 and 6 mm centered on the fovea. A 20x20° scan, with 25 scans per section, was performed. The two outer circles (inner and outer macular ring) were subdivided into four quadrants (nasal, temporal, superior, inferior). The center circle is the fovea. All images obtained had a quality of more than 15.

For evaluation of the optical disc, RNFL thickness was assessed using the protocol of glaucoma for the evaluation of "RNFL", with a scan pattern of 12° centered on the head of the optical disc. The default pattern position is 2.6° nasal and 2.1° superior from the fovea and only one scanning per section is performed. The global thickness and six areas of the peripapillary region (temporal-T, inferior-temporal-IT, inferior-nasal-IN, nasal-N, superior-nasal-SN and superior-temporal-ST) were analysed using a STINT pattern. Three images were always used, with a quality of more than 15and "ART 100 frames" of 100%. The last acquisition was always chosen.

2.4 Statistical Analysis

Statistical analysis was performed using the Statistical Package for Social Sciences (SPSS®) Version 22 (SPSS, Inc., Chicago, IL, USA). Differences between groups were analyzed using the independent samples t-test. To establish correlations, the Pearson's correlation was used. Tests were considered significant for a significance level of $\alpha=0.05$.

3. RESULTS AND DISCUSSION

3.1 Results

3.1.1 Demographic data

The population sample consisted of 40 individuals, 20 with a diagnosis of schizophrenia and 20 healthy individuals as the control group.

The two groups were age-matched (control 33.4±11.2; schizophrenic 32.9±11.9). The group of patients with schizophrenia with more than 5 years of disease duration was on average older (42.0±3.9) than the group with less years (23.8±9.9), p<0.001. Regarding gender, there were more males in both groups that was balanced between groups (Table 1). Both eyes were evaluated separately, thus each group consists of 20 individuals and 40 eyes.

Table 1. Demographic data

	Men	Women
Control	16 (80%)	4 (20%)
Schizophrenic	17 (85%)	3 (15%)

3.1.2 Statistical analysis of OCT data

Comparison of RNFL thickness in its different quadrants showed no statistically significant differences neither between the control group and the group of patients with schizophrenia, nor between the two subgroups with schizophrenia (Table 2). However, there was a negative correlation between the duration of illness and decrease of global RNFL thickness, with r=-0.338 and p=0.033 (Fig. 1).

All macular measurements, volumes and thickness, showed a statistically significant decrease between the group with schizophrenia and the control group (Table 3). Patients with schizophrenia showed a particularly statistically significant decrease, with p<0.001, of the following parameters: global macular volume, temporal macular outer ring volume, superior macular inner ring thickness and temporal macular outer ring thickness.

Comparison between the group with schizophrenia for less than five years and the group with more than 5 years, showed statistically significant differences in volume (p=0.021) and thickness (p=0.018) of the temporal macular outer ring (Table 4).

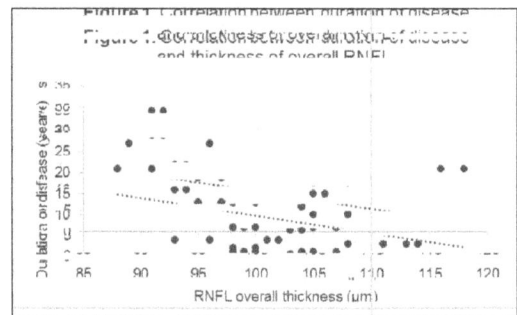

Fig. 1. Correlation between duration of diseases and thickness of overall RNFL

3.2 Discussion

Schizophrenia is a complex disease, whose pathophysiological is still being unveiled. Currently, the neuroprogressive nature of this disorder has an increasing number of supporters [2,3,6]. Therefore, imaging diagnostic methods are increasingly requested for a better understanding of the neurodegenerative component of the disease. It is in this context that OCT, being a non-invasive imaging technique that does not use radiation, becomes an attractive tool for the study of the nervous tissue.

In this study, the groups were not balanced in terms of gender, with male predominance in both groups, and the average age was higher in the subgroup of patients with schizophrenia for more than 5 years. However, these changes were expected given that schizophrenia is more prevalent in males and, as the duration of illness increases, it is also expected that patients become older [7]. Nevertheless, the schizophrenic patients group and the control group were gender- and age-matched.

Contrary to a study by Lee et al. [8] there were no statistically significant differences in the decrease of RNFL thickness between the control group and the group of patients with schizophrenia, in all studied quadrants. In the present study, as the duration of illness increases, the overall RNFL thickness shows a statistically significant decrease, which is in accordance with Lee et al. [8]. These results allow us to agree with a number of studies that have shown the existence of changes in nerve tissue as the disease progresses [2,3,9].

Table 2. Comparison of RNFL thickness (um) between schizophrenic patients and control group

	n	Mean	SD
Overall RNFL			
Control	40	101,2	9,101
Schizophrenic	40	101,05	7,338
< 5 years	20	102,6	5,698
≥ 5 years	20	99,5	8,544
ST RNFL			
Control	40	145,8	16,034
Schizophrenic	40	135,7	17,297
< 5 years	20	135,55	17,887
≥ 5 years	20	135,85	17,15
SN RNFL			
Control	40	112,5	16,954
Schizophrenic	40	120,575	23,894
< 5 years	20	124,7	25,826
≥ 5 years	20	116,45	21,659
IT RNFL			
Control	40	143,75	16,089
Schizophrenic	40	144,475	15,509
< 5 years	20	144,65	14,996
≥ 5 years	20	144,3	16,381
IN RNFL			
Control	40	112,5	11,908
Schizophrenic	40	114,475	19,931
< 5 years	20	116,95	20,516
≥ 5 years	20	112	19,534
N RNFL			
Control	40	74,9	16,445
Schizophrenic	40	76,875	10,743
< 5 years	20	79,15	11,86
≥ 5 years	20	74,8	9,288
T RNFL			
Control	40	73,3	11,305
Schizophrenic	40	69,325	7,833
< 5 years	20	69,45	7,316
≥ 5 years	20	69,2	8,508

Table 3. Comparison between macular thickness (um) and volume (mm3) between patients whit schizophrenia (1) and control group (0)

	Groups	n	Mean	SD	p
Overall thickness	0	40	271,3	22,74	0,019
	1	40	258,73	24,23	
Central volume	0	40	0,214	0,018	0,012
	1	40	0,203	0,019	
Thickness - Fovea	0	40	229,33	27,64	0,005
	1	40	213,63	20,3	
Overall volume	0	40	8,844	0,281	<0,001
	1	40	8,59	0,325	
Thickness - Superior inner ring	0	40	352,05	11,56	<0,001
	1	40	340,9	15,05	
Thickness - Inferior inner ring	0	40	344,83	12,59	0,013
	1	40	336,75	15,66	
Thickness - Nasal inner ring	0	40	348,58	13,18	0,018
	1	40	340,3	17,29	
Thickness - Temporal inner ring	0	40	334,75	12	0,029
	1	40	327,63	16,25	
Thickness - Superior outer ring	0	40	305,38	11,31	0,002
	1	40	297,35	11,41	
Thickness - Inferior outer ring	0	40	293,45	10,62	0,006
	1	40	286,78	10,29	
Thickness - Nasal outer ring	0	40	322,78	11,27	0,005
	1	40	314,33	14,57	
Thickness - Temporal outer ring	0	40	294	9,394	<0,001
	1	40	284,85	12,25	
Volume - Superior inner ring	0	40	0,553	0,018	0,001
	1	40	0,536	0,024	
Volume - Inferior inner ring	0	40	0,542	0,02	0,015
	1	40	0,529	0,025	
Volume - Nasal inner ring	0	40	0,547	0,02	0,03
	1	40	0,535	0,027	
Volume - Temporal inner ring	0	40	0,526	0,019	0,025
	1	40	0,514	0,026	
Volume - Superior outer ring	0	40	1,619	0,061	0,003
	1	40	1,577	0,061	
Volume - Inferior outer ring	0	40	1,556	0,056	0,006
	1	40	1,521	0,055	
Volume - Nasal outer ring	0	40	1,711	0,06	0,005
	1	40	1,666	0,077	
Volume - Temporal outer ring	0	40	1,559	0,052	<0,001
	1	40	1,51	0,066	

Table 4. Comparison of volume and thickness in temporal macular outer ring between schizophrenic with <5 years (0) and ≥ years of disease progression

	Groups	n	Mean	SD	p
Thickness - Temporal outer ring	0	20	289,35	12,29	0,018
	1	20	280,35	10,69	
Volume - Temporal outer ring	0	20	1,534	0,067	0,021
	1	20	1,486	0,057	

Schizophrenic patients showed a significant decrease of macular central ring thickness (control 271.30±22.74 µm; schizophrenic 258.73± 3.83 µm; p=0.019) and overall macular volume (control 0.281±8.844 µm; schizophrenic 8.589±0.325 µm; p<0.001) compared to the control group. All macular measurements, volumes and thickness, showed a statistically significant decrease in the group with schizophrenia compared to the control group (Table 3). In the study of Ascaso et al. [9] this was not verified, and may be due to the fact that, in our study, we used an OCT with greater ability of image resolution and spectral domain (OCT SPECTRALIS®, Heidelberg *versus* Stratus® OCT, Carl Zeiss), and our sample being larger.

Comparison between the group with schizophrenia for less than five years and the group with more than 5 years, showed statistically significant differences in volume and thickness of the temporal macular outer ring. The fact that significant results were only found in the temporal quadrant may be explained by this being the macular quadrant with lower thickness, second to the fovea, and therefore small changes in a layer may possibly be better evaluated in this quadrant [10] However, given the small size of our sample, this result should be interpreted with caution.

The results of this study show a significant decrease in the evaluated macular parameters in patients with schizophrenia, but this is not true for RNFL. It is known that the retina, in the peripapillary area, is mainly composed by NFL, while in the macula this layer corresponds, together with the ganglion cell layer, to around 30% to 35% of retinal thickness [11,12]. Thus, it may be concluded that the decrease in macular thickness and volume in patients with schizophrenia cannot be solely attributed to the decrease of NFL, for a similar or higher decrease of the RNFL thickness would have been observed. Therefore, other layers of the retina, such as the layer of ganglion cells, may also contribute to the differences observed in the macula between the two studied groups. In addition, the NFL not only comprises axons of the ganglion cells, but also other cell types, such asneuroglia and astrocytes, which may contribute to the loss of ganglion cells, and consequently their axons, has not been significant in the peripapillary zone [11,12]. However, it may be concluded that there is a neurodegenerative component of the disease, due to the observed significant correlation between decreased RNFL and increasing years of illness. In a study with a larger sample, Lee et al. [8] reported a significant decrease of RNFL in patients with schizophrenia. Thus, our results could benefit from a larger population sample.

Chu et al. [13] found no statistically significant differences in macular volume between the group of patients with schizophrenia and the control group. Due to these results, the authors proposed that axonal damage was less important than changes in the myelinated areas of the brain. However, results of the present study, as well as the results obtained by Lee et al., are contrary to this proposal [8,13]. This disparity in results may be due to several factors: the sample including patients with schizophrenia and schizoaffective disorder, and the OCT equipment used (Stratus® OCT, Carl Zeiss) having a lower resolution than the one used in the present study (OCT®SPECTRALIS, Heidelberg) and in the study by Lee et al. (OCT Cirrus®, Carl Zeiss).

Other recent studies on ophthalmological changes in schizophrenia also revealed changes in the visual fields of patients with schizophrenia and their family members (decreased global sensitivity), and microvascular changes in the retina of patients, thus confirming that other ophthalmological changes may exist in schizophrenia [14,15]. Further studies are warranted to understand to what extent these changes can help in monitoring and treatment of the disease.

All patients with schizophrenia were under antipsychotic medication during the study and the medication was not the same for all patients. This could be a limitation of this study, thus it is not possible to dissociate the potential effects of medication in the evaluated thicknesses and volumes. However, given medication in these patients is chronic, its withdrawal could also create a bias factor. Another limitation is that OCT is operator-dependent. However, and in order to minimize this influence, the operator was always the same, so bias due to differences between operators was removed.

4. CONCLUSION

It is increasingly recognized that ophthalmology may provide an important contribution to understanding the changes in the Nervous System in several pathologies, such as schizophrenia, but also in other neurological diseases. The eye, beyond a sensorial organ, also provides a privileged path to access nerve tissue *in vivo*, being a true open window into the brain. Thus, there is an urgent need to observe the patient in an increasingly multidisciplinary perspective, in order to understand the disease as a whole and in all its possible dimensions.

In conclusion, Optical Coherence Tomography may be a useful tool in the evaluation and follow-up of patients with schizophrenia, without exposing them to ionizing radiation, as in other imaging methods. However, further studies are still needed to understand all the possible ophthalmological changes that these patients present, as well as for the design of algorithms, so that OCT can be used both at the time of diagnosis and in monitoring disease progression. The future encompasses the acceptance of the neurodegenerative component of this disease and the development of novel therapies based on this assumption.

COMPETING INTERESTS

Authors have declared that no competing interests exist.

REFERENCES

1. Anonymous. World Health Organization; 2014.
Available:http://www.who.int/mental_health/management/schizophrenia/en/

2. Ellison-Wright I, Bullmore E. Meta-analysis of diffusion tensor imaging studies in schizophrenia. Schizophr Res. 2009; 108(1-3):3-10.

3. Srihari S Bangalore, et al. Untreated illness duration correlates with gray matter loss in First Episode Psychoses. Neuroreport. 2009;20(7):729–734.

4. Harrison, PJ. The Neurobiology of schizophrenia. New Oxford Textbook of Psychiatry, Second edition. Oxford. Oxford University. Press. 2009;561-568.

5. Fusar-Poli P, et al. Progressive brain changes in schizophrenia related to antipsychotic treatment? A meta-analysis of longitudinal MRI studies. Neurosci Biobehav. Rev. 2013;37(8):1680-1691.

6. Malaspina D. Looking schizophrenic in the eye. Am J Psychiatry. 2013;170(12):1382-4.

7. Usall J. Diferencias de género en la esquizofrenia. Rev Psiquiatría Fac Med Barna. 2003;30(5):276-287.

8. Lee WW, et al. Retinal nerve fiber layer structure abnormalities in schizophrenia and its relationship to disease state: Evidence from optical coherence tomography. Invest Ophthalmol. 2013;54: 7785-792.

9. Ascaso J, et al. Retinal nerve fiber layer thickness measured by optical coherence tomography in patients with schizophrenia: A short report. Eur. J. Psychiat. 2010;24(Nº4):227-235.

10. Annie Chan MD, et al. Normal macular thickness measurements in healthy eyes using stratus optical coherence tomography. Arch Ophthalmol. Author manuscript. Arch Ophthalmol. 2006; 124(2):193–198.

11. Greenfield D, et al. Macular thickness changes in glaucomatous optic neuropathy detected using optical coherence tomography. Arch Ophthalmol. 2003; 121(1):41-46.

12. Guedes V, et al. Optical coherence tomography measurement of macular and nerve fiber layer thickness in normal and glaucomatous human eyes. Ophthalmology. 2003;110(1).

13. Chu M, et al. A window into the brain: An in vivo study of the retina in schizophrenia using optical coherence tomography. Psychiatry Research: Neuroimaging. 2012; 203:89-94.

14. Meier MH, et al. Microvascular abnormality in schizophrenia as shown by retinal imaging. Am J Psychiatry. 2013; 170(12):1451-9.

15. Gracitelli CP. Visual field loss in schizophrenia: evaluation of magnocellular pathway dysfunction in schizophrenic patients and their parents. Clin Ophthal mol. 2013;7:1015-21.

6

Topical Steroids, HIV Status, CD4 Cells and Corneal Health

Emmanuel Olu Megbelayin[1*], Stephen Mbosowo Ekpenyong[1] and Chiedozie Kingsley Ojide[2]

[1]*Department of Ophthalmology, University of Uyo Teaching Hospital, Uyo, Akwa-Ibom State, Nigeria.*
[2]*Department of Microbiology, Federal Teaching Hospital, Abakaliki, Ebonyi State, Nigeria.*

Authors' contributions

This work was carried out in collaboration between all authors. Author EOM designed the study, wrote the protocol, and wrote the first draft of the manuscript. Author SME managed the literature searches, and author CKO carried out microbiological studies. All authors read and approved the final manuscript.

Editor(s):
(1) Ahmad M. Mansour, Department of Ophthalmology, American University of Beirut, Lebanon.
Reviewers:
(1) Maduike C. O. Ezeibe, Department of Veterinary Medicine, University of Nigeria, Nsukka, Nigeria.
(2) Philippe Genet, Department of Hematology, Unit of Immunology, Centre Hospitalier Victor Dupouy, Argenteuil, France.
(3) Tafireyi Marukutira, Centre for Disease Control and Prevention (CDC) Botswana, USA.
(4) Anonymous, China Pharmaceutical University, China.
(5) Anonymous, University of West Georgia, USA.

ABSTRACT

A 36 year old patient presented with a history of pain and progressive loss of vision in the right eye which had lasted for 2 months. He was on topical steroids for about one year before presentation with a CD4 cell of 200cells/μL. Examination reviewed a perforated cornea with a huge uveal prolapse. Topical steroids were immediately discontinued and patient placed on topical and systemic antibiotics. Following resolution of the clinical signs, Gunderson's flap was raised to cover the prolapsed uvea. By 6th week post-op, a vascularised pseudo cornea had covered the exposed uvea resulting in cessation of pain in the eye. Conclusion: Gunderson's flap is a viable option for a prolapsed uvea in an immuno-incompetent patient.

Keywords: Steroids; CD4 cells; HIV; cornea.

*Corresponding author: E-mail: favouredolu@yahoo.com

1. INTRODUCTION

Topical steroids are often used to manage many ocular surface conditions. Unfortunately these drugs are also associated with serious ocular abnormalities, especially when used injudiciously [1,2]. A lot has been documented on the propensity of topical steroids to cause corneal ulceration or perforation but little has been reported on the results of immune deficiency on corneal health. It appears reduction in number of CD4 cells makes cornea more susceptible to steroid effects. It also appears immune deficiency makes cornea succumb to steroid toxicity after shorter period of steroid treatment than it would in healthy state. The finding in this report might have been coincidental but its plausibility deserves further scientific scrutiny.

2. PRESENTATION OF CASE

A 36 year old HIV positive driver presented with a history of pain in the right eye that had lasted for 2 months and a progressive loss of vision. Prior to presentation to our centre in December 2012, he had presented at another clinic in the previous year where he was placed on guttae maxidex (dexamethasone), mydriacyl (tropicamide), spersadex (dexamethasone), ivedexone (dexamethasone), tears naturale, cipromed (ciprofloxacin), zovirax (acyclovir) eye ointment, hypotears gel, chloramphenicol eye ointment at various times during the course of the eye problem.

With deteriorating eye condition he presented to us with 3 empty bottles of dexamethasone, a bottle of atropine and a bottle of tears naturale. He has been on topical steroids for about a year. Details of initial ocular condition could not be clarified but patient sought medical attention in a primary eye care center when he developed a painful red right eye.

There was no antecedent trauma, previous eye surgery or use of refractive spectacles. He is not a known diabetic, asthmatic, hypertensive or sickle-cell patient. He was diagnosed with HIV infection 10 months before presentation to our facility and has been on lamivudine, zidovudine and efavirenz. He neither smokes nor takes alcohol. He is single and attained secondary school education

On examination, vision was light perception (PL) with inaccurate projection on the right eye. The left eye was essentially normal with a visual acuity of 6/5.

Further reports on examination are those of the right eye. There was a full range of ocular movements with a diffuse conjunctival hyperemia and muco-purulent discharge. Cornea was perforated centrally with inferotemporal extension. A huge prolapsing uvea tissue from the perforation and descemetocele precluded further view and a reliable corneal sensitivity test (Fig. 1).

Corneal swab was taken for culture on blood agar, chocolate agar, thioglycolate broth and sabouraud dextrose agar. Culture results were negative. However CD4 cell count, carried out at a government facility designated for free HIV treatment, was 200cells/µl.

Topical steroids were discontinued and patient placed on guttae atropine, ciprofloxacin topically and systemically for 1 week. He then had Gunderson's flap raised to cover the exposed uvea (Fig. 2). He was seen first day and two weeks postoperatively. He defaulted till sixth week post-operative period.

Examination on the sixth post-operative week showed a vascularised pseudo-cornea over the prolapsed uvea (Fig. 3).

3. DISCUSSION

The deleterious effects of topical steroids on the cornea are well known [1,2]. However, there is paucity of report on the combined effects of HIV, levels of CD4 cells and topical steroids on corneal health. It can be rationally hypothesized that HIV and topical steroids combine immunosuppressive activities to unleash lethal effects on the cornea. But at what stage in the spectrum of HIV-immunosuppression-AIDS is cornea most susceptible? Certain ocular conditions have been associated with declining CD4 cells. The most common ocular complication of HIV infection is a retinal microvasculopathy called HIV retinopathy. It occurs in 50-70% of patients with CD4 cell counts below 100cells/µL [3,4]. Cytomegalovirus retinitis develops in 7.5% to 30% of AIDS patients at CD4 counts less than 50cells/µL and Kaposi's sarcoma at less than 200cells/µL [5]. It is likely that these ocular complications occur earlier in HIV patients if there are co-morbidities.

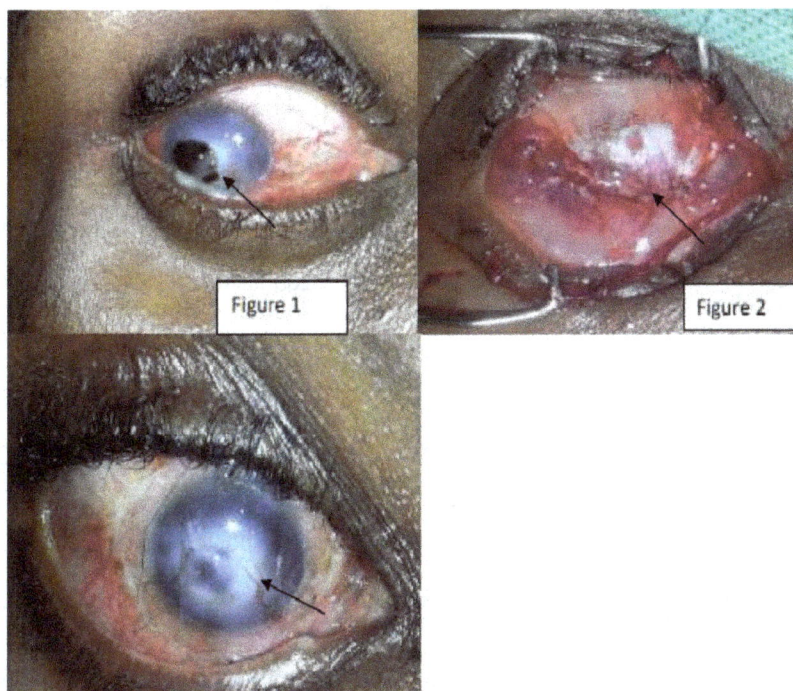

Figs. 1, 2 and 3. respectively show perforated cornea at presentation. The arrow in figure 1 shows a huge iris prolapse with associated muco-purulent discharge. The arrow in figure 2 shows Gunderson's flap raised to cover exposed uvea. The arrow in figure 3 shows a vascularised pseudo-cornea 6 weeks post-operatively

An unusual and possibly new keratopathy was reported among HIV patients by Chu et al. [6]. This indicates that the cornea may have yet to be identified unique predisposition to pathologic changes in HIV patients. This susceptibility may become pronounced with declining CD4 cells. Until such a time antigen-specific tests of T-lymphocyte function become widely available, CD4 cells remain the predicting parameter for the occurrence of specific ocular infection in patients who are HIV positive [7-9].

The pathogenesis of corneal perforation in our patient is most likely multifactorial. That the left cornea which had no topical steroid instillations was normal at presentation is instructive. Could the continued topical steroid instillations on the right eye have provided the environment for corneal melting at CD4 count of 200cells/µl? Or at what CD4 cut-off is cornea most likely to get compromised? Our patient was on anti-retroviral, could patients not on treatment at same CD4 cell counts have a different corneal susceptibility? Further studies are necessary to address some of these questions.

Patient being placed on Acyclovir ointment at the previous eye center suggested that he may have had herpes simplex keratitis which we could not confirm. In our setting, diagnosis of HSV keratitis is on clinical ground, often based on a typical dendritic corneal ulceration and loss of corneal sensation. Some patients present with geographic corneal ulcers following use of harmful traditional eye medications (HTEMs) and injudicious topical steroid use. CD4 cells are a key component of the adaptive immune system. They act as helper cells that induce cytotoxic CD8-positive T cell clones and recruit macrophages responsible for apoptosis of infected cells [10-12]. Where CD4 cells are depleted as seen in HIV infections, HSV virulence is likely to increase.

The response of our patient to discontinuation of frequent topical steroid drops, Gunderson's flap, topical and systemic antibiotic was remarkable. Only twice daily steroid ointment, 2-hourly topical and twice daily tablets 500mg ciprofloxacin were required to control postoperative inflammation and curtail infection. Since the entire cornea with the exposed uvea was covered with conjunctiva further corneal melting was unlikely despite post-operative corneal steroid ointment. Topical steroid was discontinued 2 weeks when postoperative inflammation had subsided significantly.

4. CONCLUSION

We advocate a detailed study to find the association between topical steroids and immunosuppression on corneal health and conclude that evisceration seems no immediate option for a huge iris prolapse following corneal perforation in a retro-viral positive patient with depleted CD4 cells.

CONSENT

All authors declare that written informed consent was obtained from the patient.

ETHICAL APPROVAL

All authors hereby declare that this study has been performed in accordance with the ethical standards laid down in the 1964 Declaration of Helsinki.

ACKNOWLEDGEMENTS

This was a non-funded study.

COMPETING INTERESTS

Authors have declared that no competing interests exist.

REFERENCES

1. Srinivasan M, Mascarenhas J, Rajaraman R, Ravindran M, Lalitha P, Glidden DV, et al. Corticosteroids for bacterial keratitis: The Steroids for Corneal Ulcers Trial (SCUT). Arch. Ophthalmol. 2012;130(2):143-50.

2. Carmichael TR, Gelfand Y, Welsh NH. Topical steroids in the treatment of central and paracentral corneal ulcers Br. J. Ophthalmol. 1990;74:528-31.

3. Kempen JH, Jabs DA. Ocular complications of human immunodeficiency virus infection. In: Johnson G, Minassian DC, Weale RA, West SK, editors. The Epidemiology of Eye Disease, 2nd ed. London. 2003;318-340.

4. Jabs DA. Ocular manifestations of HIV infection. Trans. Am. Ophthalmol. Soc. 1995;93:623-83.

5. Baroud JM, Haley L, Montaner JS, Murphy C, Januszewska M, Schechter MT. Quantification of the variation due to laboratory and physiologic sources in CD4 lymphocyte counts of clinically stable HIV-infected individuals. J. Acquir. Immune. Defic. Syndr. 1995;10(suppl 2):67–73.

6. David SC, Zaidman GW, Meisler DM, Lowder C, Jacobs DS, Christopher J Rapuano CJ, et al. Human immunodeficiency virus-positive patients with posterior intracorneal precipitates. Ophthalmology. 2001;108(10):1853-1857.

7. Copeland RC, Phillpotts BA, Greenfield RA. Ocular Manifestations of HIV infection. Available:http://emedicine.medscape.com/article/1216172-overview. Accessed on 14/08/2014.

8. Sabin CA, Phillips AN. Should HIV therapy be started at a CD4 cell count above 350cells/µl in asymptomatic HIV-1-infected patients? Curr Opinion Infect Dis. 2009;(2)22:191-197.

9. Mocroft A, Ledergerber B, Katlama C. Decline in the AIDS and death rates in the Euro SIDA study: An observational study. Lancet. 2003;362:22-29.

10. Mester JC, Rouse BT. The mouse model and understanding immunity to herpes simplex virus. Rev. Infect. Dis. 1991;13(Suppl11):935-45.

11. Schmid DS, Rouse BT. The role of T cell immunity in control of herpes simplex virus. Curr. Top. Microbiol. Immunol. 1992;179:57-74.

12. Ghiasi H, Cai S, Perng GC, Nesburn AB, Wechsler SL. Both CD4+ and CD8+ T cells are involved in protection against HSV-1 induced corneal scarring. Br. J. Ophthalmol. 2000;84:408–12.

7

Evaluation of Tear Secretion in Thyroid Patients in Relation to the Thyroid Status and Previous I^{131} Treatment for Thyroid Cancer

Athanasios Karamitsos[1*], Lampros Lamprogiannis[1], Kyriakos Gougoulias[2], Konstantinos Stamoulas[1], Diamantis Almaliotis[2], Athanasia Skriapa-Manta[2], Theofanis Vaseiliadis[3], Aikaterini Raptou[3] and Vasileios Karampatakis[2]

[1]*1st University Eye Clinic, AHEPA Hospital, Thessaloniki, Greece.*
[2]*Laboratory of Experimental Ophthalmology, Aristotle University of Thessaloniki, Greece.*
[3]*Department of Nuclear Medicine, "Theageneion" Cancer Hospital of Thessaloniki, Greece.*

Authors' contributions

This work was carried out in collaboration between all authors. All authors read and approved the final manuscript.

Editor(s):
(1) Rachid Tahiri Joutei Hassani, Ophthalmology Department III, XV – XX National Ophthalmologic Hospital, France.
Reviewers:
(1) Anonymous, Recep Tayyip Erdogan University, Turkey.
(2) Jose Francisco de sales chagas, Department of surgery, Campinas Catholic University, Brazil.
(3) Anonymous, Gaziantep University Medical School, Turkey.
(4) Anonymous, Semmelweis University, Hungary.

ABSTRACT

Aims: To evaluate tear secretion of thyroid patients with no clinical evidence of thyroid ophthalmopathy in relation to thyroid status and history of I^{131} treatment by the use of the 2-minute Schirmer test I (test without topical anesthesia).

Study Design: Prospective study.

Place and Duration of Study: 1st University Eye Clinic, AHEPA Hospital, Thessaloniki, Greece and Laboratory of Experimental Ophthalmology, Aristotle University of Thessaloniki, Greece, between June 2013 and July 2014.

Methodology: 128 consecutive thyroid patients, 111 females and 17 males, aged from 18 to 82 years 49.48±14.61 (mean±sd) were recruited for this study. None of the thyroid patients had clinical

---

Corresponding author: E-mail: lamproslamprogiannis@hotmail.com, karamitsos_thanos@yahoo.com

signs or symptoms of thyroid ophthalmopathy. 49 of them had history of I^{131} treatment for thyroid carcinoma. The 2-min Schirmer test I was performed on the same day the patients underwent the routine exams for thyroid hormones. As abnormal were considered Schirmer test I values <10 mm.

Results: Out of 49 thyroid patients with history of I^{131} therapeutic treatment, 35 (71.4%) had 2-minute Schirmer test I values <10 mm. However there was no statistically significant difference in relation to their thyroid status. Regarding patients, with no previous I^{131} treatment, 55 out of 79 patients (71.4%) had Schirmer test I values <10 mm and there was no statistically significant difference in relation to their thyroid status. There was no statistically significant difference in Schirmer test I values between patients who received I^{131} and those who did not.

Conclusion: Thyroid patients without clinical evidence of thyroid ophthalmopathy have impaired Schirmer test I scores irrespective of the thyroid status and previous I^{131} exposure and thus they more likely to develop ocular surface abnormalities. Patients with previous I^{131} treatment had no statistically significant differences in the tear secretion values as compared with the non-irradiated thyroid patients.

Keywords: Schirmer test I; thyroid status; tear secretion; dry eye; I^{131} treatment.

1. INTRODUCTION

Dry eye syndrome or keratoconjunctivitis sicca is a common problem among middle-aged and older adults, and very often has a serious impact on quality of life. The treatment of the condition often causes frustration to both patients and ophthalmologists [1-4]. Sjögren syndrome, thyroid disease and other autoimmune diseases are main causes of dry eye syndrome [5-8]. Recent findings suggest that there is a direct involvement of the lacrimal gland in the pathological mechanism of the dry eye syndrome in thyroid patients [9] and lacrimal glands were found to be enlarged in patients with hyperthyroid Grave's disease [10]. Furthermore, octreotide was found in the lacrimal glands of thyroid patients [11]. Octreotide is a somatostatin analogue that exclusively binds to activated lymphocytes.

As regards the thyroid tumors, they are relatively common. Differentiated thyroid cancer (DTC) accounts for approximately 90% of all thyroid cancer [12]. Initial management is surgical. A near-total thyroidectomy is favored by many [13-16]. Postoperative I^{131} therapy is effective for ablation and treatment of loco-regional or metastatic disease, while L-thyroxin therapy diminishes the recurrence and improves survival rates [17,18]. In Graves' disease, I^{131} produces thyroid ablation without the complications of surgery [19,20].

Our objective in the present study is to evaluate the tear secretion of thyroid patients with no clinical evidence of thyroid ophthalmopathy in relation to their thyroid status and previous I^{131}

treatment. The 2-minute Schirmer test I (without topical anesthesia) was performed due to the advantage of shorter duration and acceptability from the patients [21].

2. MATERIALS AND METHODS

One hundred twenty-eight thyroid patients were recruited for the study (17 males and 111 females). The age of our patients ranged from 18 to 82 years and mean age was 49.48±14.61 years. Seventy-nine patients underwent thyroid-ectomy due to cancer or hyperthyroidism and the rest forty-nine had history of I^{131} treatment. All of the patients were under substitution or suppression treatment. The therapeutic dose of the the I^{131} treatment was 100 150 mCi (3.70 to 5.55 GBq). All these patients were frequently examined (RIA methods) for their thyroid status. All patients were evaluated for possible signs and symptoms of thyroid ophthalmopathy. In order to detect and quantify the patients' symptoms of possible ocular surface complications, we administrated the Ocular Surface Disease Index (OSDI) [22]. All patients had normal OSDI values (2.08±4.2). The eyelids, eyelid margins, conjunctiva and puncti as well as the cornea and the whole ocular surface were carefully evaluated for possible changes. Furthermore, all patients were examined for soft tissue involvement including periorbital oedema, ptosis, chemosis and epibulbar injection. To exclude possible proptosis, the patients were tested with the Hertel exophthalmometer. Readings greater than 20 mm or a difference equal or greater than 2 mm between two eyes considered as abnormal and patients were excluded from the study. As regards the control group one hundred and thirty healthy individuals free of symptoms and without any known or apparent pathology affecting tear secretion or drainage were recruited for this study. The Schirmer test was performed without topical anesthesia (Schirmer test I). Only one eye of the patients was examined, so as to eliminate the patients' discomfort and the 2-minute test was preferred for the advantage of shorter duration and better acceptability by the patients. Every subject was asked to be seated, while the 5-mm-long bend-end piece of the strip was placed on the lower lid margin in a temporal position. The subject was asked to keep both eyes open looking upwards while being observed by the examiner and instructed to avoid horizontal eye movements that might cause corneal irritation and consequent tear hypersecretion.

Two minutes later, the wetted length of the strip was measured and recorded. For the statistical analysis of the results, the Kolmogorov-Smirnov test was used. Using this test, we rejected the zero hypothesis for 0.05 significance level that variables follow normal distribution. Consequently, non parametric tests were used. Abnormal values for the 2-min Schirmer test were considered values <10 mm (based upon a previous study of our laboratory in a sample of 162 individuals without dry eye symptoms and normal tear secretion) [21].

In the day of the tear secretion testing, blood samples were obtained as part of routine clinical evaluations of the thyroid patients, for serum FT3, FT4 and TSH. Blood samples were centrifuged and the sera collected were stored at -20°C. Serum FT3, FT4 and TSH were assayed by immunoradiometric (IRMA) methods (DiaSorin, Saluggia, Italy). All assays were performed in duplicate. In our laboratory, reference values for FT3 were 2.2-5.5 pg/Ml (3.4–8.5 pmol/L), for FT4 were 7.8-19.4 pg/mL (10–25 pmol/L) and for TSH were 0.30-4.0 mU/L. As concerns FT3 the detection limit of the assay

and the intraassay and interassay variation expressed as coefficients of variation were 0.73 pmol/L, 5.0%, and 4.4%, respectively, for FT4, 1.25 pmol/L, 3.4%, and 5.1%, respectively and for TSH 0.04 mU/L, 2.5%, and 4.1%, respectively.

3. RESULTS AND DISCUSSION

The distribution of normal and abnormal Schirmer test I values, in relation to the thyroid status and previous history of I^{131} treatment, in our material is deployed in Table 1.

3.1 Statistical Analysis

In the statistical analysis the variables did not reach normality (Kolmogorov-Smirnov); we used non-parametric techniques, such as Mann-Whitney U test, Kruskal Wallis test and Spearman's Rank Correlation. Statistical significance was based on alpha level of .05.

a) Mann-Whitney Test was conducted to compare the Schirmer test's I *median value* of normal individuals and patients who did and did not have history of I^{131} treatment.

Statistically significant difference was found between Schirmer test I values of normal individuals and patients with no history of I^{131} treatment ($p<.005$). Statistically significant difference was found between Schirmer test I values of normal individuals and patients with history of I^{131} treatment ($p<.005$). There was no statistical significance (sig= .741 >.05) between the *median values* of patients with and without I^{131} treatment (Table 2).

b) Chi-square test (X^2) was conducted to assess the relationship between patients with *pathological* Schirmer test I in relation to having received I^{131} treatment or not.

Table 1. Distribution of normal and abnormal Schirmer test I values in relation to the thyroid status and previous history of I^{131} treatment

	Number of Patients		
	Euthyroids	**Hypothyroids**	**Hyperthyroids**
Normal values (with I^{131} treatment)	2	12	-
Abnormal values (with I^{131} treatment)	6	29	-
Normal values (no I^{131})	12	1	11
Abnormal values (not I^{131})	24	6	25

Table 2. Schirmer test's I median value of normal individuals and patients who did and did not have history of I[131] treatment

Normal	12.5
Without I[131]Treatment	7.5
With I[131]Treatment	7

There was no statistically significant difference (*P*= .985>.05) between patients with pathological Schirmer test I and who were treated with I[131] and those who were not. However, though there is no statistical significance between the two groups, the thyroid patients who received I[131] treatment tended to have lower Schirmer test I values (Table 3).

   c) Kruskal-Wallis test was conducted to assess the difference among the *mean values* of Schirmer test I of all patients who did and did not receive I[131] treatment, in relation to their thyroid status (euthyroids and hypothyroids).

In patients who receive I[131] treatment, there was no statistically significant diference (*P*= .535>.05) in relation to their thyroid status (euthyroids and hypothyroids). In patients who did not receive iodine, no statistically significant diference (p= .867>.05) was found in relation to their thyroid status (euthyroids, hypothyroids and hyperthyroid) (Table 4).

   d) Mann-Whitney Test was conducted to compare the Schirmer test's I *median value* of hypothyroid and euthyroid patients who received I[131] treatment and those who did not.

There was no statistical significance (sig= .645 >.05) between the *median values* of hypothyroid

and euthyroid patients with and without I[131] treatment (Table 5).

Table 3. Patients with pathological Schirmer Test I in relation to having received I[131] treatment or not

N	With I[131] Treatment	Without I[131] Treatment
Pathological Schirmer test	35 (out of 49)	55 (out of 79)

Chi Square test p=.985

The above analysis indicates that thyroid patients, who receive I[131] for thyroid cancer, have statistical significant abnormal Schirmer test I values irrespective of the thyroid status on the day of the examination and also, thyroid patients who did not receive I[131] treatment have statistical significant abnormal Schirmer test I values irrespective of the thyroid status, when compared with Schirmer test values on normal individuals. Comparing the results of the two groups, there was no statistically significant difference between the Schirmer test I values of those patients.

The Schirmer test I is a simple test and one of the commonest in use in the every day practice for the evaluation of tear secretion. The 2-minute test was prefered due to the shorter duration and less discomfort for the patients. Values ≥10 mm in 2 minutes were considered as normal [21]. We use to perform the test with open eyes so as to observe the eye movements of the patients and also to give him/her a target to see and thus to eliminate undesirable eye movements which may cause irritation and tear hypersecretion. Others prefer to perform the test with closed eyes [23-25].

Table 4. Schirmer Test I values±SD and thyroid status in patients with and without I[131] treatment

	Euthyroid	Hypothyroid	Hyperthyroid	
Patients with I[131] treatment	8.437±5.447	8.908±4.848		Kruskal Wallis Test p=.385
Patients without I[131] treatment	8.902±5.332	9.000±3.719	9.097±4.823	Kruskal Wallis Test p=.867

Table 5. Schirmer Test I median score of hypothyroids and euthyroids in relation to I[131] treatment

	With I[131] treatment	Without I[131] treatment	
Hypothyroids	7	8.5	Mann-Whitney Test p=.645
Euthyroids	6	8	Mann-Whitney Test p=.645

Thyroid associated ophthalmopathy is related with impaired tear secretion and to the best of our knowledge there are no reports in the international literature investigating tear production in thyroid patients who have no clinical signs and symptoms of thyroid associated ophthalmopathy and in relation to their thyroid status. As regards patients with thyroid associated ophthalmopathy, researchers evaluated the relationship between ocular surface damage, elevated lid aperture/impaired Bell's phenomenon and reduced tear production. Investigating the possible role of autoantibodies specific for TSH receptor (TSHR), they also investigated TSHR expression in the healthy lacrimal gland (LG). They concluded that ocular surface damage in thyroid associated ophthalmopathy significantly correlates with reduced tear production and not significantly with mechanical alterations and that LG impairements seem to be a major cause of eye dryness. They also concluded that physiological expression of TSHR by LG suggests that, in thyroid disease, autoantibodies may bind to lacrimal TSHR and contribute to LG impairment [9]. It is interesting to see that other investigators, who tried to define the clinical, laboratory, and histological features of patients with dry eyes and mouth syndrome (DEMS) and patients with sicca asthenia polyalgia syndrome (SAPS), found out that these patients have positive titers of antibodies against thyroid peroxidase [26]. Other researchers also investigated thyroid associated eye disease. In a study with Schirmer test II (with topical anesthesia) 21 patients with orbital echographic findings consistent with thyroid eye disease were evaluated. Only 19% of patients had abnormal Schirmer test II values and the symptomatology of eye dryness appeared to be attributable to an underlying ocular surface inflammation [27]. Also, in a study that aimed to evaluate preoperative and postoperative tear function tests and conjunctival surface changes in multinodular goiter (MNG) patients, and to compare their results with healthy control subjects, both tear function tests (including Schirmer test I values as well) and cytology findings of the MNG cases were statistically different from the results of the control group during the pre- and postoperative period. When thyroid hormone values of MNG patients were examined, it was seen that preoperative mean fT3 and mean fT4 values were lower than the mean values of the control group. After surgery and despite treatment, fT3 values were still in normal limits but were closer to the lower limit and they were significantly lower than the preoperative values, suggesting

insufficient T4-T3 turnover in some of the patients. This is suggesting that there is a probable relationship between postoperative low fT3 and high TSH levels indicating subclinical hypothyroidism that developed after nearly total thyroid gland excision that affects tear function tests [28].

The present study recruited thyroid patients without clinical evidence of thyroid ophthalmopathy. According to our results these thyroid patients tend to have impair tear secretion. 128 patients were examined. 79 had no history of previous I^{131} treatment. 36 of them were euthyroids, 7 hypothyroids and 36 hyperthyroids. 67% of euthyroids, 86% of hypothyroids and 69% of hyperthyroids had abnormal Schirmer test I values in 2 minutes. From 49 patients, who received I^{131} treatment for thyroid cancer, 8 were euthyroids and 41 were hypothyroids on the day of tear secretion evaluation. 75% of these euthyroids and 71% of these hypothyroids had abnormal Schirmer test I values.

As regards patients who received iodine, other researchers also investigated the long term effects of high dose I^{131} therapy on tear secretion. In a study concerning 175 eyes of 88 patients with history of I^{131} treatment, all patients received at least 2.96 GBq I^{131}. Schirmer test was decreased (<10 mm in 5 minutes) in 47 out of 88 patients and it was definitely abnormal (<5 mm in 5 minutes) in 35 out of 88 patients. All participants were free of any disease and of any drug that may affect tear production [29]. In an other study concerning patients who received high dose of I^{131}, the researchers studied 100 eyes of 50 patients who were treated for differentiated thyroid carcinoma and 100 eyes of 50 unexposed patients, who consisted the control group. Both groups (exposed and unexposed to I^{131} treatment) were consisted of thyroid patients of euthyroid status and they were free of any disease and of any drug that could affect tear secretion. Lower Schirmer test values were measured in the exposed group 14.5±10.8 mm, as compared with the control group (18.2±11.0 mm) (p=0.016). Relative risk of an abnormal Schirmer test in the exposed cases to control group was 1.78±0.62. Correlation coefficient analysis showed no significant relationship between Schirmer test values and cumulative doses of administrated I^{131} [30]. In the present study no statistically significant difference was found between exposed and non exposed to I^{131} treatment thyroid patients of euthyroid status. Furthermore, no statistically significant difference was found between exposed and non exposed to I^{131} treatment of hypothyroid status. In our study, 35 out of 49 patients (71.4%), who had history of previous I^{131} treatment, had abnormal Schirmer test I(<10 mm in 2 minutes) but no statistically significant difference was found between them and the thyroid patients who had no previous history of I^{131} treatment. Our patients received 3.70 to 5.55 GBq I^{131}.

Considering all thyroid patients in the present study (patients with I^{131} treatment and patients without I^{131} treatment and without clinical evidence of thyroid ophthalmopathy) have statistically significant lower Schirmer test I values in 2 minutes when compared with normal individuals. [...*text removed...*] No statistically significant difference was found among the mean scores of Schirmer test I of euthyroids, hypothyroids and hyperthyroids. No statistically significant difference was found among the mean scores of Schirmer test I of those thyroid patients who received I^{131} treatment and those who did not and also there was no statistically significant difference of the pathological Schirmer test I values between them.

4. CONCLUSION

Conclusively, thyroid patients without clinical evidence of thyroid ophthalmopathy tend to have impaired Schirmer test scores irrespective of the thyroid status and previous I^{131} exposure and thus it is more likely to develop ocular surface abnormalities. Also, patients with history of I^{131} treatment have no statistically significant differences in the tear secretion values as compared with the non-irradiated thyroid patients.

CONSENT

All authors declare that written informed consent was obtained from the patient for publication of this research. A copy of the written consent is available for review by the Editorial office/Chief Editor/Editorial Board members of this journal.

ETHICAL APPROVAL

All authors hereby declare that all experiments have been examined and approved by the ethics committee of AHEPA Hospital and have therefore been performed in accordance with the ethical standards laid down in the 1964 Declaration of Helsinki.

COMPETING INTERESTS

Authors have declared that no competing interests exist.

REFERENCES

1. Moss SE, Klein R, Klein BE. Incidence of dry eye in an older population. Arch Ophthalmol. 2004;122:369-373.

2. Thomas E, Hay EM, Hajeer A, Silman AJ. Sjögren's syndrome: A community-based study of prevalence and impact. Br J Rheumatol. 1998;37:1069-1076.

3. Nelson JD, Helms H, Fischella R, Southwell Y, Hirsch JD. A new look at dry eye disease and its treatment. Adv Ther. 2000;17:84-93.

4. Schifmann RM, Walt JG, Jacobsen G, Doyle JJ, Lebovics G, Summer W. Utility assessment among patients with dry eye disease. Ophthalmology. 2003;110:1412-1419.

5. Moss SE, Klein R, Klein BE. Prevalence of and risk factors for dry eye syndrome. Arch Ophthalmol. 2000;118:1264-1268.

6. Schein OD, Munoz B, Tielsch JM, Bandeen-Roche K, West S. Prevalence of dry eye among the elderly. Am J Ophthalmol. 1997;124:723-728.

7. McCarty CA, Bansal AK, Livingston PM, Stanislavsky YL, Taylor HR. The epidemiology of dry eye in Melbourne, Australia. Ophthalmology. 1998;105:1114-1119.

8. Caffery BE, Richter D, Simpson T, Fonn D, Doughty M, Gordon K. Candees: The Canadian dry eye epidemiology study. Adv Exp Med Biol. 1998;438:805-806.

9. Eckstein AK, Finkenrath A, Heiligenhaus A, Renzing-Köhler K, Esser J, Krüger C et al. Dry eye syndrome in thyroid-associated ophthalmopathy: Lacrimal expression of TSH receptors suggests involvement of TSHR-specific autoantibodies. Acta Ophthalmol Scand. 2004;82:291-297.

10. Chang TC, Huang KM, Chang TJ, Lin SL. Correlation of orbital computed tomography and antibodies in patients with hyperthyroid Graves' disease. Clin Endocrinol (Oxf). 1990;32:551-558.

11. Moncayo R, Baldissera I, Decristoforo C, Kedler D, Donnermiller E. Evaluation of immunological mechanisms mediating thyroid-associated ophthalmopathy by radionuclide imaging using the

somatostatin analogue 111 In-ocreotide. Thyroid. 1997;7:21-29.

12. Tuttle RM, Leboeuf R, Martorella AJ. Papillary thyroid cancer: Monitoring and therapy. Endocrinol Metab Clin North Am. 2007;36:753-78,7.

13. Gosnell JE, Clark OH. Surgical approaches to thyroid tumors. Endocrinol Metab Clin North Am. 2008;37:437-55,10.

14. Schlumberger MJ. Papillary and follicular thyroid carcinoma. N Engl J Med. 1998; 338:297-306.

15. Al-Brahim N, Asa SL. Papillary thyroid carcinoma: An overview. Arch Pathol Lab Med. 2006;130:1057-62.

16. Pacini F, Schlumberger M, Dralle H, Elisei R, Smit JW, Wiersinga W. European thyroid cancer taskforce. European consensus for the management of patients with differentiated thyroid cancer of the follicular epithelium. Eur J Endocrinol. 2006;154:783-803.

17. Van Nostrand D, Wartofsky L. I^{131} in the treatment of thyroid cancer. Endocrinol Metab Clin North Am. 2007;36:807-22,7-8.

18. Biondi B, Filetti S, Schlumberger M. Thyroid-hormone therapy and thyroid cancer: A reassessment. Nat Clin Pract Endocrinol Metab. 2005;1:32-40.

19. Hegedus L, Bonnema SJ, Bennedbaek FN. Management of single nodular goiter: Current status and future perspectives. Endocr Rev. 2003;24:102-132.

20. Sabri O, Zimny M, Schreckenberger M, Reiartz P, Ostwald E, Buell U. I^{131} therapy in Graves' disease patients with large diffuse goiters treated with or without carbimazole at the time of I^{131} therapy. Thyroid. 1999;9:1181-1188.

21. Karampatakis V, Karamitsos A, Skriapa A, Pastiadis G. Schirmer test I in 2 and in 5 minutes in normal individuals. Cornea. 2010;29(5):497-501.

22. Ocular Surface Disease Index (OSDI). Allergan; 1995. Available:http://www.dryeyezone.com/documents/osdi.pdf

23. Kashkouli MB, Pakdel F, Amani A, Asefi M, Aqhai GH, Falavarjani KG. A modified Schirmer test in dry eye and normal subjects: Open versus closed eye and 1-minute versus 5-minute tests. Cornea. 2010;29(4):384-387.

24. Serin D, Karslioglou S, Kryan A, Alaqöz G. A simple approach to the repeatability of the Schirmer test without anesthesia. Eyes open or closed? Cornea. 2007;26:903-906.

25. Bawazzer AM, Hodge WG. One-minute Schirmer test with anesthesia. Cornea. 2003;22:285-287.

26. Mavragani CP, Skopouli FN, Moutsopoulos HM. Increased prevalence of antibodies to thyroid peroxidase in dry eyes and mouth syndrome or sicca asthenia polyalgia syndrome. J Rheeumatol. 2009;36(8): 1626-30.

27. Gupta A, Sadeghi PB, Akpek EK. Occult thyroid eye disease in patients presenting with dry eye symptoms. Am J Ophthalmol. 2009;147:919-923.

28. Cavusoglu T, Nurozler AB, Titiz C, Ustun H, Aral Y, Ozer E, Kasim R, Tezel S. Tear function and ocular surface changes in multinodular goiter patients. Ophthalmologica. 2007;221(4):264-8.

29. Zeittinig G, Hanselmayer G, Fueger BJ, Hofmann A, Pirich C, Nepp J et al. Long-term impairment of the lacrimal glands after I^{131} therapy: A cross-sectional study. Eur J Nucl Med. 2002;29:1428-1432.

30. Fard-Esfahani A, Mirsherkarpour H, Fallahi B, Eftekhari M, Saqhari M, Beiki D, et al. The effect of high-dose I^{131} treatment on lacrimal gland function in patients with differentiated thyroid carcinoma. Clin Nucl Med. 2007;32:696-699.

8

A Prospective Study of Neuro-Cognitive Enhancement with Carotenoids in Elderly Adult Males with Early Age Related Macular Degeneration

Kelly G. Hoffmann[1*], Stuart P. Richer[2], James S. Wrobel[3], Eugenia Chen[4] and Carla J Podella[5]

[1]Neuro Psychology Department, Captain James A Lovell Federal Health Care Center, 3001 Green Bay Road, IL. 60064, North Chicago, USA.
[2]Optometry/Ophthalmology, Captain James A Lovell Federal Health Care Center, 3001 Green Bay Road, IL. 60064,North Chicago, USA.
[3]Department of Internal Medicine, University of Michigan Health System, Division of Metabolism, Endocrinology & Diabetes (MEND), USA.
[4]Rosalind Franklin University of Medicine and Science, 3333 Green Bay Road, North Chicago, USA.
[5]Captain James A Lovell Federal Health Care Center, 3001 Green Bay Road, North Chicago, USA.

Authors' contributions

This work was carried out by the Zeaxanthin and Vision Function (ZVF) Study Group, FDA IND #78,973, at the Captain James A Lovell, Federal Health Care Center, North Chicago, IL. Author SPR designed ZVF and wrote the main study protocol. Author KGH wrote and conducted the sub-protocol experimental work and wrote the first draft of the manuscript. Author JSW planned and conducted the statistical analysis. Author EC managed the literature searches, and author CJP maintained the database, assuring all manuscript requirements were met. All authors read and approved the final manuscript.

Editor(s):
(1) Li Wang, Department of Ophthalmology, Cullen Eye Institute, Baylor College of Medicine, USA.
Reviewers:
(1) Angel Nava-Castañeda, Oculopastic and Orbit Department, Universidad Nacional Autónoma de México, México.
(2) Michal Szymon Nowak, Department of Ophthalmology, Medical University of Lodz, Poland.
(3) Anonymous, Finland.
(4) Rahmi Duman, Dr. A.Y. Ankara Oncology Hospital, Turkey.

ABSTRACT

Background: Diets rich in carotenoids may reduce cognitive impairment. Little is known about dietary zeaxanthin.
Objective: Evaluate zeaxanthin carotenoid supplementation against change in cognitive status.

Corresponding author: E-mail: Kelly.Hoffmann@va.gov

Methods: American Psychological Association (APA) certified cognitive evaluation from the Zeaxanthin and Vision Function Study (USFDA Investigative New DrugIND#78,973), a 1 year prospective randomized controlled trial (RCT) of elderly males with mild age related macular degeneration. Neurocognitive testing Repeatable Battery for the Assessment of Neuropsychological Status Update RBANS and Trail Making A & B. Subjects evaluated at baseline and 1 year after dietary isomer RR zeaxanthin (8 mg/d) alone or combined with lutein (9 mg/d) using one way ANOVA, ($P<0.05$) and T testing.

Results: n=50 subjects completed both study visits. Delayed memory in the zeaxanthin group improved from RBANS score of 91.8 (SD 16) to 99.4 (SD 12), $P = 0.04$.

Conclusions: Zeaxanthin, typically minimally present in the US diet, may nonetheless be important in the context of emerging relationships in primates between dietary xanthophyll carotenoids and cognitive function. Additional larger scale RCTs is indicated to investigate the clinical utility of this carotenoid in nutritional neuroscience.

Keywords: Age related macular degeneration; carotenoids; macular pigment; cognition.

1. OBJECTIVES

The ZVF primary objectives were to evaluate the visual function properties of zeaxanthin independent of lutein, and to assess the added benefit of dietary RR zeaxanthin to traditional lutein supplementation, in elderly male veterans with AMD [1]. Accordingly, for this segment of the study, the objectives were as follows:

1) Evaluate the effect of carotenoid zeaxanthin on cognitive status.
2) Evaluate the effect of 8 mg zeaxanthin combined with 9 mg lutein on cognitive status.

2. PURPOSE AND BACKGROUND

Age-related macular degeneration (AMD) and cognitive impairment are both neurodegenerative disorders associated with aging and have been hypothesized to share common pathogenic pathways [2]. In a large population based study, Wong et al showed a weak association between cognitive function and early ARM. That is, persons with severe cognitive impairment based on Word Fluency Test scores were more likely to have early AMD (odds ratio (OR: 1.6, 95% confidence interval [CI]: 1.1-2.2) and its components, soft drusen (OR: 1.6; 95% CI: 1.1-2.3) as well as pigmentary abnormalities (OR: 1.5; 95% CI: 0.9-2.5) than those without severe impairment [3]. In a later second large scale trial, persons with low Digit Symbol Substitution Test (DSST) (lowest quartile of scores, ≤ 30) were more likely to have early AMD (odds ratio, 1.38; 95%confidence interval, 1.03-1.85) [4]. The authors conclude that in older populations, cognitive impairment may share common age-related pathogenesis and risk factors with early AMD.

There is a growing body of literature to support the use of dietary carotenoids i.e. lutein and zeaxanthin in the intervention of AMD [5,1]. Research has linked vision loss greater than 20/40 with cognitive impairment [6]. In healthy older adults, macular pigment optical density (MPOD) was only related to visual-spatial and constructional abilities. More recently, for subjects with mild cognitive impairment (MCI), MPOD was shown to be broadly related to cognition including the composite score on the mini-mental state examination, visual-spatial and constructional abilities, language ability, attention and total scale on the Repeatable Battery for the Assessment of Neuropsychological Status [7]. MPOD is related to cognitive function in primates and older adults, and a biomarker of L and Z embedded in all neural tissue [8,9].

Older adults consuming the highest amounts of green leafy vegetables and cruciferous vegetables (both rich sources of lutein) have slower cognitive decline than those consuming the lowest amounts [10,11]. Supplementation with lutein has been shown to improve cognitive function in older women [12]. As well, there is increasing support for the idea that oxidative stress may play an important role in the pathogenesis of more severe cognitive impairment, specifically Alzheimer's disease (AD), the most common form of cognitive impairment.

Historical evolving evidence has suggested oxidative stress is highly implicated in diseases associated with aging, and lesions typically associated with attacks by free radicals have been found in the brains of persons with AD. The free radicals in the brain that cause oxidative stress, high vascularity and metabolism along with an abundance of fat, provide fodder for free radical attack and protection by endogenous antioxidants [13]. However, early research with the specific antioxidants A and E, thought related to beta amyloid toxicity in AD brains, were found *not associated with* cognitive decline in non-demented subjects [14].

Nonetheless, more recent studies demonstrate that dietary antioxidants may indeed help with slowing the pathogenesis and thereby the progression of cognitive impairment. Observed delays in decline of ADL status, severe dementia, institutionalization and death support this position [13]. Other large scale cross sectional studies [15] suggest that while it is unclear whether low levels of plasma carotenoids precede or are the consequence of cognitive impairment, low carotenoid levels may play a role in cognitive impairment. Plasma analysis of a broad spectrum of antioxidants including carotenoids in elderly groups with unimpaired cognition, mild cognitive impairment (MCI) and Alzheimer's Disease (AD), showed lower levels of peripheral levels and activities of antioxidants in the MCI and AD groups as compared to healthy controls [16]. Therefore, it has been hypothesized that diets rich in antioxidants or supplementation may reduce the risk of cognitive impairment. Recently in the Georgia Centenarian Study, serum lutein, zeaxanthin, and β-carotene concentrations were most consistently related to better cognition ($P < 0.05$) in the whole population as well as centenarians. Only serum lutein was significantly related to better cognition in octogenarians [17].

Obviously, a lifetime of healthy, nutritionally rich foods would be preferable to late life supplementation. Yet, studies have statistically shown significant improvements with verbal fluency and memory scores following lutein and n3 fatty acid supplementation [12], and given that supplementation yields notoriously low negative side effects, this therapy avenue has warranted continued exploration. Accordingly, this study would purport to examine protective factors in the form of dietary supplements that are found in neural tissues and their effect on both AMD and cognitive functions. While both zeaxanthin and lutein are found throughout body tissues, the highest concentration exists in central neural regions, namely the retina, as well as frontal and occipital cortical regions of the brain [8,9].

3. STUDY DESIGN

The present study was conducted as a portion of a larger, one-year, prospective randomized, double blind, intention to treat, lutein (faux-placebo) controlled study of patients with early and moderate AMD, as determined by a retinal specialist using the AREDS 1 simplified scale. [1] No patients with advanced AMD were included. The sample included 60 patients, equally assigned to one of two dietary supplement treatment carotenoid pigment arms, or the traditional 9 mg non–esterified lutein (Kemin Health, Des Moines IA) supplement control group. The groups were broken down as follows: 8mg dietary RR zeaxanthin (Chrysantis, Ball Horticulture, Inc, Chicago, IL) (n=25); 8 mg zeaxanthin + 9 mg lutein (n=25) and the faux placebo 10 mg lutein control Group (n=10).

Subjects were patients in the Optometry/ Ophthalmology Clinic at the North Chicago VAMC with early AMD retinopathy participating in the Zeaxanthin and Vision Function RCT (The ZVF Study Group (FDA IND #78,973) [1]. Those with high risk NEI AREDS retinopathy or who had taken lutein or zeaxanthin supplements or had cataract or retinal surgery within the last 6 months were excluded. Those subjects taking photosensitizing drugs, did not meet ophthalmic/visual entrance criteria, had active comorbidities such as dementia (AD and non-AD type), schizophrenia, severe diabetes, glaucoma, uveitis or optic neuritis or were taking retinotoxic medications were all excluded.

4. METHODS

Age range of patients was 54 to 93 (mean of 75.1, SD = 10.0). Education ranged from 6 years of formal education to 20 years (mean of 13.4, SD = 2.6).After subjects were deemed eligible and informed consent was obtained, several assessments were completed and subsequently published, including:

1. Demographic and Symptom Assessment
2. Ocular Physical Assessment
3. Macular Function and Visual Measure-ments
4. Neuropsychological Assessment

Macular pigment is a well known surrogate marker of plasma levels – more so as it represents end organ tissue accumulation of carotenoids following competition within the duodenum for absorption as well as lipoprotein segregation within the liver. The present article focuses only on the Neuropsychological Assessment portion of the study at baseline and final study visit. Neurocognitive testing consisted of Repeatable Battery for the Assessment of Neuropsychological Status (RBANS) and the Trail Making Test A & B. RBANS is a brief and comprehensive cognitive assessment tool with age stratified norms, which provides a more global assessment of neuropsychological functioning for adults age 20 and older. Specifically, neurocognitive domains evaluated include immediate and delayed memory, attention, language and visuospatial/ constructional abilities. Trail Making Test A & B is a portion of the larger Halstead Reitan Neuropsychological Battery and measures simple and divided attention respectively. This test also taps speed of information processing, sequencing and visual scanning abilities. Norms from Tombaugh [18] were employed for the Trail Making Test, and norms published with the RBANS were used to interpret those scores.

RBANS and Trail Making Test A & B were administered at baseline and one year, at the conclusion of ZVF, by an APA certified neuropsychologist (KG-H) and her team.

5. STATISTICS

Data were determined to be normally distributed using the Kolmogorov-Smirnoff and Shapiro-Wilk tests. Analysis of variance (ANOVA) was used to assess for between group differences and the test of Scheffe was used to assess specific comparisons. Bartlett's Test was also used to test ANOVA's equal variances assumption. Differential scores were taken (baseline pre-test - 1 year post-test) and placed in a correlation matrix. Within the group, changes over time were assessed using a two sample, T test using an equal variances assumption. For all tests an alpha level of 0.05 was considered statistically significant. All calculations were made using STATA™ version 10.1 (College Station, Texas, USA).

6. RESULTS

In ZVF, 90% of subjects completed ≥ 2 visits with an initial Age Related Eye Disease Study (AREDS report #18) retinopathy score of 1.4 (1.0 SD) /4.0 (mild macular degeneration), pill intake compliance of 96% and no adverse effects. [1]All testing was administered by the ZVF study

neuropsychologist or trained and supervised technicians. Of 60 patients recruited, 60 completed the initial assessment, and 50 completed the second assessment. Data from deceased subjects (n = 2), those who dropped out (n = 7) or those who refused retesting (n = 1) were not analyzed. Therefore, the control group was comprised of 7 subjects of the original 10, 21 of 25 zeaxanthin only, and 22 of 25 in the lutein + zeaxanthin group.

In Table 1 appear the mean (SD) descriptive statistics (age, education), neurocognitive baseline and final RBANS and Trail Making A, B status. There was initial unequal variance for the RBANS variables 'Attention" and "Trail Making Factors B" which failed to sustain statistical significance, by study end.

As there was no true placebo in the ZVF design, one way analysis of variance (ANOVA) was performed on the entire data set to determine an effect from carotenoid supplementation. The RBANS mean sample index and Z scores indicated that, with the exception of immediate memory, the scores for simple and divided attention, delayed memory, visuospatial/ constructional abilities and language were all in the average range. Immediate memory fell within the low average range, in comparison with age and educationally matched normative samples:

- Immediate Memory ANOVA yielded $F_{(2, 49)} = 1.58$ with $p=0.22$.
- Visuospatial / constructional ANOVA yielded $F_{(2, 49)} = 0.731$ with $p=0.49$.
- Language ANOVA yielded $F_{(2, 49)} =0.052$ with $p=0.95$.
- Attention ANOVA yielded $F_{(2, 49)} = 1.35$ with $p=0.87$.
- Delayed Memory ANOVA yielded $F_{(2, 49)} = 0.067$ with $p=0.96$.
- Total RBANS Score ANOVA yielded $F_{(2, 49)} = 0.383$ with $p=0.68$.
- Trails A ANOVA yielded $F_{(2, 49)} = 1.429$ with $p=0.25$.
- Trails B ANOVA yielded $F_{(2, 49)} =0.039$ with $p=0.96$.

In Table 2, changes in neurocognitive status over time, for each of the 3 intervention groups is presented with a T test $P< 0.05$ considered significant. Individual and Total RBANS parameters as well as Trails A and B were all non-significant with the exception of zeaxanthin, RBANS delayed memory. Delayed memory in

Table 1. Mean (sd)ZVF population descriptive statistics (age, education) and neurocognitive baseline and final RBANS and Trail Making A, B scores. Initial baseline unequal variance for the variables "Attention" and "Trail Making Factors B" failed to sustain statistical significance, by study end

Variable	Baseline			Baseline Bartlett's test for equal variance between groups	Final			Final Bartlett's test for equal variance between groups
	N	Mean	(sd)		N	Mean	(sd)	
Age (yrs)	60	75.1	10.0	NS				NS
Education (yrs)	60	13.4	2.6	NS				NS
Immediate memory	60	88.3	15.3	NS	50	93.9	14.0	NS
Trails making factors b	60	-0.8	1.7	0.05	50	-0.9	2.3	NS
Visual spatial construction	60	98.4	19.7	NS	50	91.0	17.6	NS
Language	60	97.0	9.9	NS	50	99.1	8.6	NS
Attention	60	93.2	15.5	0.02	50	96.5	14.0	NS
Delayed memory	60	92.5	14.7	NS	50	95.4	16.0	NS
Total	60	91.6	13.3	NS	50	93.1	13.5	NS
Trails making factors a	60	0.1	0.9	NS	50	-0.1	1.3	NS

the zeaxanthin group improved from a RBANS score of 91.8 (SD 16) to 99.4 (SD 12), one way ANOVA, P = 0.04.

7. DISCUSSION

No significant differences were found between the groups except for "Delayed Memory", suggesting no broad multi factorial effect was seen by supplementing with zeaxanthin or by adding zeaxanthin to lutein. A larger sample size may have been able to show an effect size. Notably, subjects did however maintain their cognitive function during the duration of the study, lending at least modest support for the hypothesis that xanthophyll carotenoids can slow the progression of oxidative stress by containing free radicals and preserving neural tissue, over the 1 year ZVF study period, in elderly adult male veterans.

The strengths of this study are randomization, double masking and sensitive instruments. The weaknesses were no true placebo and non – generalizable to other populations such as the young, females and those without AMD. Differences with other studies were subtle, and may have been enhanced by subject selection and placement in groups with graded levels of

dementia (i.e., unimpaired, mild moderate and severe), that may have highlighted subtle effect(s). Subjects may have also been 'pre-screened for dementia' or other comorbid conditions adversely affecting cognitive performance.

The presence of a true 'control group' receiving a placebo instead of one of three treatment groups may have been useful to underscore any difference that might have been correlated with supplement use. As such, study design or subject selection procedures may have been a factor in masking additional benefit(s). Some studies actually stratify subjects' education-level [14], which is a known protective factor in the development of cognitive impairment. Since ZVF veterans manifested a broad range of education levels between 6 and 20 years, but overall a higher than average mean level at 13.2 years, this may have had a veiling effect on outcome.

Quite recently, serum markers of both oxidation and inflammation have been found to predate the onset of AD [19,20]. It follows that dietary modification / supplementation with carotenoids may take more than 1 year to mount an effect size measurable by our selected instruments.

Table 2. Change in Neurocognitive status over time, for 3 intervention groups: faux placebo lutein (left column); zeaxanthin (central column) and zeaxanthin + lutein (right column). 1 way ANOVA, $P<0.05$ considered significant

	n=	Lutein mean (SD)	P value	n =	Zeaxanthin mean (SD)	P value	n =	L + Zmean (SD)	P value
Immediate Memory	Baseline = 10 / Final = 7	84.7 (16.5) / 91.7 (17.5)	NS	Baseline = 25 / Final = 21	89.8 (16.0) / 96.5 (10.4)	NS	Baseline = 25 / Final = 22	88.3 (14.5) / 92.0 (16.1)	NS
Visual Spatial Construction	Baseline = 10 / Final = 7	102.6 (19.1) / 99.1 (19.2)	NS	Baseline = 25 / Final = 21	99.0 (18.0) / 93.6 (15.9)	NS	Baseline = 25 / Final = 22	96.1 (22.0) / 85.9 (17.8)	NS
Language	Baseline = 10 / Final = 7	91.8 (10.9) / 98.0 (5.2)	NS	Baseline = 25 / Final = 21	98.6 (9.5) / 98.0 (9.4)	NS	Baseline = 25 / Final = 22	97.4 (9.6) / 100.5 (8.9)	NS
Attention	Baseline = 10 / Final = 7	85.7 (18.2) / 97.9 (17.9)	NS	Baseline = 25 / Final = 21	90.2 (15.9) / 94.5 (14.2)	NS	Baseline = 25 / Final = 22	99.3 (11.8) / 98.0 (12.8)	NS
Delayed Memory	Baseline = 10 / Final = 7	93.1 (19.2) / 97.9 (20.7)	NS	Baseline = 25 / Final = 21	91.8 (12.3) / 99.4 (11.8)	0.04	Baseline = 25 / Final = 22	93.0 (15.5) / 90.7 (17.0)	NS
RBAN TOTAL	Baseline = 10 / Final = 7	89.0 (16.8) / 96.0 (17.9)	NS	Baseline = 25 / Final = 21	91.4 (11.6) / 93.7 (11.4)	NS	Baseline = 25 / Final = 22	93.0 (13.8) / 91.6 (14.3)	NS
Trails Making A	Baseline = 10 / Final = 7	-0.50 (1.2) / -0.99 (1.2)	NS	Baseline = 25 / Final = 21	0.10 (0.8) / -0.18 (1.5)	NS	Baseline = 25 / Final = 22	0.4 (0.9) / 0.2 (1.0)	NS
Trails Making B	Baseline = 10 / Final = 7	-1.2 (1.7) / -1.3 (1.8)	NS	Baseline = 25 / Final = 21	-0.74 (1.7) / -0.65 (1.4)	NS	Baseline = 25 / Final = 22	-0.65 (1.8) / -0.99 (3.2)	NS

Future studies may also do well to pair serum markers with cognitive screening tools completed by patients or their surrogates, functional visual assessment measures and new objective structural measures of the human lens and retina. This would yield data that could illuminate any relationship between plasma levels, cognitive performance, objective ocular tissue biomarkers and patient/family observations regarding functional cognitive capacity. Such a global data set would enable researchers to evaluate cognitive performance and ocular functional/structural improvements, enhancing the ecological validity of evaluating the eye and brain together.

4. CONCLUSION

Cognitive decline and visual decline remain major comorbidities among the aging population, with incidence increasing exponentially from 65 years of age to 85 years of age [21]. With the significant increase in both the number and longevity of older persons, it becomes necessary to identify universal lifestyle choices and treatment options that might stabilize or reduce the effects of aging on both visual and cognitive disability. Dietary xanthophyll carotenoids will surely play a role.

INFORMED CONSENT AND ETHICAL APPROVAL

The ZVF study (FDA IND # 78,973) obtained and secured informed consent, protection of privacy, and other human rights through the Institutional Review Board and Human Subjects Committees at Hines, VA (Chicago, IL). "All authors hereby declare that all experiments have been examined and approved by the appropriate ethics committee and have therefore been performed in accordance with the ethical standards laid down in the 1964 "Declaration of Helsinki."

ACKNOWLEDGEMENTS

This work was supported by the Optometry/Ophthalmology sections of Captain James Lovell Federal Health Care Facility, DVA-Naval Medical Center, North Chicago, IL, USA. Thanks also to EJ Johnson, PhD - Tufts University, for thoughtful review and comments.

COMPETING INTERESTS

Authors have declared that no competing interests exist.

REFERENCES

1. Richer SP, Stiles WR, Graham-HoffmannK, Levin MR, Ruskin D, Wrobel J, et al. Randomized, double-blind, placebo-controlled study of zeaxanthin and visual function in patients with atrophic age-related macular degeneration: the zeaxanthin and visual function study (ZVF) FDA IND#78,973. Optometry. 2011;82(11): 667-680.e6.
DOI: 10.1016/j.optm.2011.08.008.

2. Nolan JM, Loskutova E, Howard AN, Moran R, Mulcahy R, Stack J, et al. Macular pigment, visual function, and macular disease among subjects with Alzheimer's disease: an exploratory study. JAlzheimers Dis. 2014;42(4):1191-202.
DOI: 10.3233/JAD-140507.

3. Wong TY, Klein R, Nieto FJ, Moraes SA, Mosley TH. Is early age-related maculopathy related to cognitive function? The atherosclerosis risk in communities study. Am J Ophthalmol. 2002;134(6):828-35.

4. Baker ML, Wang JJ, Rogers S, Klein R, Kuller LH, Larsen EK, et al. Early age-related macular degeneration, cognitive function, and dementiathe cardiovascular health study. Arch Ophthalmol. 2009;127(5):667-673.
DOI: 10.1001/archophthalmol.2009.30.

5. Richer SP, Stiles W, Statkute L, Pulido J, Frankowski J, Rudy D, et al. A placebo-controlled, double blind, randomized trial of lutein and antioxidant supplementation for the treatment of age related macular degeneration: the Lutein Antioxidant Supplementation Trial. Optometry. 2004;75: 216-30.

6. AREDS Research Group. Cognitive impairment in the age related eye disease study (AREDS report number 16). Archives of Ophthalmology. 2006;124(4):537-43.

7. Renzi LM, Dengler MJ, Puente A, Miller LS, Hammond BR Jr. Relationships between macular pigment optical density and cognitive function in unimpaired and mildly cognitively impaired older adults. Neurobiol Aging. 2014;35(7):1695-9.
DOI:10.1016/j.neurobiolaging.2013.12.024. Epub 2013 Dec 27.

8. Vishwanathan R, Neuringer M, Snodderly DM, Schalch W, Johnson EJ. Macular lutein and zeaxanthin are related to brain lutein and zeaxanthin in primates. Nutr Neurosci. 2013;16(1):21-9.

DOI: 10.1179/1476830512Y.0000000024. Epub 2012 Jul 9.

9. Vishwanathan R, Iannaccone A, Scott TM, Kritchevsky SB, Jennings BJ, Carboni G, et al. Macular pigment optical density is related to cognitive function in older people. Age Ageing. 2014;43(2):271-5. DOI:10.1093/ageing/aft210. Epub 2014 Jan 15

10. Kang JH, Ascherio A, Grodstein F. Fruit and vegetable consumption and cognitive decline in aging women. Ann Neurol. 2005;57(5):713-20.

11. Morris MC, Evans DA, Tangney CC, Bienias JL, Wilson RS. Associations of vegetable and fruit consumption with age-related cognitive change. Neurology. 2006;67(8):1370-6.

12. Johnson, EJ, McDonald, K, Caldarella, S, Chung H, Troen AM, Snodderly DM. Cognitive findings of an exploratory trial of docosahexaenoic acid and lutein supplementation in older women. Nutr Neur. 2008;11(2):75-83. DOI: 10.1179/147683008X301450.

13. Christen Y. Oxidative stress and Alzheimer's disease. Amer J ClinNutr. 2000;71(2):621S-9S.

14. Engelhart MJ, Ruitenberg A, Meijer J, Kiliaan A, van Swieten JC, Hofman A, Witteman JC, et al. Plasma levels of antioxidants are not associated with Alzheimer's disease or cognitive decline. Dement Geriatr Cogn Disord. 2005;19(2-3):134-9. Epub 2004 Dec 23.

15. Akbaraly NT, Faure H, GourletV, Favier A, Berr C. Plasma carotenoid levels and cognitive performance in an elderly population: results of the EVA study. J Gerontol A BiolSci Med Sci. 2007;62(3): 308-16.

16. Rinaldi P, Polidori MC, Metastasio A, Mariani E, Mattoli P, Cherubini A, et al. Plasma antioxidants are similarly depleted in mild cognitive impairment and in Alzheimer's disease 2003. Nov (the cochrane controlled trials register – cctr/central) Neuro Aging. 2003;915:915-9.

17. Johnson EJ, Vishwanathan R, Johnson MA, Hausman DB, Davey A, Scott TM, et al. Relationship between Serum and Brain Carotenoids, α-Tocopherol, and Retinol Concentrations and Cognitive Performance in the Oldest Old from the Georgia Centenarian Study. J Aging Res. 2013;2013:951786. DOI: 10.1155/2013/951786. Epub 2013 Jun 9

18. Tombaugh TN. Trail making test a and b: normative data stratified by age and education. Arc Clin Neur. 2004;19:203-14.

19. Nguyen JC, Killcross AS, Jenkins TA. Obesity and cognitive decline: role of inflammation and vascular changes. Front Neurosci. 2014;8:375. DOI:10.3389/fnins.2014.00375. eCollection 2014.

20. Clarke JR, LyraESilva NM, Figueiredo CP, Frozza RL, Ledo JH, Beckman D, Katashima CK, et al. Alzheimer-associated Aβ oligomers impact the central nervous system to induce peripheral metabolic deregulation. EMBO MolDed. 2015;7(2):190-210. DOI: 10.15252/emmm.201404183.

21. Bernstein AB, Remsburg RE. Estimated prevalence of people with cognitive impairment. Results from a nationally representative community and institutional surveys. Gerontologist. 2007;47:350-4.

9

Therapeutic Efficacy of Intravitreal Bevacizumab (Avastin)® in Patients with Parafoveal Telangiectasia Type II Complicated by Choroidal Neovascular Membrane and/or Cystoid Macular Edema

Achyut N. Pandey[1*], Anil Kakde[2], Parul Singh[1], Amit Vikram Raina[1] and Ameeta Kaul[1]

[1]*Departement of Ophthalmology, VCSG Medical College and Research Institute, Srinagar Garhwal, Uttarakhand, 246174, India.*
[2]*Eye Q Super Speciality Hospital, Gurgaon, India.*

Authors' contributions

This work was carried out in collaboration between all authors. All authors read and approved the final manuscript.

Editor(s):
(1) Ahmad M Mansour, Department of Ophthalmology, American University of Beirut, Lebanon.
Reviewers:
(1) Brian C Joondeph, Colorado Retina Associates, Denver, CO, USA.
(2) Asaad Ahmed Ghanem, Mansoura ophthalmic center, Mansoura University, Egypt.

ABSTRACT

Aim: To evaluate the therapeutic efficacy of intravitreal bevacizumab (Avastin)® on visual acuity and macular edema in patients with parafoveal telangiectasia type II complicated by choroidal neovascular membrane and/or cystoid macular edema.

Methods: Study conducted over a period of 12 months, at a tertiary eye care hospital including forty eyes of 25 patients (11 male, 14 female) suffering from type II parafoveal telangiectasia with choroidal neovascular membrane and/or cystoid macular edema who fulfilled the inclusion criteria. These were treated with intravitreal bevacizumab (Avastin). Each of the 40 eyes was enrolled into one of two groups, namely group 1: Eyes with parafoveal telangiectasia type II with choroidal neovascular membrane and group 2: Eyes with parafoveal telangiectasia type II with

---

*Corresponding author: E-mail: achyutpandey@gmail.com

presence of cystoid macular edema but without choroidal neovascular membrane .All the patients underwent best corrected visual acuity slit lamp bimicroscopy, direct and indirect ophthalmoscopy, intra ocular pressure (IOP), clinical fundus photography, fundus fluorescein angiography (FFA) and optical coherence tomography (OCT). Follow up of patients was done at the first, third and sixth months after presentation.

Results: 2 groups, in group1-11 patients with equal male and female ratio, mean age 56.27±8.49 years, group 2-18 patients with female preponderance, mean age 53.5±7.18 years. In group1, no significant improvement in mean BCVA before inj. Bevacizumab 0.121±0.06 and after injection 0.147±0.06 (P=0.051), while statistically significant improvement noticed in mean CFT, before inj. 469±89.67 and after injection 310.78±85.61 (P=0.001). Similarly in group 2, no significant improvement in mean BCVA before inj. Bevacizumab 0.224±0.16 and after injection 0.254±0.09 (P=0.453), while statistically significant improvement noticed in mean CFT, before inj. 356.77±43.22 and after injection 253±42.59 (P=0.001). Transient hyperemia and subconjunctival hemorrhage were noticed in 2 patients in both group 1 and 2, while increase in blood pressure were observed in 2 patients in group 1 and 4 in group 2. None of the patients reported deterioration of vision following the injection.

Conclusion: In parafoveal telangiectasis type II complicated by choroidal neovascular membrane there is definite short-term improvement in the visual acuity (approaching statistical significance) and definite significant reduction of central foveal thickness following intravitreal injection of bevacizumab. In patients suffering from parafoveal telangiectasis type II complicated by cystoid macular oedema, there is definite significant reduction of central foveal thickness but no significant improvement in the visual acuity following intravitreal injection of bevacizumab. Bevacizumab is safe and well tolerated in eyes with parafoveal telangiectasis type II complicated by choroidal neovascular membrane and/or cystoid macular edema. No severe ocular or systemic adverse effects were encountered in this study.

Keywords: Parafoveal telangiectasia; choroid neovascular membrane; cystoids macular edema; bevacizumab; central foveal thickness.

1. INTRODUCTION

Retinal telangiectasia refers to a developmental retinal vascular disorder characterized by an ectasia of capillaries of the retina, in which irregular capillary dilatation and incompetence occur in the retinal periphery or the macula [1-3]. When only the capillaries of the foveal avascular zone are involved it is known as "parafoveal telangiectasia". Idiopathic juxtafoveolar retinal telangiectasis is also known as parafoveal telangiectasia or idiopathic macular telangiectasia [4,5].

The term "retinal telangiectasis" was first coined by Reese to describe the developmental vascular anomalies seen in patients with Coat's disease and Leber's military aneurysms. The term "parafoveal telangiectasis" was first used by Gass who observed that only the parafoveal retinal capillaries showed telangiectasia and fluorescein angiography (FA) was required to diagnose these cases [2]. Gass and Oyakawa proposed the first classification of these entities into four groups based largely on their clinical and fluorescein angiographic (FA) features [2,6-8].

In parafoveal telangiectasia type II, vascular endothelial growth factor has been implicated as the major angiogenic stimulus responsible for neovascularization. Several case series in the literature have investigated bevacizumab or ranibizumab for the treatment of parafoveal telangiectasia type II with choroidal neovascularization but with limited follow-up (12 months or less) [3-7]. However, only a few studies have been done thus far regarding the use of intravitreal bevacizumab (Avastin)® in parafoveal telangiectasia type II with or without choroidal neovascularization [7-11]. Moreover, no prospective study has been performed thus for on Indian patients regarding use of intravitreal bevacizumab in parafoveal telangiectasia type II.

The purpose of the current study was to evaluate the anatomical and functional efficacy of intravitreal bevacizumab (Avastin)® in Indian patients suffering from parafoveal telangiectasia type II with or without choroidal neovascularisation in a prospective manner.

To evaluate the therapeutic efficacy of intravitreal bevacizumab (Avastin)® on visual acuity and macular edema in patients with parafoveal telangiectasia type II complicated by choroidal neovascular membrane and/or cystoid macular edema.

2. SUBJECTS AND METHODS

This Investigative, open label, prospective, interventional study was performed at the retina department of tertiary eye care institute over a period of 12 months.

2.1 Study Groups

Group1: parafoveal telangiectasia (PFT) type II with choroidal neovascular membrane (CNVM); Group 2: Parafoveal telangiectasia (PFT) type II with cystoid macular edema (CME).

Interventional group 1 consisted of 11 patients (18 eyes) and interventional group 2 consisted of 14 patients (22 eyes).

Inclusion Criteria Patients were enrolled if they satisfied the inclusion criteria, namely: 1) Presented with type II parafoveal telangiectasia with choroidal neovascular membrane (CNVM) and/or cystoid macular edema (confirmed by fundus photography, fluorescein angiography, and optical coherence tomography); 2) Were males or females aged 40 years and above; 3) Were willing to provide signed written informed consent to participate in the study.

Exclusion Criteria Patients were not considered for enrolment in the study if they had any one of the following exclusion criteria: 1) Additional eye disease that could compromise visual acuity (VA); 2) Ocular inflammation; 3) Intraocular surgery had been performed ≤1 month before presentation; 4) Patient had received prior treatment with laser photocoagulation or other interventions for macular edema; 5) Media opacities that prevented clear visualization of the fundus and OCT examination; 6) Patient was pregnant; 7) Patients not willing to provide signed written informed consent to participate in the study.

Sample Size and Sample Technique Based on frequency of presentation of patients with parafoveal telangiectasis at the Study Place in previous years, it was estimated that, at the rate of five new patients per month, approximately 120 new patients (population size) would be seen during the study period of one year (August 2010 to July 2011). Expecting a response distribution of 20% and

taking into account a confidence level of 95% and margin of error of 5%, the recommended sample size in each arm of the study was calculated to be 49 patients (on-line sample size calculation, raosoft.com), using the formula $n=Nx/[(N-1)E^2 +x]$, where 'n' refers to the calculated sample size, 'N' refers to the population size, 'E' refers to the margin of error and 'x' refers to the response distribution(percentage).

Due to various constraints, in particular the reluctance of patients to receive an intraocular injection and to be enrolled in a formal study with regular follow-up, it was finally possible to enroll only a smaller number of patients.

Forty eyes of 25 patients (11 male, 14 female) suffering from type II parafoveal telangiectasia with choroidal neovascular membrane and/or cystoid macular edema who fulfilled the inclusion criteria and did not have any exclusion criteria, were enrolled. These were treated with intravitreal bevacizumab (Avastin)® 2.50 mg (0.10 mL volume of solvent). Each of the 40 eyes was enrolled into one of two groups, namely:_1) Group 1: eyes with parafoveal telangiectasia type II with choroidal neovascular membrane; 2) Group 2: eyes with parafoveal telangiectasia type II with presence of cystoid macular edema but without choroidal neovascular membrane.

2.2 Efficacy Parameters

Improvement of one line or more in best corrected visual acuity (BCVA) and reduction of central foveal thickness (CFT) by 50 microns or more at intervals of one month were taken to indicate acceptable criteria (value) of clinical efficacy of intravitreal bevacizumab in the present study. Due to the inherent time constraint of the current study, sustenance of the improved BCVA or reduced CFT over a longer time period was not possible.

2.3 Safety and Tolerability

Safety and tolerability assessments (both ocular and systemic) of intravitreal bevacizumab administration were monitored by subjective evaluation of patients (complaints, detailed history and relevant examination), ocular examination and systemic evaluation (including relevant laboratory investigations). The greatest importance was given to all-cause mortality and serious adverse events, validated visual acuity measures and effects on activities of daily living and quality of life .Severe ocular adverse events sought included retinal tear, endophthalmitis, lenticular opacity, vitreous hemorrhage, glaucoma, retinal detachment and specific complications including anterior chamber reactions and fibrous proliferation retinal, pigment epithelial tear, submacular haemorrhage, progression of tractional retinal detachment and visual hallucinations. Systemic adverse events sought included increased blood pressure, myocardial infarction, stroke, transient ischemic attacks, deep vein thrombosis, angina, renal disorders, gastrointestinal bleeding, skin rash or redness and menstrual irregularities within 1 month of intravitreal bevacizumab injection.

2.4 Statistical Methods

Data pertaining to age of patients are presented as proportions (percentage of patients in specific age ranges) as well as mean age (in years)±standard deviation. Data pertaining to BCVA (pre-treatment and post-treatment) in individual eyes are presented as decimal values and data pertaining to CFT (pre-treatment and post-treatment) in individual eyes are presented asμm (micrometers). Data pertaining to mean BCVA and mean CFT values are presented as mean±standard deviation.

The statistical significance of intergroup differences between mean age, mean BCVA (pre-treatment and post-treatment) and mean CFT (pre-treatment and post-treatment) in Group 1 eyes versus Group 2 eyes was calculated by the Student 't' test using SPSS software package for Windows (Version 16.0; SPSS Inc, Chicago, IL, USA). The statistical significance of intragroup differences between pre-treatment and post-treatment mean BCVA values and mean CFT values were also calculated by the Student 't' test Values were considered statistically significant when $P<0.05$.

3. RESULTS

This investigative, open-label, prospective, interventional study was performed at the retina clinic of a tertiary eye care facility in southern India over a period of 12 months. Twenty five patients (40 eyes), comprising 11 males and 14 females (age range 40 to 70 years), who presented with parafoveal telangiectasia type II during the study period, who satisfied the inclusion criteria and who provided consent for participation, were included in the study. This study was approved

by the Institutional Ethics Committee of the eye care facility. Upon presentation (baseline) and after ensuring that all investigational requirements were satisfied, patients were divided into two interventional groups:

Group 1: Parafoveal telangiectasia (PFT) type II with choroidal neovascular membrane (CNVM);
Group 2: Parafoveal telangiectasia (PFT) type II with cystoid macular edem (CME).

Interventional group 1 consisted of 11 patient (18 eyes) and interventional group 2 consisted of 14 patients (22 eyes). Patient demographics and baseline ocular characteristics are listed in Tables 1-4.

Table 1. Gender of patients who presented with parafoveal telangiectasia type 2 with choroidal neovascular membrane (Group 1)

Gender	No. of patients
Male	6
Female	5
Total	11

Table 2. Age of patients who presented with parafoveal telangiectasia type 2 with choroidal neovascular membrane (Group 1)

Age group (years)	No. of patients	Percentage (%)
40 – 50	3	27.27%
51 – 60	3	27.27%
61 – 70	5	45.45%
Total	11	100

The mean age was 56.27±8.49 years (range=45 years to 70 years)

3.1 Evaluation of Efficacy of Intravitreal Bevacizumab in Patients with Parafoveal Telangiectasia Type 2

3.1.1 a) Group 1 (PFT type II witn CNVM) (Fig. 1)

This group included 11 patients (18 eyes) with PFT type II with CNVM who were treated with an intravitreal injection of bevacizumab 2.50 mg (0.1 mL) under aseptic conditions. Of these 11 patients six were males (55%) and five were females (45%). The age distribution ranged between 45 to 70 years (mean age=56.27±8.5 years; median age=54 years); 45.45% of the patients belonged to the 61-70 year age group. Two patients had both diabetes mellitus (DM) and hypertension (HTN), whereas one patient had both DM and ischemic heart disease (IHD).

Table 3. Gender of patients who presented with parafoveal telangiectasia type 2 with cystoid macular edema (Group 2)

Gender	No. of patients
Male	5
Female	9
Total	14

Table 4. Age of patients who presented with parafoveal telangiectasia type 2 with cystoid macular edema (Group 2)

Age group (years)	No. of patients	Percentage (%)
40 – 50	5	36%
51 – 60	6	43%
61 – 70	3	21%
Total	14	100

The mean age of the patients was 53.5±7.18 years (range=40 years to 65 years)

Details about the pre-treatment and post-treatment best corrected visual acuity (BCVA in decimals) and central foveal thickness (in μm) values in each individual eye in this group are shown in Fig. 1. The mean BCVA at presentation was 0.121 (approximately 6/60)±0.06 decimals, which was not significantly different (P=0.051) from the post-bevacizumab injection BCVA value of 0.147 (approximately 6/36)±0.06 decimals.

However, there was a significant difference (P=0.001) between the mean central foveal thickness at presentation (469.17±89.67 μm) and the mean central foveal thickness (310.78±85.61 μm) after the intravitreal injection of bevacizumab. One eye showed a decreased BCVA (from 6/60 to 3/60) following intravitreal bevacizumab; however, the same eye exhibited a reduction in central foveal thickness (from 417 μm to 313 μm) following the injection. Ten eyes did not exhibit any change in BCVA, but showed a significant reduction in central foveal thickness.

3.1.2 b) Group 2 (PFT type II with CME) (Fig. 2)

This group included 14 patients with PFT type II and CME who were treated with an intravitreal injection of bevacizumab 2.50 mg (0.1 mL) under aseptic conditions. Out of 14 patients, five were males (36%) and nine were females (64%). The age distribution ranged from 40 to 65 years (mean age 54.0±7.18 years), six patients belonged to the 51-60 year age group. Four patients had DM and HTN as associated systemic illnesses, two patients had only HTN, two patients had only DM and one patient had bronchial asthma.

Details about the pre-treatment and post-treatment BCVA and central foveal thickness values in each individual eye in this group are shown in Fig. 2.

The mean BCVA at presentation was 0.224 (approximately 6/24)±0.16 decimals which was not significantly different (P=0.453) from the post-bevacizumab injection BCVA value of 0.2545 (approximately 6/24)±0.09 decimals.

There was a significant difference (P=0.001) between the mean central foveal thickness at presentation (356.77±43.22 μ) and the mean central foveal thickness (253±42.59 μ) after the intravitreal injection of bevacizumab. One eye showed a decreased BCVA (from 6/36 to 3/60) following intravitreal bevacizumab; however, the same eye exhibited a reduction in central foveal thickness (from 410 μ to 298 μ) following the injection. Six eyes did not exhibit any change in BCVA, but showed a significant reduction in central foveal thickness.

3.1.3 c) Comparison between different parameters in Group 1 and Group 2

The mean age of the 11 patients in Group 1 (parafoveal telangiectasia type II [PFT] with choroidal neovascular membrane [CNVM]) was 56.27±8.8 years and the mean age of the 14 patients in Group 2 (PFT with cystoid macular edema [CME]) was 53.5±7.2 years (Table 5); this difference was not statistically significant (unpaired 't' test value=0.88 [degree of freedom {df}]=23); P=0.39).

Males comprised six of 11 (55%) patients in Group 1 and five of 14 (36%) patients in Group 2; this difference was not statistically significant (χ^2 (d.f.=1)=0.6; P>0.05).

The pre-treatment mean best corrected visual acuity (BCVA) in Group 1 (18 eyes) was 0.121±0.06 decimals while that in 22 Group 2 eyes was 0.22±0.16 decimals (Table 5; this difference was statistically significant (unpaired 't' test value=2.31[df=38]; 2-tailed P=0.03).

Table 5. Comparison of mean age, pre-treatment and post-treatment best corrected visual acuity and pre-treatment and post-treatment central foveal thickness in patients and eyes with parafoveal telangiectasis type II

Parameter	Group 1	Group 2
Age (years)	56.27±8.50 (11 patients)	53.5±7.18 (14 patients)
Pre- treatment Visual acuity (decimals	0.121±0.07 (18 eyes)	0.224±0.16 (22 eyes)
Post- treatment Visual acuity (decimals)	0.147±0.064 (18 eyes)	0.254±0.098 (22 eyes)
Pre-treatment central foveal thickness (µ)	469.17±89.67 (18 eyes)	360.73±43.32 (22 eyes)
Post-treatment central foveal thickness (µ)	310.78±85.61 (18 eyes)	253.45 ±42.6 (22 eyes)

Group 1: 11 patients (18 eyes) with parafoveal telangiectasis with choroidal neovascular membrane
Group 2: 14 patients (22 eyes) with parafoveal telangiectasis with cystoid macular edema

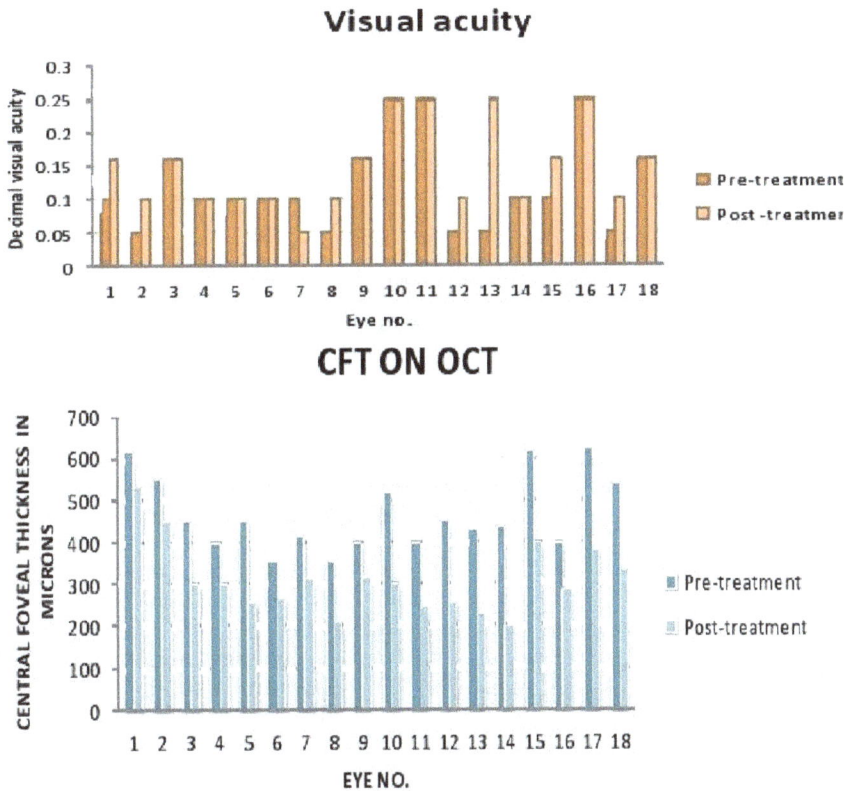

Fig. 1. Comparison of pre-treatment and post-treatment
a) Best corrected visual acuity (in decimals) and b) central foveal thickness (µm) in 18 eyes with parafoveal telangiectasia type 2 with choroidal neovascular membrane (group 1)

The post-treatment mean BCVA in Group 1 eyes (18 eyes) was 0.147±0.06 decimals while the post-treatment mean BCVA in Group 2 eyes (22 eyes) was 0.254±0.098 decimals (Table 5); this difference was highly statistically significant (unpaired `t' test value=4.51 [df=38]; 2-tailed P<0.0001).

The pre-treatment mean central foveal thickness (CFT) in 18 Group 1 eyes was 469.17±89.67 µm while that in 22 Group 2 eyes was 360.73±43.3 µm (Table 5); this difference was highly statistically significant (unpaired `t' test value=5.01 [df=38]; 2-tailed P<0.0001).

The post-treatment mean CFT in 18 Group 1 eyes was 310.78±85.61 µm while the post-treatment mean CFT in 22 Group 2 eyes was 253.0±42.6 µm (Table 5); this difference was statistically significant (unpaired `t' test value=2.78 [df=38]; 2-tailed P=0.0084).

Visual acuity

CFT ON OCT

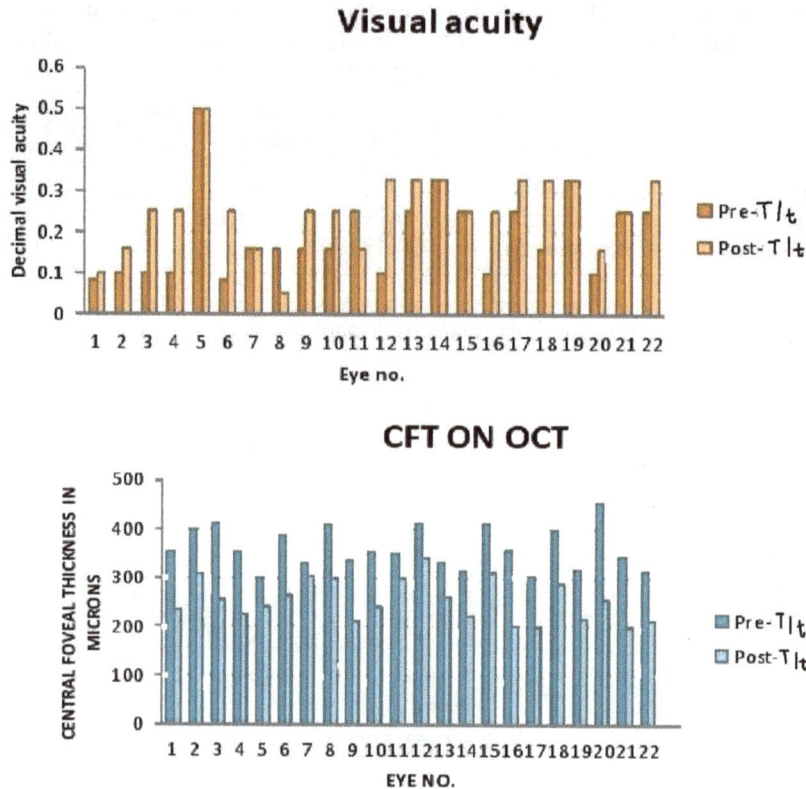

Fig. 2. Comparison of pre-treatment and post-treatment
a) Best corrected visual acuity and b) central foveal thickness in 22 eyes with parafoveal telangiectasia type 2 with cystoid macular edema

3.2 Statistical Analysis

a) Mean age of patients in Group 1 *vs* Group 2; Unpaired `t' test value=0.88 (degree of freedom [df]=23); P=0.39 (not significant);

b) Pre-treatment mean best corrected visual acuity (BCVA) in Group 1 *vs* Group 2 eyes; Unpaired `t' test value=2.31(df=38); 2-tailed P=0.03 (significant);

c) Post-treatment mean BCVA in Group 1 eyes *vs* Group 2 eyes; Unpaired `t' test value=4.51 (df=38); 2-tailed P<0.0001 (very significant);

d) Pre-treatment mean central foveal thickness (CFT) in Group 1 eyes *vs* Group 2 eyes; Unpaired `t' test value=5.01 (df=38); 2-tailed P<0.0001 (very significant);

e) Post-treatment mean CFT in Group 1 eyes *vs* Group 2 eyes; Unpaired `t' test value=2.78 (df=38); 2-tailed P=0.0084 (significant);

f) In Group 1 eyes, pretreatment mean BCVA *vs* post-treatment mean BCVA; Unpaired `t' test value=1.16 (df=34); 2 tailed P=0.051 (not significant);

g) In Group 2 eyes, pretreatment mean BCVA *vs* post-treatment mean BCVA; Unpaired `t' test value=0.75 (df=42); 2 tailed P=0.46 (not significant);

h) In Group 1 eyes, pretreatment mean CFT *vs* post-treatment mean CFT; Unpaired `t' test value=5.4 (df=34); 2 tailed P=0.001 (very significant);

i) In Group 2 eyes, pretreatment mean CFT *vs* post-treatment mean CFT; Unpaired `t' test value=8.28 (df=42); 2 tailed P=0.001 (very significant).

3.3 Evaluation of Safety and Tolerability of Intravitreal Bevacizumab When Used to Treat Parafoveal Telangiectasia Type 2

Safety and tolerability assessments (both ocular and systemic) of intravitreal bevacizumab administration were monitored by subjective evaluation of patients (complaints, detailed history and relevant examination), ocular examination and systemic evaluation (including relevant laboratory investigations).

In the current study, severe ocular adverse events were not noted in any of the enrolled patient eyes. Only transient hyperaemia and subconjuctival hemorrhage were noted in 2 eyes in group 1 and 2 eyes in group 2.

In the current study, increase in blood pressure were observed in few enrolled patients (in group 1-2 patients and group 2–4 patients).

In the current study, none of the patients reported marked deterioration of vision following intravitreal bevacizumab administration.

In the current study, none of the patients reported persistent adverse effects on activities of daily living or quality of life after intravitreal bevacizumab administration. Interestingly, some of the patients reported beneficial effects on activities of daily living and quality of life due to improvement in the BCVA.

4. DISCUSSION

In the present investigation, 25 patients were enrolled; 11 (44%) were males and 14 (56%) were females. The patients ranged in age from 40 to 70 years. Eight patients were between 40 to 50 years of age, nine patients were between 51 to 60 years of age and eight patients were between 61 to 70 years of age (Tables 1 and 3). In this study, 40 eyes of the 25 patients were studied.

Gass [2] found that the long-term prognosis for patients with parafoveal telangiectasia II is poor, so that argon laser photocoagulation was not recommended by Gass for parafoveal telangiectasia type II. De Lahitte et al. [12] who evaluated the short-term effect of verteporfin photodynamic therapy in parafoveal telangiectasia Type II patients, found that there was no improvement in vision and no effect on permeability of vessels.

Alldredge et al. [13] reported that intravitreal triamcinolone acetonide is not effective in patients with parafoveal telangiectasia type II, but provides only mild improvement of visual acuity [14]. A study done by Wu et al. [15] also showed that intravitreal triamcinolone acetonide, in a dose of 4mg, does not improve visual acuity in most eyes with parafoveal telangiectasia type II.

The natural history of untreated choroidal neovascular membrane in parafoveal telangiectasia type II is generally poor, with 80% of eyes in a series of 26 eyes having a final visual acuity of 20/200 or worse [15,16]. Before the advent of VEGF antagonists, therapeutic options for subretinal neovascular membrane associated with parafoveal telangiectasia type II included laser photocoagulation, photodynamic therapy with or without intravitreal triamcinolone acetonide, transpupillary thermotherapy and surgical removal of the membrane [16-24].

In the present investigation, in eyes with parafoveal telangiectasia type II with choroidal neovascular membrane, the mean best corrected visual acuity (BCVA) at presentation was 0.121 (approximately 6/60)±0.06 decimals, which did not differ significantly ($P=0.051$) from the post-bevacizumab injection mean BCVA value of 0.147 (approximately 6/36)±0.06 decimals. However, there was a significant difference ($P=0.001$) between the mean central foveal thickness at presentation (469.17±89.67 µm) and the mean central foveal thickness (310.78±85.61 µm) after intravitreal bevacizumab. In this group, one eye exhibited a decrease in BCVA (from 6/60 to 3/60) but also a reduction in central foveal thickness (from 417 µm to 313 µm) following intravitreal bevacizumab. In addition, nine eyes did not exhibit any change in BCVA, but showed a significant reduction in central foveal thickness. These results suggest that in this group of eyes (parafoveal telangiectasia type II with choroidal neovascular membrane) that received intravitreal bevacizumab, visual acuity was improved (although not significantly) in some of the eyes whereas there was a significant reduction in mean central foveal thickness in many of the eyes.

In the present investigation, in eyes with parafoveal telangiectasia type II with cystoid macular edema, the mean BCVA at presentation (0.224 [approximately 6/24]±0.16 decimals) was not significantly different ($P=0.453$) from the post-bevacizumab injection mean BCVA value (0.2545 [approximately 6/24]±0.09 decimals). However there was a significant ($P=0.001$) reduction in the central foveal thickness from 356.77±43.22 µm at presentation to 253±42.59 µm after intravitreal administration of bevacizumab. In this group, one eye showed a decreased BCVA (from 6/36 to 3/60) but also a reduction in central foveal thickness (from 410 µm to 298 µm) following intravitreal bevacizumab. While six eyes did not exhibit any change in BCVA, but showed a significant reduction in central foveal thickness.

No significant ocular or systemic side-effects were observed in patients who received intravitreal injections of bevacizumab. The safety of anti VEGF agents has been documented in other studies also [25-26]. However, any intravitreal injection follows a small but definite risk of complications such as retinal tears, endophthalmitis and cataract and it would seem wise to limit the number of intravitreal injections to the barest required. Thus in the present study, where 25 patients received anti-VEGF agents (11 patients in group 1 and 14 patients in group 2), the true rate of the adverse event in question in the population is about 3/25 or 12%. Hence, more detailed studies on larger number of patients is needed to confirm the safety of these anti-VEGF agents. However, the results of the present study are certainly promising, since the confidence in the efficacy of a treatment or management approach is enhanced if the results are based on a prospective randomized trial as in the case of the present study [26].

The results of the present investigation suggest that in eyes with parafoveal telangiectasia type 2 complicated by cystoid macular edema, the mean visual acuity and mean central foveal thickness values are significantly better than the same values in eyes with parafoveal telangiectasis type 2 complicated by choroidal neovascular membrane. In both groups of eyes, there is definite (although not statistically significant) short-term improvement in the best corrected visual acuity and statistically significant reduction in the central foveal thickness following intravitreal injection of bevacizumab.

In the present study, no complications occurred following intravitreal bevacizumab injection. Similarly, no apparent or serious ocular or systemic adverse events were observed in patients who had received intravitreal injections of bevacizumab. None of the patients died following injection of bevacizumab or during the course of the study.

In the current study, severe ocular adverse events were not noted in any of the enrolled patient eyes. (Only Hyperaemia and Subconjuctival hemorrhage were reported in a few patients).

In the current study high blood pressure was noted in 6 enrolled patients after injection. No other systemic adverse event was noted in any of the patients.

In the current study, none of the patients reported marked deterioration of vision following intravitreal bevacizumab administration.

In the current study, none of the patients reported persistent adverse effects on activities of daily living or quality of life after intravitreal bevacizumab administration. Interestingly, some of the patients reported beneficial effects on activities of daily living and quality of life due to improvement in the BCVA.

Micieli et al. [23] reviewed systemic adverse events associated with intravitreal bevacizumab in patients with ocular disease; 22 studies (12,902 eyes of 12,699 patients) were included in their review, which included prospective and retrospective clinical studies and safety studies. The duration of follow-up ranged from one to 25 months. The most common side-effect reported was increased blood pressure (in 59 patients [0.46% of all patients]). Other reported adverse events included cerebrovascular accidents, myocardial infarction, transient ischemic attacks and angina, deep vein thrombosis, angina, renal disorders, gastrointestinal bleeding, skin rash or redness and menstrual irregularities. There were 23 deaths (0.18% of total). These authors concluded that the results of their review suggested that the systemic risk of bevacizumab was low; however, they opined that more active surveillance was needed to study the long-term safety of this drug in larger populations and to better evaluate the effects of bevacizumab on blood pressure. In another review, it was concluded that there was insufficient evidence to draw conclusions on the effects of intravitreal bevacizumab on mortality, serious morbidity, activities of daily living and quality of life. [26]

An interesting aspect of the present investigation was the observation that while intravitreal bevacizumab may marginally improve BCVA in patients with parafoveal telangiectasis that is complicated by cystoid macular edema or choroidal neovascular membrane, it emphatically and significantly reduces central foveal thickness in eyes of parafoveal telangiectasia with these complications. Further studies of a longer duration and on a larger sample size of patients are required to confirm the initial results obtained in the present investigation.

One limitation of the present investigation was the short time-duration of the study; the results may have been different if the patients had been followed up for a longer duration of time. Another limitation of the present study was the limited sample size in each of the groups, with the number not reaching that required for unequivocal statistical analysis.

5. CONCLUSION

In parafoveal telangiectasis type II complicated by choroidal neovascular membrane there is definite short-term improvement in the visual acuity (approaching statistical significance) and definite significant reduction of central foveal thickness following intravitreal injection of bevacizumab. In patients suffering from parafoveal telangiectasis type II complicated by cystoid macular oedema, there is definite significant reduction of central foveal thickness but no significant improvement in the visual acuity following intravitreal injection of bevacizumab. Bevacizumab is safe and well tolerated in eyes with parafoveal telangiectasis type II complicated by choroidal neovascular membrane and/or cystoid macular edema. No severe ocular or systemic adverse effects were encountered in this study.

ETHICS

The design and methodology of the study were reviewed and approved by the Institutional Review Board prior to the start of the investigation. In addition, written informed consent was obtained from each individual patient prior to enrolment in the study.

Methodology all eligible patients were followed for 12 months from baseline. The Primary end point in this study was to assess the efficacy of bevacizumab (Avastin)® 2.50 mg (in a 0.10 mL volume of solvent), by evaluating mean change from baseline in best-corrected visual acuity (BCVA) and central foveal thickness (CFT). Secondary endpoints in this study included the evaluation of tolerability and safety of bevacizumab (Avastin®) 2.50 mg (0.10 mL volume of solvent) and the Best Corrected Visual Acuity (BCVA) on Snellen's chart and intra-retinal thickness changes in Optical Coherence Tomography (OCT). Higher dose of avastin has been used to see whether more improvement in visual acuity and CFT, as it has already been mentioned in other studies where 2.5 mg dose used.
Visit Schedule at Visit 1 (baseline, week 0), the following information was collected to allow adequate characterization of the disease and the patient's medical history;

WORKUP PARAMETERS (BASELINE)

1) Best corrected visual acuity; 2) Slit lamp bimicroscopy; 3) Direct and indirect ophthalmoscopy; 4) Intra ocular pressure (IOP); 5) Clinical fundus photography; 6) Fundus fluorescein angiography (FFA); 7) Optical coherence tomography (OCT). Follow up of patients was done at the first, third and sixth months after presentation.

COMPETING INTERESTS

Authors have declared that no competing interests exist.

REFERENCES

1. Yannuzzi LA, Bardal AM, Freund KB, Chen KJ, Eandi CM, Blodi B. Idiopathic macular telangiectasia. Arch Ophthalmol. 2006;124:450–60.

2. Gass JD. Histopathologic study of presumed parafoveal telangiectasis. Retina. 2000;20:226–7.

3. Watzke RC, Klein ML, Folk JC, Farmer SG, Munsen RS, Champfer RJ. Long-term juxtafoveal retinal telangiectasia. Retina. 2005;25:727–35.

4. Surguch V, Gamulescu MA, Gabel VP. Optical coherence tomography findings in idiopathic juxtafoveal retinal telangiectasis. Graefes Arch Clin Exp. Ophthalmol. 2007;245:783–8.

5. Paunescu LA, Ko TH, Duker JS, Chan A, Drexler W, Schuman JS. Idiopathic juxtafoveal retinal telangiectasis: New findings by ultrahigh-resolution optical coherence tomography. Ophthalmology. 2006;113:48–57.

6. Bottoni F, Eandi CM, Pedenovi S, Staurenghi G. Integrated clinical evaluation of Type 2A idiopathic juxtafoveolar retinal telangiectasis. Retina. 2010;30:317–26.

7. Albini TA, Benz MS, Coffee RE, Westfall AC, Lakhanpal RR, McPherson AR. Optical coherence tomography of idiopathic juxtafoveolar telangiectasia. Ophthalmic Surg Lasers Imaging. 2006;37:120–8.

8. Cohen SM, Cohen ML, El-Jabali F, Pautler SE. Optical coherence tomography findings in nonproliferative group 2a idiopathic juxtafoveal retinal telangiectasis.

Retina. 2007;27:59–66.

9.   Charbel Issa P, Helb HM, Rohrschneider K, Holz FG, Scholl HP. Microperimetric assessment of patients with type 2 idiopathic macular telangiectasia. Invest Ophthalmol Vis Sci. 2007;48:3788–95.

10. Charbel Issa P, Holz FG, Scholl HP. Metamorphopsia in patients with macular telangiectasia type 2. Doc Ophthalmol. 2009;119:133–40.

11. The national eye institute visual function questionnaire in the macular telangiectasia (MacTel) project. The national eye institute visual function questionnaire in the macular telangiectasia (MacTel) project. Invest Ophthalmol Vis Sci. 2008;49:4340–6.

12. De Lahitte GD, Cohen SY, Gaudric A. Lack of apparent short-term benefit of photodynamic therapy in bilateral, acquired, parafoveal telangiectasis without subretinal neovascularization. Am J. Ophthalmol. 2004;138:892–4.

13. Alldredge CD, Garretson BR. Intravitreal triamcinolone for the treatment of idiopathic juxtafoveal telangiectasis. Retina. 2003;23:113–6.

14. Wu L, Evans T, Arévalo JF, Berrocal MH, Rodríguez FJ, Hsu M. Long-term effect of intravitreal triamcinolone in the nonproliferative stage of type II idiopathic parafoveal telangiectasia. Retina. 2008;28:314–9.

15. Moon SJ, Berger AS, Tolentino MJ, Misch DM. Intravitreal bevacizumab for macular edema from idiopathic juxtafoveal retinal telangiectasis. Ophthalmic Surg Lasers Imaging. 2007;38:164–6.

16. Charbel Issa P, Finger RP, Holz FG, Scholl HP. Eighteen-month follow-up of intravitreal bevacizumab in type 2 idiopathic macular telangiectasia. Br J. Ophthalmol. 2008;927:941–5.

17. Charbel Issa P, Holz FG, Scholl HP. Findings in fluorescein angiography and optical coherence tomography after intravitreal bevacizumab in type 2 idiopathic macular telangiectasia. Ophthalmology. 2007;114(9):1736-42.

18. Gamulescu MA. Bevacizumab in the treatment of idiopathic macular telangiectasia. Graefes Arch Clin Exp. Ophthalmol. 2008;246:1189–93.

19. Kovach JL, Rosenfeld PJ. Bevacizumab (Avastin) therapy for idiopathic macular telangiectasia type II. Retina. 2009;29:27–32.

20. Nachiappan K, Shanmugam MP. Treatment of CNVM secondary to idiopathic juxtafoveal retinal telangiectasis by transpupillary thermotherapy. Am J Ophthalmol. 2005;139:577–8.

21. Gordon M, Morales-Canton V, Solis-Vivanco A. Complications after intravitreal bevacizumab (Avastin): Analysis of 1910 injections. Invest Ophthalmol Vis Sci. 2007;48:A88.

22. Aggio FB, Farah ME, de Melo GB, d'Azevedo PA, Pignatari AC, Hofling-Lima AL. Acute endophthalmitis following intravitreal bevacizumab (Avastin) injection. Eye. 2007;21:408–9.

23. Prager F, Michels S, Kriechbaum K, Georgopoulos M, Funk M, Geitzenauer W, Polak K, Schmidt-Erfurth U. Intravitreal bevacizumab (Avastin) for macular oedema secondary to retinal vein occlusion: 12-month results of a prospective clinical trial. Br J. Ophthalmol. 2009;93(4):452-6.

24. Haritoglou C, Kook D, Neubauer A, Wolf A, Priglinger S, Strauss R, Gandorfer A, Ulbig M, Kampik A. Intravitreal bevacizumab (Avastin) therapy for persistent diffuse diabetic macular edema.Retina. 2006;26(9):999-100.

25. Fortin P, Mintzes B, Innes M. A systematic review of intravitreal bevacizumab for the treatment of diabetic macular edema. Ottawa: Canadian Agency for Drugs and Technologies in Health; 2012.

26. Mandal S, Venkatesh P, Abbas Z, Vohra R, Garg S. Intravitreal bevacizumab (Avastin) for subretinal neovascularization secondary to type 2A idiopathic juxtafoveal telangiectasia. Graefes Arch Clin Exp. Ophthalmol. 2007;245:1825–9.

10

Conjunctiva Histology in Long-standing Esotropia

Miguel Paciuc-Beja[1*], Victor Hugo Galicia-Alfaro[2], Myriam Retchkiman-Bret[2], Ryan Phan[3] and Hugo Quiroz-Mercado[1]

[1]*Department of Ophthalmology, University of Colorado School of Medicine, Denver Health Medical Center, USA.*
[2]*Department of Ophthalmology, American British Cowdray Medical Center, Mexico City, Mexico.*
[3]*School of Medicine, University of Colorado, USA.*

Authors' contributions

This work was carried out in collaboration between all authors. Author MPB designed the study, wrote the protocol and wrote the first draft of the manuscript. Authors VHGA, MRB, RP and HQM managed the literature searches and author MPB carried out microbiological studies. All authors read and approved the final manuscript.

<u>Editor(s):</u>
(1) Tatsuya Mimura, Department of Ophthalmology, Tokyo Women's Medical University Medical Center East, Japan.
<u>Reviewers:</u>
(1) Anonymous, Mansoura University, Egypt.
(2) Prabhakar Srinivasapuram, Ophthalmology, JSS University, India.
(3) Rahmi Duman, Şevket Yılmaz Training and Research Hospital, Turkey.

ABSTRACT

Background: Conjunctiva can be restrictive in long-standing strabismus. To date, there are no reports in the literature describing the histology of the conjunctiva in these patients.
Methods: Conjunctiva biopsies over the medial and lateral rectus were taken at the time of strabismus surgery in 3 patients with restrictive large angle long-standing esotropia.
Results: The conjunctiva overlying the medial rectus has a much more condensed, organized lamina propria compared to the conjunctiva of the contralateral lateral rectus. The medial conjunctiva has scattered small-diameter vessels and numerous clusters of plasmatic cells. The lateral conjunctiva has large blood vessels with occasional scattered plasmatic cells and the lamina propria present a lax structure.
Conclusions: These new findings reinforce the clinical understanding that conjunctiva can become more restrictive over the medial rectus in long-standing esotropia.

Keywords: Strabismus; esotropia; conjunctiva; histology.

*Corresponding author: E-mail: visualkids@aol.com

1. INTRODUCTION

It has long been recognized that the conjunctiva can be restrictive in long-standing strabismus [1,2]. Recessing the conjunctiva in such situations increases the amount of prismatic diopters corrected postoperatively [3,4].

The microscopic structure of the restrictive conjunctiva has not been described. We present the conjunctiva histology findings on 3 patients with large angle long-standing esotropia.

2. MATERIALS AND METHODS

In this case series, we look at the histologic aspect of the conjunctiva of 3 patients that have had long-standing horizontal strabismus, specifically, esotropia. For this study, we define large angle long-standing esotropia as esotropia of 50 prismatic diopters (PD) or more and esotropia that has been persistent for more than 20 years. We excluded patients with previous strabismus surgery or conjunctiva pathology. Every patient included in the case series tested positive on forced duction test on attempted abduction. All the patients were male and Hispanic. Patient 1, 58 year old, with esotropia of 60 PD on left eye. Visual acuity 20/20 OD, 20/100 OS. Patient 2, 45 year old, alternating esotropia of 50 PD. Patient 3, 27 year old with alternating esotropia of 50 PD. The two patients that presented alternating esotropia had uncorrected visual acuity of 20/30 in both eyes.

The surgical technique utilized was a conjunctiva limbal approach. Recession of the medial rectus with recession of the conjunctiva allowing a forced duction test on abduction to be negative and resection of the opposite lateral rectus. Biopsies of conjunctiva overlying the medial and lateral rectus muscles from the operated eye were taken at the time of surgery.

Informed consent was obtained from all individual participants included in the study. All procedures performed were in accordance with the ethical standards of the institutional national research committee and with the 1964 Helsinki declaration and its later amendments or comparable ethical standards.

3. RESULTS

The changes found on histology were consistent among all patients. On H&E staining, we found that the conjunctiva overlying the medial rectus have a much more condensed organized lamina propria compared to the conjunctiva of the contralateral lateral rectus muscle. The medial conjunctiva has scattered small-diameter vessels and numerous clusters of plasmatic cells (Fig. 1). In contrast, the lateral conjunctiva has large, abundant blood vessels with occasional scattered plasmatic cells. The lamina propria itself is poorly organized in a lax structure (Fig. 2). The conjunctiva epithelium overlying the lateral rectus muscle has fewer cells in comparison to the normal looking epithelium of the medial conjunctiva.

4. DISCUSSION

Several studies have addressed the role of recessing the conjunctiva to increase success rate in strabismus surgery [2-4]. Although fornix conjunctiva incision is favored by most surgeons for primary horizontal rectus muscle surgery [5], a limbal approach has been shown to allow recession of restrictive conjunctiva along with medial rectus muscle recession. Studies have shown that recessing conjunctiva along with the medial rectus results in consistently increased correction of diopters postoperatively compared to recession of rectus alone [4]. The conjunctiva over the opposite resected rectus muscle is often loose and sometimes needs to be trimmed in order to have a good cosmetic appearance. Clinically, the medial conjunctiva is different from the lateral conjunctiva in large angle long-standing esotropia. The question is: are there histologic differences between the medial and lateral conjunctiva in large angle long-standing strabismus? Yes, they are.

The main histologic findings are on the lamina propria. The "increased density" of the lamina propria over the medial rectus could explain the small-diameter vessels as well as the increased relative number of plasmatic cells. The "tight" lamina propria could make the plasmatic cells to be close to one another, not necessarily increasing the absolute number of cells. The dense lamina propria could "compress" the vessels making them look smaller in diameter. In practice, a tight conjunctiva is able to restrict a muscle recession, and that could explain why recessing the conjunctiva consistently increased correction of diopters postoperatively compared to recession of rectus alone [4]. There have been no studies to date that look at the histologic changes on the overlying conjunctiva in strabismus. Our study is limited by our small cohort, but the histologic findings were consistent among all our patients.

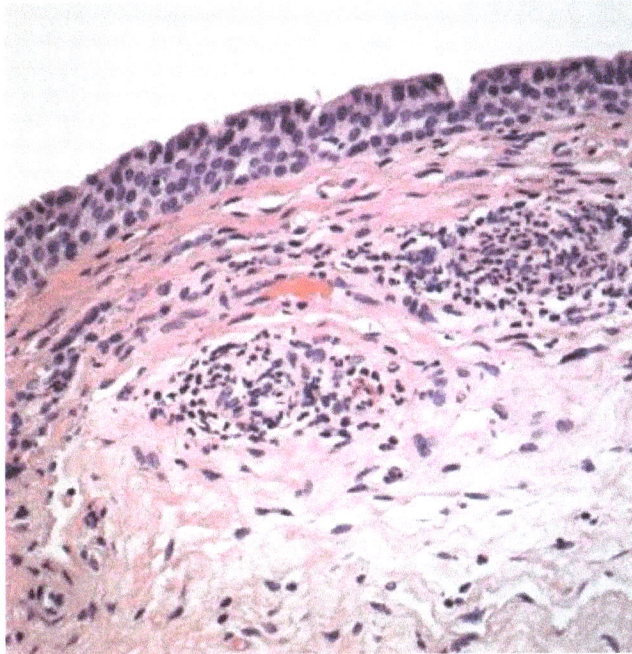

Fig. 1. H & E 40X the conjunctiva over medial rectus in large angle long-standing Esotropia. Condensed organized lamina propria. Scattered small-diameter vessels and numerous clusters of plasmatic cells

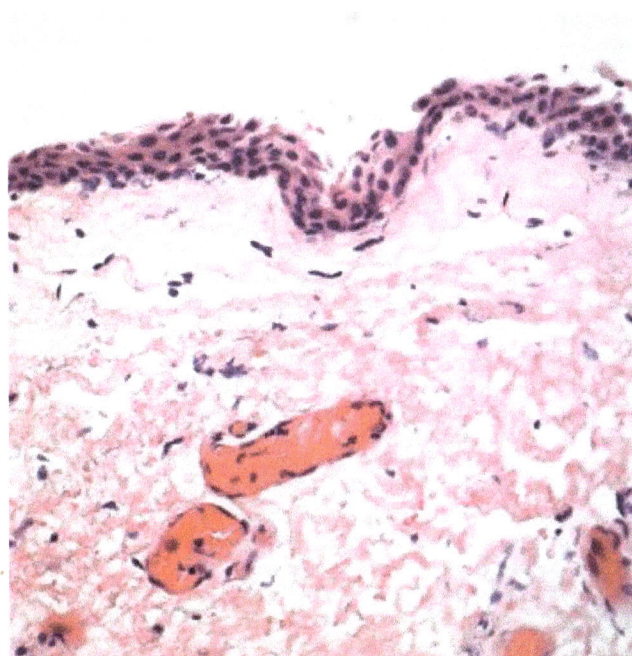

Fig. 2. H & E 40X large blood vessels with occasional scattered plasmatic cells. The lamina propria itself is poorly organized in a lax structure. The conjunctiva epithelium overlying the lateral rectus muscle has fewer cells in comparison to the normal looking epithelium of the medial conjunctiva

5. CONCLUSION

This is the first study to look at the histologic changes in the conjunctiva overlying the rectus muscles of patients with long-standing large angle esotropia. Conjunctiva overlying the medial and lateral rectus muscles in long-standing esotropia undergo histologic changes that may affect the structure of the conjunctiva. These new findings reinforce the clinical understanding that conjunctiva can become more restrictive over the medial rectus in long-standing esotropia. This description warrants further studies regarding the role of the conjunctiva in long-standing strabismus.

COMPETING INTERESTS

Authors have declared that no competing interests exist.

REFERENCES

1. Cole JG, Cole HG. Recession of the conjunctiva in complicated eye muscle operations. Am J Ophthalmol. 1962; 52:618-22.

2. Mazow M. Recession of the conjunctiva in esotropia surgery. Int Ophthalmol Clin. 1976;16(3):91-5.

3. Helveston EM, Ellis FD, Patterson JH, Weber J. Augmented recession of the medial recti. Ophthalmology. 1978; 85(5):507-11.

4. Willshaw HE, Mashhoudi N, Powell. Augmented medial rectus recession in the management of esotropia. Br J Ophthalmol. 1986;70(11):840-843.

5. Mikhail M, Verran R, Farrokhyar F, Sabri K. Choice of conjunctival incisions for horizontal rectus muscle surgery-a survey of American Association for Pediatric Ophthalmology and Strabismus Members. J AAPOS. 2013;17:184-187.

11

Collagen Matrix Implant (Ologen)™ in Glaucoma Surgeries; Precautions for a Better Control of Intraocular Pressure

Momen Mahmoud Hamdi[1*] and Islam Mahmoud Hamdi[1]

[1]Department of Ophthalmology, Ain Shams University, Cairo, Egypt.

Authors' contributions

This work was carried out in collaboration between both authors. Author MMH designed the study, performed the surgeries and the follow up, wrote the protocol, and wrote the first draft of the manuscript. Author IMH managed the literature searches. Both authors read and approved the final manuscript.

Editor(s):
(1) Tatsuya Mimura, Department of Ophthalmology, Tokyo Women's Medical University Medical Center East, Japan.
Reviewers:
(1) Anonymous, Egypt.
(2) Barbara Giambene, SOD Oculistica – AOUC - University of Firenze, Italy.

ABSTRACT

Background: Collagen matrix implant (CM) is used in glaucoma surgery to regulate healing under the conjunctiva.

Purpose: To highlight the precautions that should be taken for a better intraocular pressure (IOP) control with CM in different glaucoma surgeries during and after the operation.

Methods: Thirty five cases of glaucoma were treated surgically with adjunctive Ologen™.

a) Fifteen subscleral trabeculectomies (SST): for adult Primary Open Angle Glaucoma (POAG).

b) Five SST's for Primary Congenital Glaucoma (PCG).

c) Fifteen Phaco-trabeculectomies for advanced POAG with cataract. One was converted to extracapsular cataract extraction with SST because of a subluxated (270 degree) cataractous lens with advanced glaucoma.

The number of 10/0 nylon stitches to close the scleral flap, the method of closure of the fornix based conjunctival flap and injection of Na hyaluronate at the end of the surgery were evaluated. Postoperatively: Anterior chamber(AC) depth, the need for ocular massage, any additional medications or further surgical intervention were assessed.

Results: Better IOP control was obtained with slightly shallow AC postoperatively and tight

*Corresponding author: E-mail: mo2_76@hotmail.com

conjunctival closure. Ocular massage may be needed as well as medications for cases which experienced tight closures of the scleral flap. Three SST´s and four phaco-trabeculectomies needed supplemental medications after surgeries. Failure in one SST (PCG) and two phacotrabeculectomies was due to presence of additional risk factors in the patients. The rest of cases went successfully with IOP < 21 mm Hg without medications.

Conclusion: CM is a successful adjunct to glaucoma surgeries, intraoperative and postoperative precautions should be taken to maintain proper aqueous drainage and functioning blebs to improve the degree of success.

Keywords: Trabeculectomy; collagen matrix implant; phacotrabeculectomy; congenital glaucoma.

1. INTODUCTION

Glaucoma filtering surgery fails because of scarring of the filtering bleb. Fibroblasts proliferation from the episclera and Tenon's capsule play an important role in the scarring process. The use of antimetabolites in glaucoma filtering surgery has a beneficial effect on the lowering of intraocular pressure (IOP) especially in eyes at poor surgery prognosis. They inhibit the fibroblasts proliferation and subsequent scarring of filtering bleb [1].

Mitomycin C (MMC) is currently the preferred antiproliferative agent [2]. In addition to affecting DNA, it also affects RNA and protein synthesis. It thereby inhibits fibroblast proliferation and is toxic to endothelial cells. It introduces new complications of its own, including chronic hypotony with maculopathy, cystic avascular blebs, bleb leakage, bleb failure, bleb infections and endophthalmitis [3].

Ologen^{TM} is an artificial porcine extracellular matrix, which is made of atelocollagen cross-linked with glycosaminoglycan. It is a biodegradable scaffolding matrix that induces a regenerative wound-healingprocess in the absence of antifibrotic agents.It is designed to prevent episcleral fibrosis and subconjunctival scarring and minimize the random growth of fibroblasts, instead promoting their growth through the pores in the matrix. This implant is found to be biodegradable within 90–180 days [4]. After degradation, this collagen matrix implant (CM) leaves behind a loose alignment of collagen fibers inside the bleb, which are remarkably similar to normal tissues [5].

Two types of CM (Ologen, Aeon Astron Europe B.V., Leiden, The Netherlands) are used in glaucoma surgery, as per the manufacturer's design: the first is a disc of 6 mm diameter × 2 mm thickness and the second is a disc of 12 mm diameter × 1 mm thickness (Figs. 1a, b).

The advantages are claimed to be preventing episcleral fibrosis, subconjunctival scarring, risks of MMC (epithelial toxicity, hypotony, avascular blebs, late endophthalmitis).CM ensures as well a stable vascular bleb.

CM acts as a three dimensional porous scaffolding matrix. It promotes regenerative wound healing by allowing organized fibroblasts growth and physiological regeneration. Thus, a loosely structured filtering vascular bleb is formed. It has also a tamponading effect in the early postoperative course. This may promote long term IOP control.

CM is widely used in SST; according to Marey and co-workers, SST gave comparable successful results when assisted by Ologen^{TM} as with adjunctive MMC [6].

Ologen is getting to be assessed in phacotrabeculectomy by many surgeons, Narayana Swamy and his colleagues found it to be suboptimal in performance as compared with MMC in combined glaucoma and phacoemulsification [7]. Biodegradable CM (Ologen) can be used to reduce the surgical risks and complications of SST with MMC in infants [8].

2. PATIENTS AND METHODS

This is a retrospective study conducted from January 2011 to December 2013. It is considered as a collective overview on all cases in which Ologen^{TM} was used. All of them were done in the Department of Ophthalmology in Ain Shams University Hospitals and in Magrabi Eye Hospital in Cairo. All cases were operated upon by a single surgeon (the first author). The primary objective was to highlight the precautions that should be taken for a better intraocular pressure (IOP) control with CM in different glaucoma surgeries during and after the operation; this would help to evaluate the efficacy and safety of CM (Ologen, Aeon Astron Europe B.V., Leiden, The Netherlands) in order to reach the target IOP and stabilize the changes in the optic nerve head and visual field.

The authors have no financial interest with this product.

All patients were operated upon after taking informed consent from them if adults or from their parents in cases with PCG.

Thirty-five cases were studied including the following:

- Fifteen subscleral trabeculectomies (SST): for adult Primary Open Angle Glaucoma (POAG).
- Five SST's: for Primary congenital glaucoma (PCG).
- Fifteen phaco-trabeculectomies:

  o Fourteen for advanced POAG with cataract.
  o One converted to extracapsular cataract extraction with SST (asubluxated (270 degree) cataractous lens with advanced pseudo- exfoliative glaucoma).

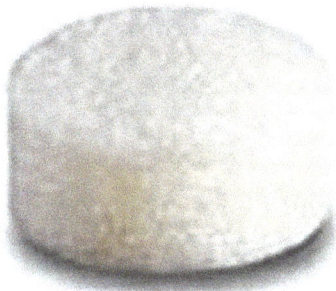

(a)

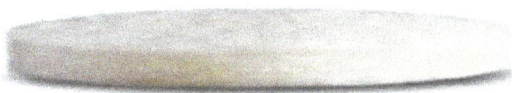

(b)

Fig. 1. Types of Ologen

2.1 Inclusion Criteria For

2.1.1 A- SST for adults

- POAG confirmed by gonioscopy with IOP>21 mm Hg despite maximally tolerated anti glaucoma treatment and/or progressive visual field changes.

2.1.2 B- SST's for Primary congenital glaucoma (PCG)

- Age from newborn to 5 years.
- Corneal diameter>13 mm with cloudy cornea.
- IOP>21 mmHg.
- Both unoperated or previously operated eyes.

2.1.3 C- phaco-trabeculectomies

- Visually significant cataract with BCVA worse than 20/40 associated with POAG confirmed by gonioscopy with IOP>21 mm Hg despite maximally tolerated anti glaucoma treatment and/or progressive visual field changes.

2.2 Exclusion Criteria

2.2.1 A- SST for adults

- Primary Angle Closure Glaucoma
- Secondary glaucoma (neovascular, uveitic, traumatic).
- Previous glaucoma surgery or other ocular operations.

2.2.2 B- SST's for Primary congenital glaucoma (PCG)

- Secondary congenital glaucoma e.g (retinoblastoma, Peter's anomaly, nanophthalmous).

2.2.3 C- phaco-trabeculectomie

Same as SST for POAG.

2.3 A-Subscleral Trabeculectomy (SST)

A fornix based conjunctival flap was done then the episcleral blood vessels were cauterized. A scleral flap measuring 3 mm × 4 mm was performed. The latter was sutured with one or two loose 10.0 nylon stitches and CM was placed over it. A watertight closure of the fornix based conjunctival flap with buried 10.0 nylon stitches at the limbus was performed(2 peripheral stitches or 2 peripheral+1 middle continuous stitch). A combination of steroid–antibiotics (dexamethasone–tobramycin) eye drops q.i.d. was prescribed for six weeks then tapering over the following two weeks.

2.4 B-phacotrabeculectomy

Phacotrabeculectomy was performed using two different sites: a temporal clear corneal incision for the phacoemulsification and a superior scleral flap measuring 2 mm x 3 mm. Fornix based conjunctival flap was used and episcleral blood vessels were cauterized. The scleralflap was sutured with one or two loose 10.0 nylon stitches and CM was placed over it. A watertight closure of the fornix based conjunctival flap with buried 10.0 nylon stitches at the limbuswas performed (2 peripheral stitches or 2 peripheral+1 middle continuous stitch).* A combination of steroid–antibiotics (dexamethasone–tobramycin) eye drops q.i.d. was prescribed for 6 weeks, tapering over the following two weeks.

One phacotrabeculectomy was converted to extracapsular cataract extraction with SST (a subluxated (270 degree) cataractous lens with advanced glaucoma).The capsulorrhexis failed, the cataractous lens was retrieved by a scoop after enlarging the temporal corneal incision, limited anterior vitrectomy was done. Anterior chamber IOL was implanted and the corneal incision was closed by four interrupted 10.0 nylon stitches. The glaucoma surgery was continued as described.

2.5 Intraoperative measures to be evaluated

- Number and tightness of 10/0 nylon stitches to close the scleral flap (one or two).
- Method of closure of the fornix based conjunctival flap with buried 10/0 nylon stitches (2 peripheral stitches or 2 peripheral+1 middle continuous stitch).
- Na hyaluronate injection in AC at the end of surgery.

*As the cases enrolled in this study were considered the beginning of the learning curve using CM, closure of the scleral flap was done by one loose stitch in some cases or two in others. The variation in closure of the fornix based conjunctival flap as well by two or three stitches was due to the same reason.

2.6 Postoperative Evaluation Included

- Anterior chamber (AC) depth.
- Need for ocular massage.
- Need for supplemental steroids.
- Additional IOP lowering medication(s).

2.7 The definition of success was as follow for SST treating POAG and phacotrabeculectomies

- Complete success (IOP < 21 mm Hg without medications).
- Qualified success (IOP<21 mm Hg with IOP lowering medication(s)).
- Failure (IOP >21 mm Hg not responding to medications).

The previous definition of success has been frequently used in the literature by many researchers [9-11].

2.8 The definition of success for PCG**

2.8.1 (**Based on a study by the first author that was published in 2013.(8)

- Full success: IOP less than 15 mmHg without medications; clear cornea.***
- Satisfactory success: IOP less than 21 mmHg without medications; clear cornea.
- Poor success: IOP less than 21 mmHg with medications.
- Failure: IOP more than 21 mmHg.

*** Complete success in PCG was considered 15 mmHg rather than 17 mmHg as this level might be more suitable for better corneal clarity and the target IOP for such young age group should be lower than adults with POAG.

3. RESULTS

3.1 A-SST for POAG

Ragarding the fifteen SST's with CM done for POAG the following remarks and results were noted:

- Flat AC and hypotony occurred in fou rcases (26.6%) in early postoperative period. In two of them, one10/0 nylon stitch was applied for closure of the scleral flap (overfiltration). In the two other cases, loose conjunctival closure was done with only two10/0 nylon stitches(aqueous leakage).
- Two cases (13.3%) needed supplemental medications to lower IOP. Tight closure of the scleral flap was done by two 10/0 nylon stitches. Ocular massage and frequent topicalsteroids were needed for few weeks postoperatively.

- Five cases (33.3%) showed very stable postoperative AC with Na hyaluronate injection at the end of the surgery, one loose 10/0 nylon stitch for closure of the scleral flap but with tight closure of the conjunctiva with three 10/0 nylon stitches.
- Bleb morphology was monitored by frequent photography, vascularity of the bleb was more intense in the first two weeks after the operation, and gradually faded in the following weeks under frequent topical dexamethasone eye drops to be nearly the same vascularity as the neighboring conjunctiva after four months. (Figs. 2 a, b,c).
- The success rate was: 13 cases (86.6%) with complete success and two cases (13.4%) with qualified success.

3.2 B-SST for PCG

Regarding the five cases of SST with CM for PCG, the following was noted:

- One case (20%) showed flat AC and hypotony in the early postoperative period; one very loose 10/0 nylon stitch was applied for closure of scleral flap.
- One case (20%) needed supplemental medications to lower IOP. The last two cases had more risk factor as they were recurrent PCG after previous SST.
- Bleb morphology revealed normal vascularity and flattened bled at 4-6 months follow up both in superiorly located bleb as in Fig. 3 and in temporally located bleb as in Fig. 4.

The success rate was: one case (20%) full success, two cases (40%) with satisfactory success, one (20%) case with poor success and one case (20%)with failure for which glaucoma drainage implant was planned.

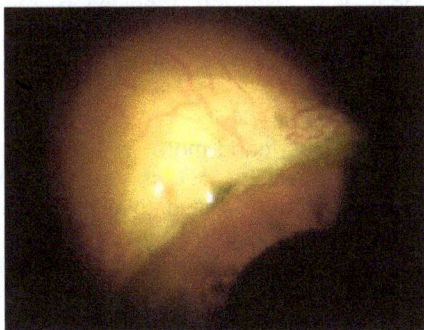

(a) Bleb at 2 weeks postop

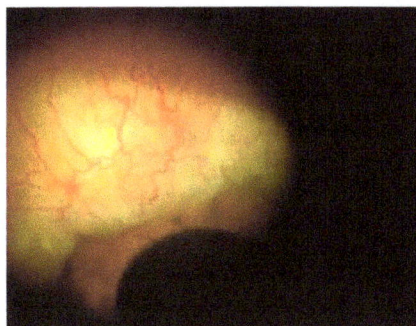

(b) Bleb at 6 weeks postop

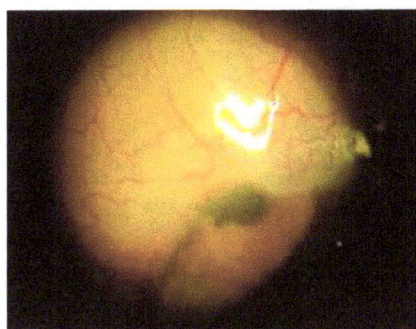

(c) Bleb at 4 months postop

Fig. 2. Bleb morphology in SST

3.3 C-Phaco-trabeculectomies

Regarding the fifteen cases of phacotrabeculectomies with CM, the following was noted:

- Four cases (26.6%) showed flat AC and hypotony in early postoperative period due to loose closure of the conjunctiva with two10/0 nylon stitches.
- Four cases (26.6%) needed supplemental medications to lower IOP. In these cases, tight closure of the scleral flap with two 10/0 nylon stitches was used and concurrently deep AC was noted in first week. Ocular massage and frequent topical steroids (dexamethasone) were needed few weeks postoperatively.
- Five cases (33.3%) showed very stable postoperative AC with Na hyaluronate injection at the end of the surgery, one loose 10/0 nylon stitch for closure of the scleral flap but with tight closure of the conjunctiva with three 10/0 nylon stitches.
- Tortuous vascluarized bleb was frequently noted four weeks after phacotrabeculectomy with corck screw

vessels (Fig. 5); which improved after three months with more intensive topical steroids and ocular massage (Fig. 6).

The success rate was: nine cases (60%) with complete success, four cases (26.6%) with qualified success and two cases (13.4%) with failure for which glaucoma drainage implant was planned.

SST in PCG with superior bleb

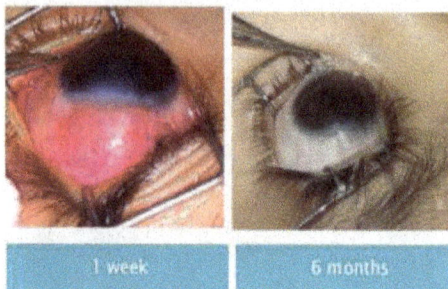

Fig. 3. shows successful SST in PCG with a superior bleb

SST in PCG with temporally located bleb

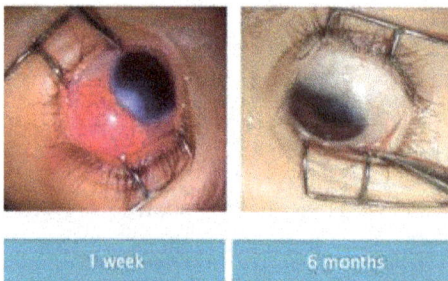

Fig. 4. shows successful SST in PCG with temporally located bleb

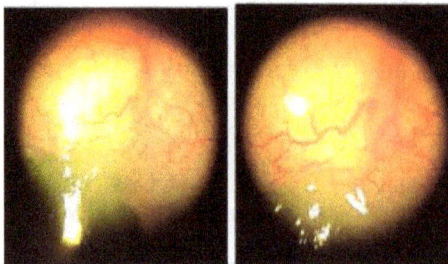

Fig. 5. tortuous vascluarized bleb 4 weeks after phacotrabecuctomy

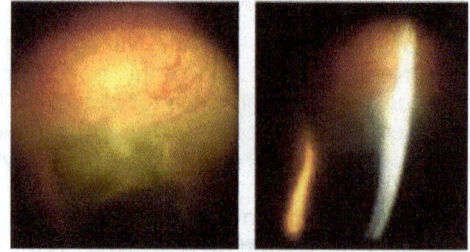

Fig. 6. Improved vascularization after 3 months with more topical steroids and ocular massage

4. DISCUSSION AND CONCLUSION

CM is a successful adjunct to glaucoma surgeries. Intraoperative and postoperative precautions should be taken to maintain :proper aqueous drainage, functioning blebs, and better degree of success; thus, reaching the desired target IOP. The latter would stop optic nerve head changes and allow for stable visual field changes in the long term follow up.

Operative precautions to ensure filtration entail mainly loose closure of the scleral flap by two 10/0 nylon stitches. This should be supported by avoiding leakage through tight closure of the fornix based conjunctiva flap by two peripheral and one middle continuous 10/0 nylon stitches buried at the limbus. Na hyaluronate injection in AC at the end of the surgery promote a stable AC in the early few days following the operation; which is likely to resist hypotony and prevent production of plasmoid aqueous that may block the trabeculectomy. Closure of the scleral flap by one loose 10/0 nylon stitch can be done but with more experience regarding the degree of looseness at the end of the learning curve of CM use.
Post operative precautions include frequent ocular massage in the first few weeks, more frequent topical steroids for up to three months. Additional IOP lowering medication may be needed with some cases not achieving the planned target IOP.

Complete success (IOP < 21 mm Hg without medications) was found more with cases which had slightly shallow AC in the 1st week postoperatively with raised bleb. This would promote filtration and smooth incorporation of the CM into the bleb. Proper filtration necessitates loose scleral flap closure with tight conjunctival closure.

Qualified success (IOP<21 mm Hg with IOP lowering medication) was encountered with cases in which there was tight closure of scleral flap, very deep AC in day-1 postoperative.Ocular massage and frequent steroids were needed few weeks postoperatively up to three months to normalize the IOP.

Failure (IOP >21 mm Hg not responding to medications) occurred in the presence of one or more additional risk factors mainly ocular surface disease, dark race, younger age etc. These cases were candidates for glaucoma drainage implants later.

The relatively smaller number of cases with primary congenital glaucoma (PCG) can be justified by two reasons: 1st this study is a collective overview on all cases in which Ologen^{TM} was used rather than specifically for PCG, 2nd PCG cases are rare and unfortunately a very few number was available with big difficulty in scheduling the follow up visits with the parents living usually far from our center.

The relative disadvantages of CM is the need for experience with the implant to adjust filtration, as well as possible infection and shallow AC (as any SST complication).

The most peculiar finding which had to be managed vigorously was the foreign body like reaction and encapsulation around the CM as manifested by vcorck-screw vessels; which occurred few weeks postoperatively risking failure. The latter happened in phacotrabeculectomies mainly due to the severe postoperative inflammation and breakdown of blood aqueous barrier that accompanies phacoemulsification; the release of inflammatory mediators leads to reduced bleb function [12].

It can be also explained by the indolent episcleral fibrosis that produces a dense coat around an extrascleral foreign body such as a scleral buckle [13].

Phacotrabeculectomies in general are considered less effective in reducing IOP than SST as demonstrated by Lochhead and his colleagues [14].

There is evidence in the literature to suggest that IOP control is not as great in combined procedures as with trabeculectomy alone and that blebs from combined procedures tend not to be as well established at 6 months. The prospective studies that have looked at this suggest that there is a 1.7-8.1-mmHg further decrease in IOP with trabeculectomy relative to combined procedures [15-17].

In a research work by Rosentreter in 2012 to study the reaction of the subconjunctival tissue and the histopathologic findings in explanted Ologen Implant, Ologen matrices and scar tissue were explanted in revision surgery in case of failed trabeculectomies or after glaucoma drainage device surgery. Histological sections were studied by hematoxylin-eosin (HE) staining. Further immunohistochemic stainings were performed for α-smooth muscle actin (α-SMA),

Table 1. Success rate with CM use

	Complete success	Qualified success	Failure
SST for POAG (n=15)	13 (86.6%)	2 (13.4%)	0
SST for PCG (n=5)	3 (1 full +2 satisfactory) (60%)	1 (20%)	1 (20%)
Phacotrabeculectomy(n=15)	9 (60%)	4 (26.6%)	2 (13.4%)

*Success rate is briefly shown in Table 1.

Table 2. Postoperative Problems

	Flat AC and hypotony	Supplemental medications	Others
SST for POAG	4 (26.6%)	2 (13.4%)	vascularity of the bleb was more intense in the first two weeks
SST for PCG	1 (20%)	1 (20%)	Bleb morphology revealed normal vascularity and flattened bled at 4-6 months follow up
Phacotrabeculectomy	4 (26.6%)	4 (26.6%)	Tortuous vascluarized bleb at four weeks with corck screw vessels

**postoperative problems in Table 2

fibronectin (FN), collagen III (COL3) and CD68.9 In case of failed trabeculectomies, HE staining of the explanted Ologen revealed an invasion of fibroblasts into the implant. The implants were enclosed by a collagenous pseudocapsule and surrounded by a loose connective tissue. α-SMA staining showed an accumulation of myofibroblasts predominantly in the ologen implant, whereas COL3 was mainly detected at the border area of the implant and the pseudocapsule around the implant. Immunehistochemistry for FN showed an intensive staining inside the implant and at the pseudocapsule [18].

Based on the last study by Rosentreter and the close follow up of our cases, CM should be "floating" within the bleb. CM would not "float" unless ample aqueous is being filtered from underneath the scleral flap within a tightly closed conjunctiva. In such a condition, there will not be direct strong contact between the implant and the conjunctiva; thus, minimizing the previously mentioned foreign body reaction which manifest by corck screw vessels as in Figure 6. These tortuous vessels are more encountered with phacotrabeculectomies in which postoperative reaction are more intense than SST. This explains also the need for prolonged topical steroids to inhibit inflammation and ocular massage to break any possible fibrous threads or pseudo capsule around the implant to promote aqueous filtration.

This study focuses mainly on the operative and postoperative precautions with CM in glaucoma surgeries. These tips are important in the learning curve of using this product. Other studies on Ologen[TM] focused on the final IOP results only. Modification of some steps in glaucoma surgery and special postoperative care are essential for the success of CM to smoothly reach the target IOP. Longer follow up period and larger number of cases are needed to consolidate the conclusion.

CONCLUSION

Ologen is a promising product in assisting different glaucoma surgeries, the success of its use could be reached with both intraoperative and postoperative precautions

ETHICAL APPROVAL

All authors hereby declare that all manouvers have been examined and approved by the appropriate ethics committee and have therefore been performed in accordance with the ethical standards laid down in the 1964 Declaration of Helsinki.

COMPETING INTERESTS

Authors have declared that no competing interests exist.

REFERENCES

1. Collignon-Brach J. Mitomycin C in glaucoma surgery. Bull Soc Belge Ophtalmol. 1993;247(1):79-86 .
2. Skuta GL. Cataract surgery in the glaucoma patient. Part2: a glaucoma surgeon's perspective. Focal points: Clinical modules for Ophthalmologists. San Francisco: American Academy of Ophthalmology. 1998;4:221. American Academy –Cataract .
3. Lama PJ, Fechtner RD. Antifibrotics and wound healing in glaucoma surgery. Surv Ophthalmol. 2003;48:314-46 .
4. Sarkisian SR. A replacement for antimetabolites? Ologen is a new product that modulates wound healing in glaucoma surgery. Glaucoma Today. 2010;8:22–24.
5. Ritch R. Using bioengineered collagen matrix during trabeculectomy: biodegradable polymer implants show promise for improving the functioning of filtering blebs. Glaucoma Today. 2007; 1:14–15.
6. Marey HM, Mandour SS, Ellakwa AF. Subscleral Trabeculectomy with Mitomycin-CVersus ologen for treatment of glaucoma. J Ocul Pharmacol Ther. 2013;29(3):330-334.
7. Narayanaswamy A1, Perera SA, Htoon HM, Hoh ST, Seah SK, Wong TT, Aung T. Efficacy and safety of collagen matrix implants in phacotrabeculectomy and comparison with mitomycin C augmented phacotrabeculectomy at 1 year. Clin Experiment Ophthalmol. 2013;41(6):552-60.
8. Hamdi MM. Trabeculectomy assisted by collagen matrix implant (Ologen) in primary congenital glaucoma. Journal of Egyptian Ophthalmological Society. 2013;106:188–193.
9. Edmunds B, Thompson JR, Salmon JF, Wormald RP. The National Survey of Trabeculectomy. II. Variations in operative technique and outcome. Eye. 2001;15(Pt 4):441- 448.

10. Cankaya AB, Elgin U. Comparison of the outcome of repeat trabeculectomy with adjunctive Mitomycin C and initial trabeculectomy. Korean J Ophthalmol. 2011;25(6):401-408.

11. Ehrnrooth P, Lehto I, Puska P, Laatikainen L. Long-term outcome of trabeculectomy in terms of intraocular pressure. Acta Ophthalmol. Scand. 2002;80:267–271.

12. Siriwardena D, Kotecha A, Minassian D, Dart JKG, Khaw PT. Anterior chamber flare after trabeculectomy and after phacoemulsification. Br J Ophthalmol. 2000;84:1056–1057.

13. Liesegang TJ, Skuta GL, Cantor LB. Wound repair, from American Academy of Ophthalmology Basic and Clinical Science Course; 2004. San Francisco; section 4, chapter 2, page 22.

14. Lochhead J, Casson RJ, Salmon JF. Long term effect on intraocular pressure of phacotrabeculectomy compared to trabeculectomy. Br J Ophthalmol. 2003; 87(7):850-852.

15. Caprioli J, Park HJ, Weitzman M. Temporal corneal phacoemulsification combined with superior trabeculectomy: a controlled study. Trans Am Ophthalmol Soc. 1996;94:451-63; discussion 463-468.

16. Bellucci R, Perfetti S, Babighian S, et al. Filtration and complications after trabeculectomy and after phacotrabeculectomy. Acta Ophthalmol ScandSuppl. 1997;44-5.

17. Derick RJ, Evans J, Baker ND. Combined phacoemulsification and trabeculectomy versus trabeculectomy alone: a comparison study using mitomycin-C. Ophthalmic Surg Lasers. 1998;29:707-13.

18. Rosentreter A, Konen W, Dietlein TS, Hermann MM. Histopathologic findings in explanted ologen implants. Presentation in ARVO; 2012. Session Title: Surgical Wound Healing.

12

Wolfram Syndrome: Report of Three Siblings with Early Vision Loss and Documented Lesion of the Entire Visual Pathway

Brunella Maria Pavan Taffner[1*], Patricia Grativol Costa Saraiva[2] and Fábio Petersen Saraiva[1]

[1]*Departamento de Medicina Especializada/CCS/UFES, Federal University of Espírito Santo, Av. Marechal Campos, 1468, Maruipe, Vitória-ES, Brazil.*
[2]*Pesquisa e Extensão AS – Multivix, Rua José Alves, 301, Goiabeiras, Vitória-ES, Brazil.*

Authors' contributions

This work was carried out in collaboration between all authors. Authors FPS and PGCS designed the study, wrote the protocol, and reviewed the manuscript. Author BMPT managed the literature searches, acquired digital images and wrote the first draft of the manuscript. All authors read and approved the final manuscript.

<u>Editor(s):</u>
(1) Stephen G Schwartz, Department of Clinical Ophthalmology, Bascom Palmer Eye Institute, University of Miami Miller School of Medicine, USA.
<u>Reviewers:</u>
(1) Anonymous, Mansoura University, Egypt.
(2) Anton Terasmaa, University of Tartu, Tartu, Estonia.

ABSTRACT

Objective: Report and document in images the presence of WFS1 in three of four siblings, with loss of visual acuity as the initial clinical presentation.
Design: Case series study.
Participants: Three of four siblings with WFS born to consanguineous parents.
Methods: All patients had diagnostic imaging with contrast-enhanced brain magnetic resonance imaging (MRI) and digital retinography.
Results: The patients and their father reported vision loss since before the age of seven, backed up by reports of multiple unsuccessful prescriptions for glasses and poor first-grade school performance due to visual deficit. Diabetes mellitus was diagnosed at seven years of age. All patients presented bilateral neurosensory deafness, atrophy of the posterior pituitary lobe,

*Corresponding author: E-mail: brunellapavan@hotmail.com

cerebellum, nerve, chiasma, optic tract and optic disc (bilateral), as well as urological changes and gait and balance disorders. One patient is epileptic and another suffers from a combination of anxiety and depression.

Conclusion: Three unique cases of WFS due to early loss of visual acuity, lesion of the entire visual pathway documented in images, and an unusually high level of familial penetrance.

Keywords: Wolfram syndrom; optic atrophy; rare diseases.

1. AIMS

Wolfram syndrome (WFS) is a rare, progressive, neurodegenerative autosomal recessive disorder with incomplete penetrance characterized by the association of non-autoimmune insulin-dependent juvenile diabetes mellitus and optic atrophy [1-3]. The prevalence of WFS has been estimated at 1/100,000 pop in the US [1] and 1/770,000 pop in the UK [2].

WFS was first described by Dr. D. J. Wolfram in a report of four siblings from 1938 [3]. Later reports added diabetes insipidus (observed in 73%) and deafness (observed in 62%) to the syndrome [2,4], leading to the adoption of the acronym DIDMOAD (Diabetes Insipidus, Diabetes Mellitus, Optic Atrophy, Deafness).[2] Approximately 50% express the complete phenotype [5]. Insulin deficiency, the classic initial manifestation of WFS, tends to occur at about seven years of age, followed by optic atrophy at eleven [2]. In the second decade of life, many patients develop central diabetes insipidus and neurosensory deafness [6]. Manifestations may also include atonal bladder, ataxia, myoclonia, peripheral neuropathy, hypogonadism, depression and WFS-related psychotic behavior [6,7]. Death occurs between 25 and 49 years of age (median: 30), usually due to central respiratory failure [8].

Wolfram syndrome is usually caused by mutations in the WFS1 gene. The recent discovery WFS2, a phenotypical and genotypical variant of the syndrome, requires diabetes mellitus and optic atrophy as minimum criteria for diagnosis. WFS2 is caused by a dysfunction of the CISD2 gene. The clinical phenotype of WFS2 differs from that of WFS1 by the absence of diabetes insipidus and psychiatric disorders and by the presence of bleeding from upper intestinal ulcers and platelet aggregation defects [9].

To our knowledge, this is the first report of WFS with anterior visual pathway dysfunction manifesting well before the onset of diabetes symptoms. The familial penetrance is also unusually high. The purpose of the study was to report and document in images the presence of WFS1 in three of four siblings, with loss of visual acuity as the initial clinical presentation.

2. PRESENTATION OF CASE

Our three patients (A=42 years, male; B=40 years, male; C=32 years, female) were born to consanguineous parents (third cousins) from Southeastern Brazil. The family history included a grandfather with type II diabetes mellitus, but no reports of genetic disorders.

The first consultations were conducted at another service. The father and the three patients reported vision loss since before the age of seven. These statements were backed up by reports of multiple unsuccessful prescriptions for glasses and poor first-grade school performance due to visual deficit. At the time, visual acuity was <20/400 in both eyes. Patient A has proliferative diabetic retinopathy and Patient B has nonproliferative diabetic retinopathy, both of which diagnosed in their twenties.

Type I diabetes mellitus was diagnosed at seven years of age after which the patients were started on insulin. Bilateral sensorineural deafness with a downward curve in the audiometry forums was evidenced in the second decade of life in all three brothers.

All patients presented bilateral atrophy of the posterior pituitary lobe, cerebellum, nerve, chiasma, optic tract and optic disc documented by cranial magnetic resonance and retinography (Figs. 1, 2, 3 and 4) in addition to urological changes (A=hyperactive bladder; B & C=pyelocalyceal dilation) and gait and balance disorders. Patient A has been epileptic since age 22, with EEG-confirmed complex partial and absence seizures and upward ocular deviation lasting 10-30 seconds. Patient B suffers from a combination of anxiety and depression diagnosed at age 38.

Table 1 provides additional information on the patients' WFS 1 phenotype. However, our hospital laboratory is not presently equipped to carry out the genetic tests required to sequence the WFS1 from this family.

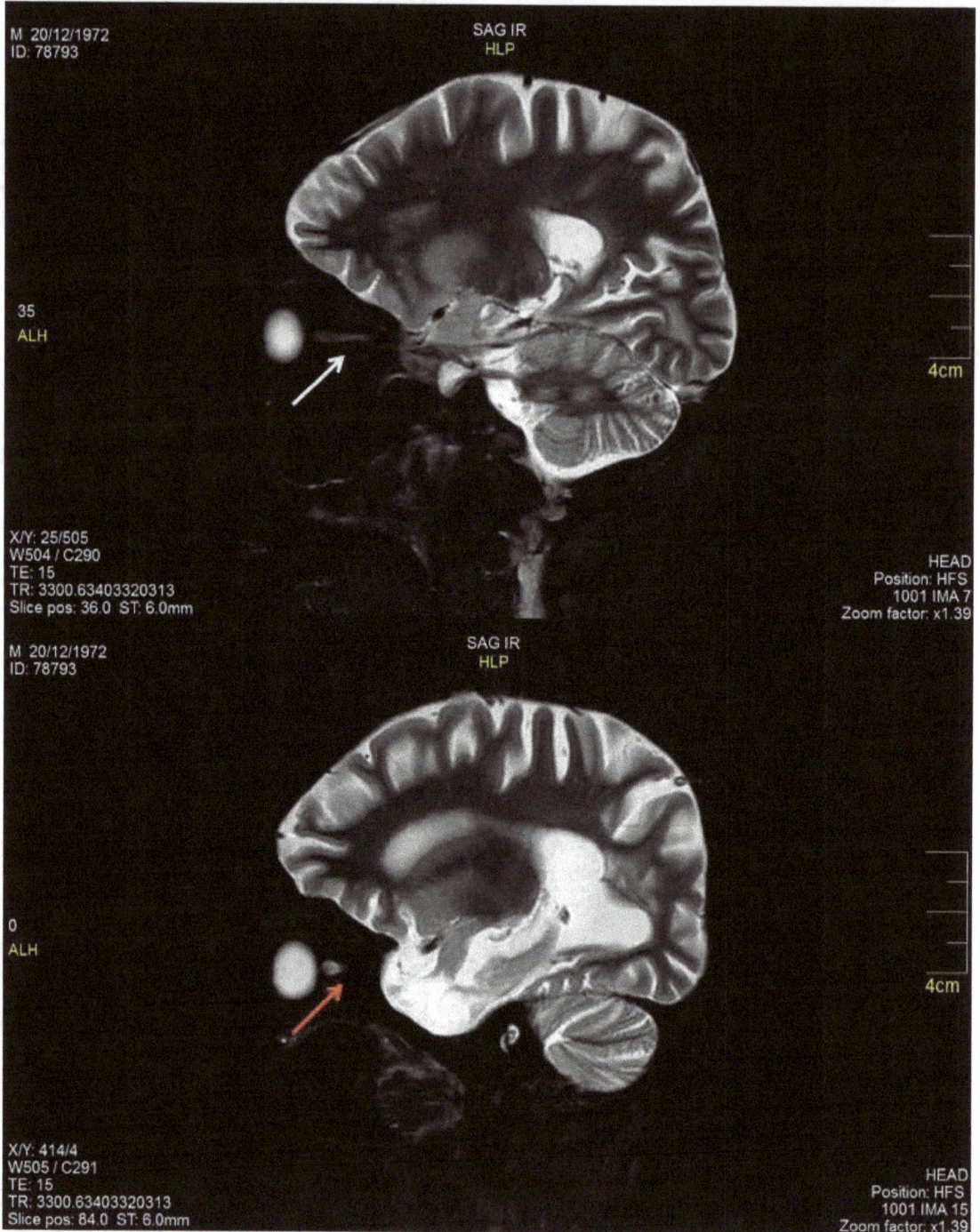

Fig. 1. Cranial magnetic resonance imaging scan of patient A

T2-weighted saggital sequence showing accentuated atrophy of the optic nerve on the right (white arrow) and left (red arrow) side

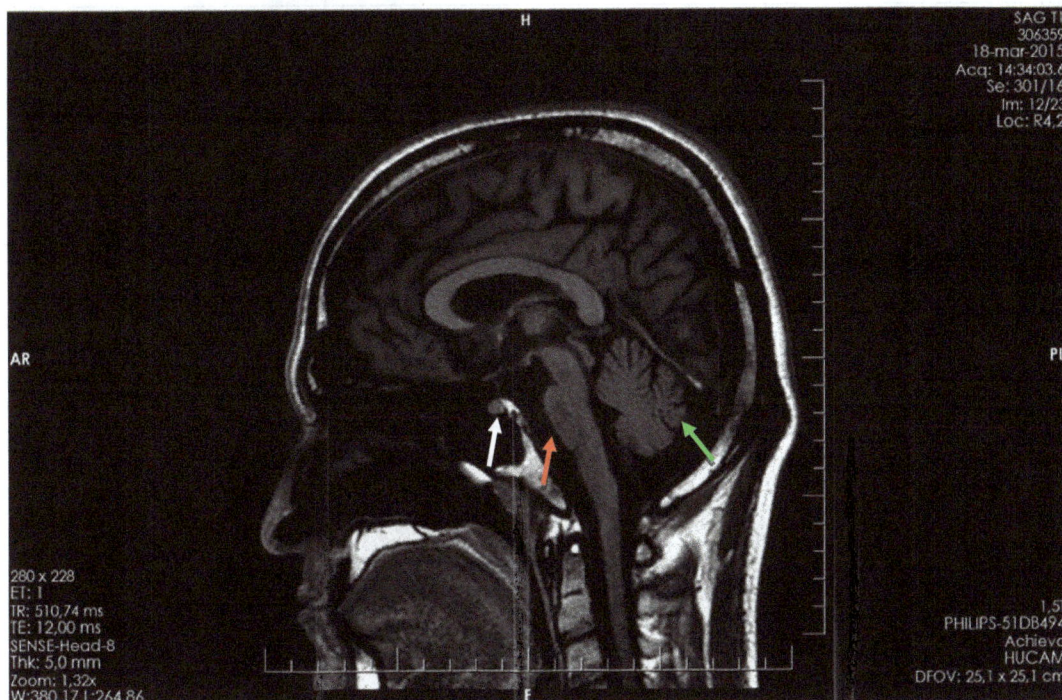

Fig. 2. Cranial magnetic resonance imaging scan of patient B

T1-weighted saggital sequence with absence of the hypersignal of the posterior pituitary lobe habitually observed in patients with diabetes insipidus (white arrow). Note hyperechoic area posterior to the pituitary gland representing the dorsum sellae, with hyperechoic fatty bone marrow in T1. Note mild atrophy of pontina anterior portion characterized by reduction of the protuberance (red arrow). Note atrophy of vermis and cerebellar hemispheres (green arrow)

Table 1. Clinical findings of patients A, B and C

Patient	A	B	C
Birth date	20/12/1972	31/05/1975	22/09/1983
Weight	70 Kg	71 kg	56 Kg
Height	1.68 m	1.73 m	1.66 m
Skin color	White	White	White
Diagnosis type I diabetes mellitus	At 7 years of age	At 7 years of age	At 7 years of age
Symptoms of vision loss	Before 7 years of age	Before 7 years of age	At 6 years of age
Otological changes	Audiometry: bilateral sensorineural hearing loss.	Audiometry: bilateral sensorineural hearing loss.	Audiometry: bilateral sensorineural hearing loss.
Urological changes	Complaints of incontinence. Urodynamic study: detrusor overactivity (overactive bladder).	Ultrasound of the urinary tract: pyelocaliceal dilation and bilateral ureteral ectasia.	Ultrasound of the urinary tract: mild dilation of the right pyelocaliceal system.
Best-corrected visual acuity in 1994	Counting fingers: 2 meters in both eyes.	Counting fingers: 3 meters in both eyes.	20/100 in both eyes.
Best-corrected visual acuity in January 2015	<20/400	<20/400	<20/400
Eye examination in January 2015	Bilateral papillary atrophy. Proliferative diabetic retinopathy stabilized with laser panretinal photocoagulation.	Bilateral papillary atrophy. Nonproliferative diabetic retinopathy. Mild bilateral cortical cataracts.	Bilateral papillary atrophy. Absence of diabetic retinopathy.

Patient	A	B	C
Neurological disorders	Epileptic absence and complex partial seizures confirmed by EEG. Trunk ataxia with unstable gait and falls. Mild muscular hypertension. Diminished patellar and Achilles reflexes.	Mixed anxiety and depression disorder. Trunk ataxia with unstable gait and falls.	Trunk ataxia with unstable gait and falls.
Diagnosis diabetes insipitus	Absence of diabetes insipitus.	At 40 years of age	At 32 years of age
Medication	Insulin + Simvastatin 50mg/day + Losartan 50 mg/day + Lamotrigine 300 mg/day + Carbamazepine 1200 mg/day	Insulin +Desmopressin + Losartan 50 mg/day +Fluoxetine 20 mg/day +Clonazepam 2mg/night	Insulin + Desmopressin

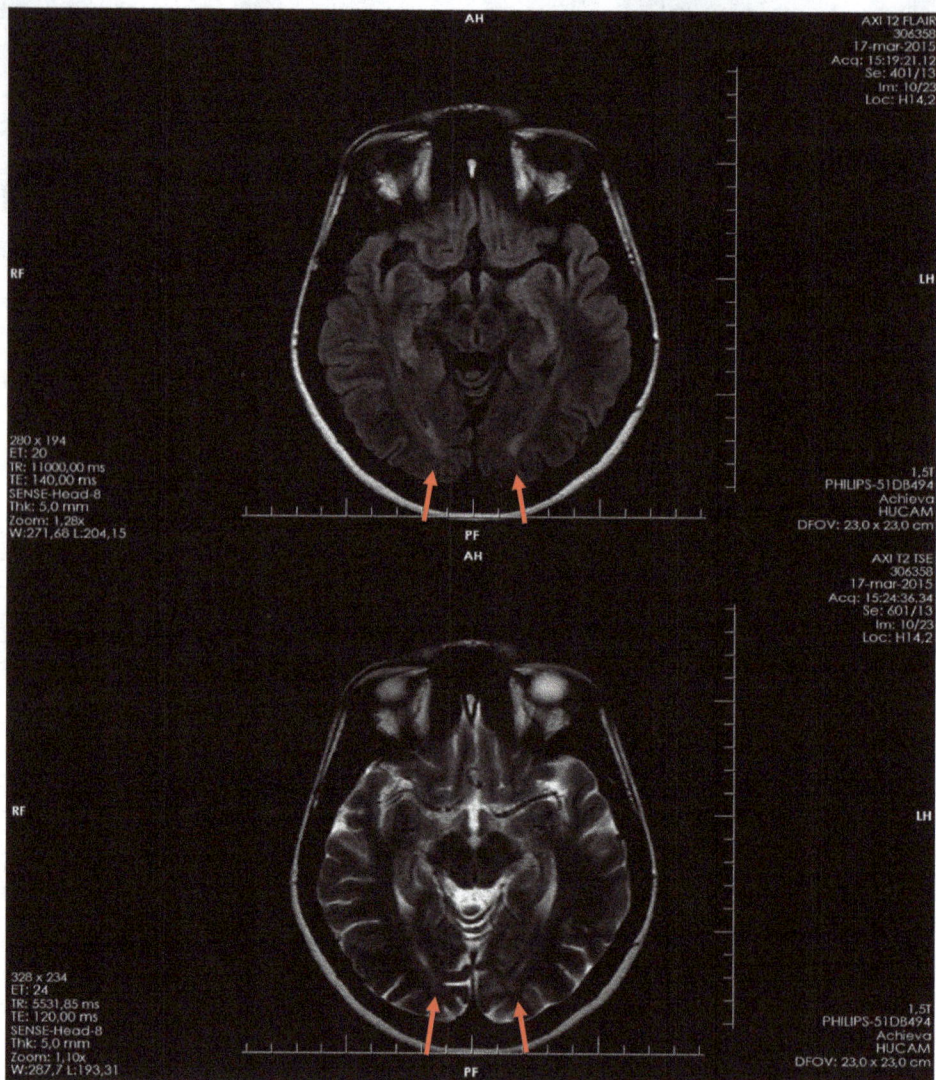

Fig. 3. Cranial magnetic resonance imaging scan of patient C
Axial FLAIR sequence showing an attenuated hypersignal in the white matter adjacent to the trigone of the lateral ventricles, and optic tracts (red arrows)

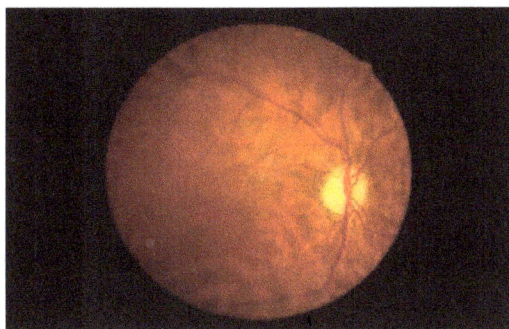

Fig. 4. Digital retinography of patient C
Optic atrophy in the right eye

3. DISCUSSION

The gene for WFS was identified on the short arm of chromosome 4 (4p16) by linkage analysis [5]. The primary genetic defect was attributed to the WFS1 gene, which accounts for symptoms in 90% of cases [10]. The gene encodes a transmembrane protein (wolframin) in the endoplasmic reticulum found in neurons, pancreatic β-cells and other tissues, such as the heart, placenta, inner ear, lung and liver. The function of wolframin is not known, but wolframin deficiency is believed to increase the tension inside the endoplasmic reticulum, with negative impacts on the cell cycle and calcium homeostasis [4,11].

In 2000, a second locus, WFS2, was mapped in chromosome 4q22-q24 after linkage analysis of four consanguineous Jordanian families. The ZCD2-encoded protein ERIS (endoplasmic reticulum intermembrane small protein) is also located in the endoplasmic reticulum but does not interact directly with wolframin [12].

The incidence of WFS is reported to be higher in children of consanguineous parents [1]. In the three cases reported here, the time of diagnosis of diabetes mellitus was compatible with the literature, but WFS-related reduced visual acuity in early childhood, prior to the onset of diabetes symptoms, to the extent of interfering with the acquisition of literacy, has to our knowledge not been described before. Likewise, The high familial penetrance of WFS (three out of four siblings), with more severe ophthalmological and neurological symptoms in the male siblings, is very unusual.

Neurological symptoms tend to occur later in the evolution of WFS.[2] However, Patient A started having epileptic seizures in the first decade of

life, and Patient B presented a combination of anxiety and depression as early as the second decade.

The MRI changes observed in our patients match descriptions of WFS patients with atrophy of the brainstem, visual pathways, hypothalamus and posterior pituitary gland [13-15].

4. CONCLUSION

The occurrence of WFS in 3 of 4 brothers born to consanguineous parents represents an unusually high level of familial penetrance. WFS is a rare syndrome, with few well described and image-documented cases in the literature. In addition, visual complaints preceding the manifestation of diabetes mellitus had not been described before.

CONSENT

All authors declare that 'written informed consent was obtained from the patient (or other approved parties) for publication of this case report and accompanying images.

ETHICAL APPROVAL

All authors hereby declare that the study´s protocol have been examined and approved by the appropriate ethics committee and have therefore been performed in accordance with the ethical standards laid down in the 1964 Declaration of Helsinki.

ACKNOWLEDGMENTS / DISCLOSURE

The authors have no competing interests to disclose.

All authors contributed substantially to the development of the study.

The authors declare that they have no additional contributions.

The authors received no financial support.

COMPETING INTERESTS

Authors have declared that no competing interests exist.

REFERENCES

1.   Fraser FC, Gunn T. Diabetes mellitus, diabetes insipidus, and optic atrophy. An

autosomal recessive syndrome? J Med Genet. 1977;14(3):190–3.

2. Barrett TG, Bundey SE, Macleod AF. Neurodegeneration and diabetes: UK nationwide study of Wolfram (DIDMOAD) syndrome. Lancet. 1995;346(8988): 1458-63.

3. Wolfram DJ. Diabetes mellitus and simple optic atrophy among siblings: Report of four cases. Mayo Clin Proc. 1938;13: 715-18.

4. Shannon P, Becker L, Deck J. Evidence of widespread axonal pathology in Wolfram syndrome. Acta Neuropathol. 1999;98(3): 304–8.

5. Polymeropoulos MH, Swift RG, Swift M. Linkage of the gene for Wolfram syndrome to markers on the short arm of chromosome 4. Nat Genet. 1994;8(1):95-7.

6. Scolding NJ, Kellar-Wood HF, Shaw C, Shneerson JM, Antoun N. Wolfram syndrome: Hereditary diabetes mellitus with brainstem and optic atrophy. Ann Neurol. 1996;39(3):352-60.

7. Swift RG, Sadler DB, Swift M. Psychiatric findings in Wolfram syndrome homozygotes. Lancet. 1990;336(8716): 667-9.

8. Domenech E, Gomez-Zaera M, Nunes V. Wolfram / DIDMOAD syndrome, a heterogenic and molecularly complex neurodegenerative disease. Pediatr Endocrinol Rev. 2006;3(3):249–257.

9. Ajlouni K, Jarrah N, El-Khateeb M, El-Zaheri M, El Shanti H, Lidral A. A Wolfram syndrome: Identification of a phenotypic and genotypic variant from Jordan. Am J Med Genet. 2002;115(1): 61–65.

10. Inoue H, Tanizawa Y, Wasson J, et al. A gene encoding a transmembrane protein is mutated in patients with diabetes mellitus and optic atrophy (Wolfram syndrome). Nat Genet. 1998;20(2):143-8.

11. Zatyka M, RickMinton J, Fenton S, et al. Sodium–potassium ATPase 1 subunit is a molecular partner of Wolframin, an endoplasmic reticulum protein involved in ER stress. Hum Mol Genet. 2008;17(2): 190–200.

12. El-Shanti H, Lidral AC, Jarrah N, Druhan L, Ajlouni K. Homozygosity mapping identifies an additional locus for Wolfram syndrome on chromosome 4q. Am J Hum Genet. 2000;66(4):1229–1236.

13. Ganie MA, et al. Presentation and clinical course of Wolfram (DIDMOAD) syndrome from North India. Diabet Med. 2011;28(11): 1337–42.

14. Hershey T, et al. Early Brain Vulnerability in Wolfram Syndrome. PLoS One. 2012; 7(7):e40604.

15. Galluzzi P, Filosomi G, Vallone IM, Bardelli AM, Venturi C. MRI of Wolfram syndrome (DIDMOAD). Neuroradiology. 1999;41(10): 729–731.

13

Peculiar Case of Orbital Emphysema Caused by High-pressure Water Jet

Y. W. Jeremy Hu[1] and Srinivasan Sanjay[1,2*]

[1]Department of Ophthalmology and Visual Sciences, Khoo Teck Puat Hospital, Singapore.
[2]Yong Loo Lin School of Medicine, National University of Singapore, Singapore.

Authors' contributions

This work was carried out in collaboration between both authors. Author YWJH managed the literature search and wrote the first draft of the manuscript. Author SS managed the literature search and edited the draft. Both authors read and approved the final manuscript.

<u>Editor(s):</u>
(1) Ahmad M Mansour, Department of Ophthalmology, American University of Beirut, Lebanon.
<u>Reviewers:</u>
(1) Jera Kruja, University of Medicine, Tirana, Albania.
(2) Anonymous, Tokyo Medical University Hachioji Medical Center, Japan.
(3) Anirudh Bhattacharya, Facial Trauma and Implantology, India.
(4) Anonymous, Mansoura University, Egypt.
(5) Rahmi Duman, Şevket Yılmaz Training and Research Hospital, Turkey.
(6) Anonymous, Asahikawa Medical University, Japan.

ABSTRACT

Aim: To report an unusual case of orbital emphysema secondary to high pressure water jet injury.
Presentation of Case: A 26-year-old Indian male sustained a two-centimeter facial laceration after a compressed water jet hit the left infra-orbital region. Ophthalmic examination showed extensive inferior commotio retinae without any clinical signs of conjunctival laceration or globe rupture. Computed tomography showed orbital emphysema with undisplaced fracture of the orbital floor. Follow-up examination 1 month after the injury showed total resolution of orbital emphysema.
Discussion and Conclusion: Our case illustrates the dangers of water jet injuries and the unique injury provides supporting evidence of our current existing orbital fracture theory. This injury is most peculiar and to our knowledge, not previously reported in the literature.

Keywords: Orbital emphysema; water jet injuries; orbital floor fracture; commotio retinae.

*Corresponding author: E-mail: sanjay_s@alexandrahealth.sg, hujeremy@hotmail.com

1. INTRODUCTION

High-pressure water jet is commonly used for surface cleaning of driveways, walls and drains. Our case presents a unique mechanism in which a high-pressure water system caused a penetrating injury of the orbit resulting in an orbital fracture and emphysema without significant globe injury.

We describe a case of orbital and subcutaneous emphysema with orbital floor fracture following penetrating water jet injury. This injury, to our knowledge, has not been reported in literature.

2. PRESENTATION OF CASE

A 26-year-old Indian male, with no past medical or surgical history of note, presented to our centre with a left lower eyelid laceration with blurring of vision after he was hit over his face accidentally by a high-pressure water jet used for floor cleaning 2 hours earlier. He was standing opposite a friend holding the water hose and was hit momentarily over the face by the water jet inadvertently. He denies blowing his nose after the incident. Best-corrected visual acuity (BCVA) was 6/6 in the right eye and 6/12 over the left eye. Color vision tested on Ishihara chart was full in both eyes. There was no relative afferent pupillary defect. There was a linear 2 cm laceration 0.5 cm below the left lower lid margin (Fig. 1a) with fullness over the lower lid. There was subconjunctival hemorrhage over the lateral part of eye without any laceration. Rest of the anterior segment examination was within normal limits. There was no limitation in eye movements.

Fundal examination revealed extensive inferior commotio retinae with Berlin's edema (Fig. 1b).

Computed tomography (CT) of the orbits revealed extensive subcutaneous and orbital emphysema extending from the laceration. There was a small, un-displaced anterior, inferior orbital floor fracture with fluid in the maxillary sinus (Fig. 2).

Left lower lid wound was sutured. Patient was treated with oral Amoxicillin/clavulanic acid and tetracycline skin ointment to the lid laceration. He was monitored daily for the first 48 hours with improvement of left BCVA to 6/6.

A repeat CT of the orbits was done 1 month after injury that showed complete resolution of the orbital emphysema (Fig. 3). Visual acuity remained 6/6 and commotio retinae resolved.

3. DISCUSSION

Orbital emphysema with or without orbital fracture due to compressed air has been reported a number of times [1-4]. High-pressure water jet orbital injury, on the other hand is relatively uncommon, and it causing orbital emphysema is, to the best of our knowledge, not been reported before. A search on Scopus, MEDLINE, EMBASE and Cochrane library using the following keywords "water jet injuries", "orbital emphysema", "water jet injury", "orbital fracture" did not show any case reports of water jet injury causing orbital emphysema.

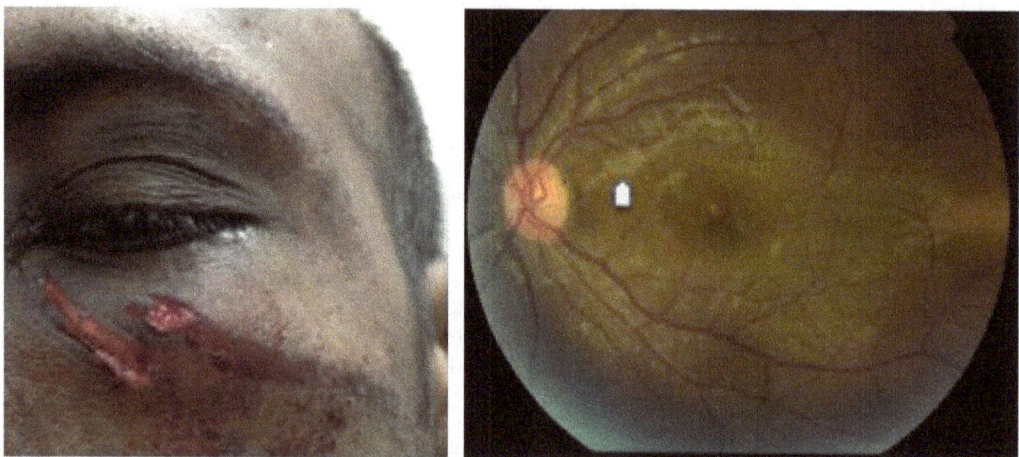

Fig. 1a. (left) showing 1cm infra-orbital laceration; 1b. (right) showing extensive commotio retinae (arrowhead)

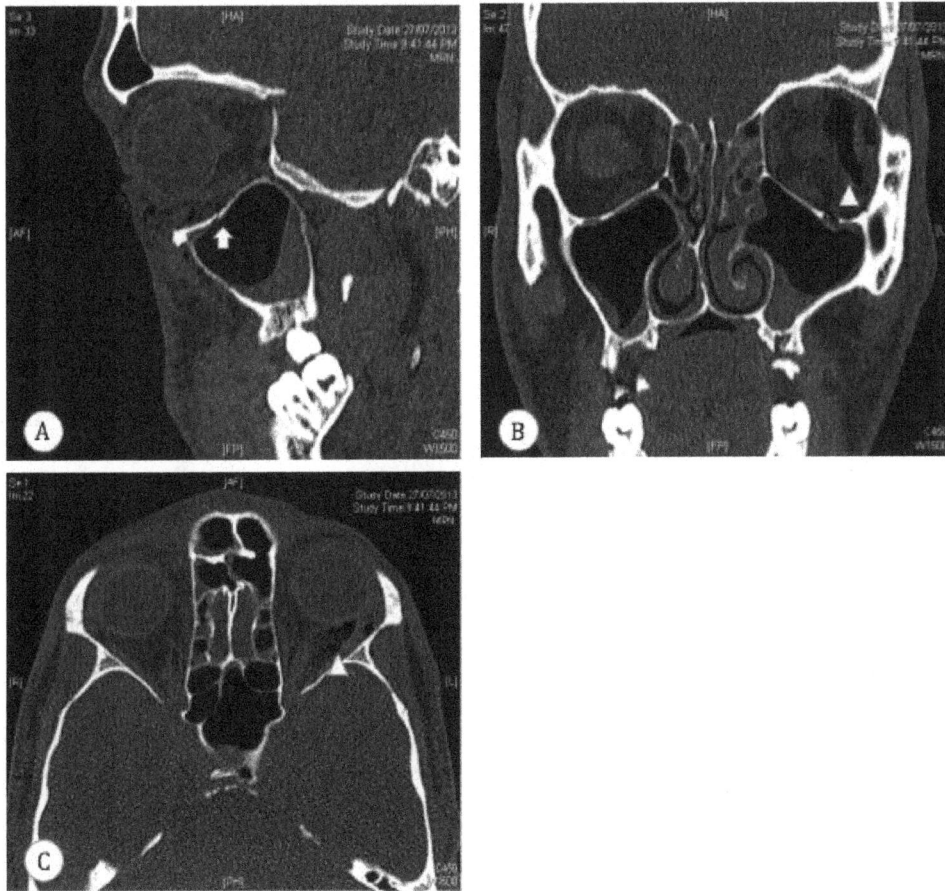

Fig. 2A. shows a fracture of orbital floor (arrow), 2B, 2C. shows presence of orbital emphysema (arrowhead)

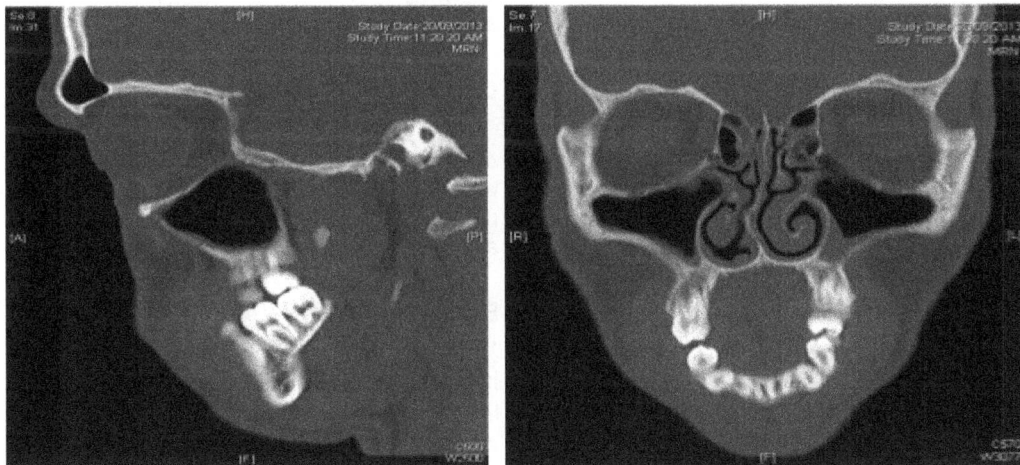

Fig. 3. shows interval resolution of orbital emphysema

The mechanism of orbital fractures has been a source of debate in many journal articles. Three theories have emerged, the "buckling", the "hydraulic" mechanism and the "globe-to-wall" contact" mechanism. The former two theories were the more known and accepted of the three.

The buckling theory, first proposed by Le Fort, suggests that trauma to the infraorbital rim may transmit force directly to the thinner orbital floor, causing disruption of the floor without fracture of the rim [5]. In contrast, Pfeifer, who first propose the hydraulic theory, contends that trauma directed to the globe results in transmission of hydraulic pressure to the walls of the orbit, which tends to fracture medially [6]. In addition, first espoused by Pfeiffer in 1943 [6], the "globe-to-wall" mechanism results in a fracture in the inferomedial orbital wall via direct contact with the globe due to posterior movement of the globe in response to an external force.

Biomechanical studies [7,8] from cadavers and theoretical models have shown that predominant buckling mechanism results in a small fracture usually confined to anterior to mid-medial wall of the orbit, and herniation of orbital contents is unusual. Rarely does impact to the living eye occur in isolation to attribute the injury to one particular mechanism; usually both hydraulic and buckling mechanisms exist. Our case, with the lack of significant globe injury, as well as the presence of lower lid laceration indicating the main force of impact, suggests that the inferior orbital rim received the bulk of the force from the water jet. The pattern of the injury and the location of fracture lead the authors to postulate that the buckling mechanism is predominantly the cause of fracture in this case.

In a review of the literature on orbital emphysema following high-pressure compressed air jet by Hiraoka et al. [9], the authors reported that of the 15 cases reported to date, 14 cases had direct entry of air into the orbit via the conjunctiva, and 1 case via the eyelid. All of the cases had conjunctival chemosis / emphysema. In contrast, our case did not have any conjunctiva laceration or chemosis, likely due to the main impact of the water jet hitting the inferior orbital rim, providing a route of entry for air. The ocular injuries associated with air jet injuries were mostly limited to anterior segment injuries (10 out of the 15 cases). Only 4 of the cases had commotio retinae and 1 case developed optic atrophy. Of the high-pressure water jet injuries reported to our knowledge, the injuries were

more severe [10-14]. All of the cases had posterior segment injuries. Our case also illustrates the possibility of orbital emphysema caused by high-pressure water jet injuries, which was not previously reported.

The source of orbital emphysema may be the result of nose blowing with resultant passage of air from the paranasal sinuses through the floor fracture into orbit. However, given the close promixity of the site of laceration to the floor fracture, it is likely that air from the paranasal passages would exit from the site of laceration instead of going retrobulbarly. The involvement of orbital emphysema from the wound of entry into the orbit in an upward fashion (Fig. 2a) leads the authors to also postulate that the air may have been introduced together with the water jet.

High-pressure water jet injuries provide an entry for potential pathogens. Fairley C et al. [15] reported a case of rhino-orbital-cerebral mucormycosis following high-pressure water jet injury in an immunocompetent patient occurring 12 hours following injury. The authors recommend a close follow-up following initial trauma to watch for any signs of orbital infection and high index of suspicion for non-bacterial pathogens should the infection not respond to antibiotics.

4. CONCLUSION

Our case illustrates the dangers of water jet injuries. Infra-orbital trauma caused by a water-jet can cause orbital emphysema. Close early follow-up is necessary to watch for any signs of orbital infection following trauma.

CONSENT

All authors declare that written informed consent was obtained from the patient (or other approved parties) for publication of this case report and accompanying images.

ETHICAL APPROVAL

It is not applicable.

COMPETING INTERESTS

Authors have declared that no competing interests exist.

REFERENCES

1. Alimehmeti R, Gjika A, Kruja J. Orbital emphysema after nose blowing. Neurology. 2011;76(14):1274.

2. Garcia de Marcos JA, del Castillo-Pardo de Vera JL, Calderon-Polanco J. Orbital floor fracture and emphysema after nose blowing. Oral and Maxillofacial Surgery. 2008;12(3):163-5.

3. Hwang K Fau - Kim DH, Kim Dh Fau - Lee HS, Lee HS. Orbital fracture due to high-pressure air injection; 2011. 20110722 DCOM- 20111229(1536-3732(Electronic)). eng.

4. Lee SL, Mills DM, Meyer DR, Silver SM. Orbital emphysema. Ophthalmology. 2006; 113(11):2113 e1-2.

5. Tessier P. The classic reprint. Experimental study of fractures of the upper jaw. I and II. Rene Le Fort, M.D. Plastic and reconstructive surgery. 1972; 50(5):497-506 contd.

6. Pfeiffer RL. Traumatic Enophthalmos. Transactions of the American Ophthalmological Society. 1943;41:293-306.

7. Ahmad F, Kirkpatrick NA, Lyne J, Urdang M, Waterhouse N. Buckling and hydraulic mechanisms in orbital blowout fractures: fact or fiction? The Journal of Craniofacial Surgery. 2006;17(3):438-41.

8. Nagasao T, Miyamoto J, Shimizu Y, Jiang H, Nakajima T. What happens between pure hydraulic and buckling mechanisms of blowout fractures? Journal of Cranio-Maxillofacial Surgery. 2010;38(4):306-13.

9. Hiraoka T, Ogami T, Okamoto F, Oshika T. Compressed air blast injury with palpebral, orbital, facial, cervical, and mediastinal emphysema through an eyelid laceration: A case report and review of literature. BMC Ophthalmology. 2013;13:68.

10. DeAngelis DD, Oestreicher JH. Traumatic enucleation from a high-pressure water jet. Archives of Ophthalmology. 1999;117(1): 127-8.

11. Georgalas I, Ladas I, Taliantzis S, Rouvas A, Koutsandrea C. Severe intraocular trauma in a fireman caused by a high-pressure water jet. Clinical & Experimental Ophthalmology. 2011;39(4):370-1.

12. Gracner B, Pahor D. Bilateral eye injury caused by a high-pressure water jet from a fire hose. Wiener klinische Wochenschrift. 2001;113(Suppl 3):62-4.

13. Salminen L, Ranta A. Orbital laceration caused by a blast of water: Report of 2 cases. The British Journal of Ophthalmology. 1983;67(12):840-1.

14. Kyoya M, Takayama A, Kashiwagi S, Saitou C, Tanaka M, Uchinuma E. A foreign body in the orbital caused by a waterjet cleaning machine. Japanese Journal of Plastic and Reconstructive Surgery. 2006;49(2):227-30.

15. Fairley C, Sullivan TJ, Bartley P, Allworth T, Lewandowski R. Survival after rhino-orbital-cerebral mucormycosis in an immunocompetent patient. Ophthalmology. 2000;107(3):555-8.

14

Visual Impairment Following Stroke - The Impact on Quality of Life: A Systematic Review

Lauren R. Hepworth[1] and Fiona J. Rowe[1*]

[1]Department of Health Services Research, University of Liverpool, Liverpool L69 3GB, United Kingdom.

Authors' contributions

This work was carried out in collaboration between both authors. Author LRH ran searches, identified relevant studies, acted as first review author, extracted data, entered data, provided content expertise and co-wrote the final drafts. Author FJR led this review, provided methodological expertise, acted as a second review author. Both authors read and approved the final manuscript.

<u>Editor(s):</u>
(1) Ahmad M. Mansour, Department of Ophthalmology, American University of Beirut, Lebanon.
<u>Reviewers:</u>
(1) Sagili Chandrasekhara Reddy, National Defence University of Malaysia, Malaysia.
(2) Elliot M. Kirstein, Western College of Optometry, USA.
(3) Anonymous, University of Eastern Finland, Finland.
(4) Asaad Ahmed Ghanem, Mansoura University, Egypt.

ABSTRACT

Background: The visual impairments caused by stroke have the potential to affect the ability of an individual to perform activities of daily living. An individual with visual impairment may also have reduced level of independence. The purpose of this review was to investigate the impact on quality of life from stroke related visual impairment, using subjective patient reported outcome measures.
Methods: A systematic search of the literature was performed. The inclusion criteria required studies to have adult participants (aged 18 years or over) with a diagnosis of a visual impairment directly resulting from a stroke. Studies which included visual impairment as a result of other intra-cranial aetiology, were included if over half of the participants were stroke survivors. Multiple scholarly online databases and registers of published, unpublished and ongoing trials were searched, in addition articles were hand searched. MESH terms and alternatives in relation to stroke and visual conditions were used. Study selection was performed by two authors independently. Data was extracted by one author and verified by a second. The quality of the evidence was assessed using a quality appraisal tool and reporting guidelines.

---

*Corresponding author: E-mail: rowef@liverpool.ac.uk

Results: This review included 11 studies which involved 5646 participants, the studies used a mixture of generic and vision-specific instruments. The seven instruments used by the included studies were the EQ-5D, LIFE-H, SF-36, NEI VFQ-25, VA LV VFQ-48, SRA-VFP and DLTV. **Conclusion:** A reduction in quality of life was reported by all studies in stroke survivors with visual impairment. Some studies used generic instruments, therefore making it difficult to extract the specific impact of the visual impairment as opposed to the other deficits caused by stroke. The majority of studies (8/11) primarily had participants with visual field loss. This skew towards visual field loss and no studies investigating the impact ocular motility prevented a comparison of the effects on quality of life due to different visual impairments caused by stroke. In order to fully understand the impact of visual impairment following stroke on quality of life, further studies need to use an appropriate vision-specific outcome measure and include all types of visual impairment which can result from a stroke.

Keywords: Stroke; visual impairment; quality of life; impact; review.

1. BACKGROUND

Visual impairment as a result of a stroke takes many different guises across four main categories: Central vision loss, visual field loss, visual perception problems and ocular motility defects. All these impairments have the potential to affect the ability of an individual to perform activities of daily living (ADLs) for example mobility, social interaction and self-care. An individual with visual impairment may also have reduced level of independence. A combination of limitations has the potential to have an effect on an individual's mood and motivation. These effects have been reported in populations with visual impairment [1-4].

The World Health Organisation (WHO) defines health as "a state of complete physical, mental and social well-being and not merely the absence of disease or infirmity" [5]. The assessment of quality of life could be seen as a measurement of the subjective perceptions of an individual of how they are effected by their health state [1].

The analysis of utility values of diabetic retinopathy and age-related macular degeneration revealed the impact on quality of life was associated with the severity of impairment rather than the cause [6]. However, it has also been shown that there is not a consistent trend between severity of symptoms and reduction in quality of life. The individuals with the most severe visual impairment may not report the poorest quality of life but those with a slight impairment may [7]. This highlights the importance of patient reported outcomes as part of clinical and research assessments.

Stroke is a complex condition; an individual can be affected by a wide range of problems, for example physical disability (hemiplegia), communication disability (aphasia), feeding disability (dysphagia), cognitive disability, and visual impairment. It is important to establish the impact of the various components of stroke in order to evaluate interventions which are aimed at one of the specific disabilities [8].

The aim of this review is to summarise the impact of stroke related visual impairment on quality of life.

2. METHODS

We conducted an integrative review, aiming to bring together all evidence relating to impact of stroke-related visual problems.

2.1 Inclusion Criteria for Considering Studies for this Review

2.1.1 Types of studies

The following types of studies were included: randomised controlled trials, controlled trials, prospective and retrospective cohort studies and observational studies. Case reports were excluded. All languages were included and translations obtained when necessary.

2.1.2 Types of participants

We included studies of adult participants (aged 18 years or over) diagnosed with a visual impairment as a direct result of a stroke. Studies which included mixed populations were included if over 50% of the participants had a diagnosis of stroke and data were available for this subgroup.

2.1.3 Types of outcome and data

A formal quality of life assessment using a patient reported outcome measure (PROM). Studies which are assessing an intervention and have used a PROMs before and after, were included if the results prior to treatment were available for comparison to other studies.

2.2 Search Methods for Identification of Studies

We used systematic strategies to search key electronic databases and contacted known individuals conducting research in stroke and visual impairment. We searched Cochrane registers and electronic bibliographic databases (Appendix 1). In an effort to identify further published, unpublished and ongoing trials, we searched registers of ongoing trials, hand-searched journals and conference transactions, performed citation tracking using Web of Science Cited Reference Search for all included studies, searched the reference lists of included trials and review articles about vision after acquired brain injury and contacted experts in the field (including authors of included trials, and excluded studies identified as possible preliminary or pilot work). Search terms included a comprehensive range of MeSH terms and alternatives in relation to stroke and visual conditions (Appendix 1).

2.3 Selection of Studies

The titles and abstracts identified from the search were independently screened by the two authors using the pre-stated inclusion criteria. The full papers of any studies considered potentially relevant were then considered and the selection criteria applied independently by the two authors.

2.4 Data Extraction

A pre-designed data extraction form was used which gathered information on sample size, study design, quality of life instrument used, visual conditions reported and population type. Data was extracted and documented by one researcher (LH) and verified by another (FR).

2.5 Quality Assessment

To assess the quality of the studies included in this review, an adapted version of a checklist was used: The STROBE (Strengthening the Reporting of Observational Studies in Epidemiology) checklist [9,10]. The checklist was adapted as the original was designed to assess the quality of reporting rather than the potential for bias within a study. There is currently no 'gold standard' quality assessment tool for observational studies [11]. The STROBE Statement covers 22 items covering introduction, method, results and discussion of observation studies (including cohort, case-control and cross-sectional studies) (Appendix 2). The adapted version used in this review included 18 items, only the information which is pertinent to quality appraisal of the studies was included. The items exclude which were not considered relevant information, such as the title, abstract, background, setting and funding.

3. RESULTS AND DISCUSSION

3.1 Results of the Search

The search results are outlined in Fig. 1. Eleven studies (5646 participants) were included. Of the 11 included studies, ten were prospective observational studies and one was a retrospective analyses. Seven different questionnaires were used in the included studies to report quality of life in stroke survivors with visual impairment.

3.2 Quality of the Evidence

Two of the eleven papers reported 100% of the items requested by the STROBE checklist [12]. Eight of the eleven papers reported 90% or more of the requested items, ten of the eleven papers reported 75% or more. All eleven papers reported 73% or more. The majority of papers (81%) reported limitations of their studies. Results from all papers were reported and the individual results for each paper are outlined in Table 1.

3.3 Quality of Life Assessment for Stroke Survivors with Visual Impairment

Eight studies investigating quality of life following stroke were focused on patients with visual field loss [12-19]. Homonymous hemianopia is the most common type of visual field loss following stroke. Other types of defect are possible including homonymous quadrantanopia, general constriction and scotomas [19]. Of the remaining studies, Ali et al. [20] and Rowe et al. [21] address a combination of visual impairments following stroke while Beaudoin et al. [22] focused on visual perception problems.

The included studies used both generic health-related instruments and/or vision specific instruments which were administered to stroke survivors.

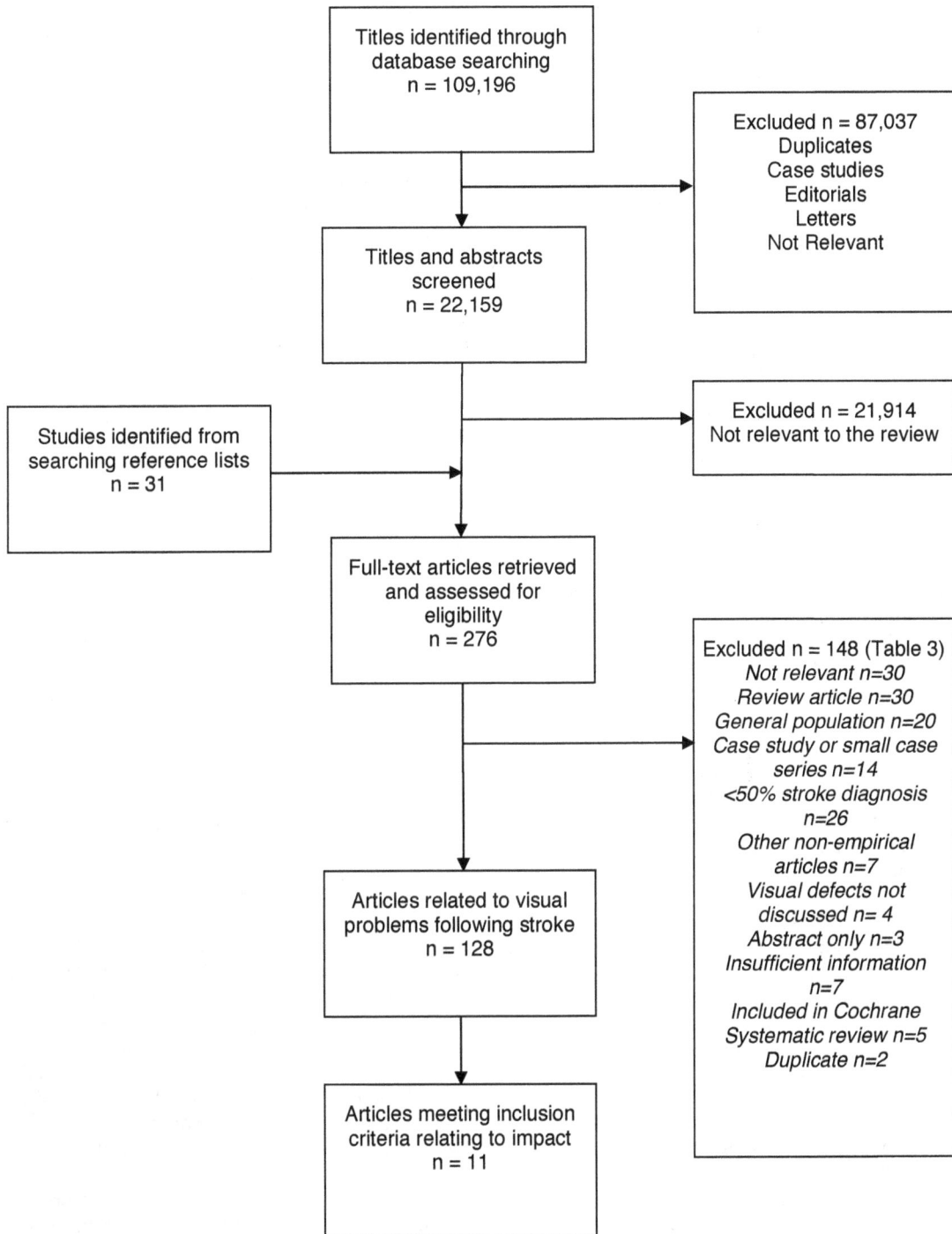

```
┌──────────────────────────┐
│ Titles identified through │
│   database searching      │
│     n = 109,196           │
└──────────────────────────┘           ┌──────────────────────────┐
            │                           │ Excluded n = 87,037       │
            ├──────────────────────────▶│ Duplicates                │
            │                           │ Case studies              │
            ▼                           │ Editorials                │
┌──────────────────────────┐           │ Letters                   │
│ Titles and abstracts      │           │ Not Relevant              │
│   screened                │           └──────────────────────────┘
│     n = 22,159            │
└──────────────────────────┘
            │                           ┌──────────────────────────┐
            │                           │ Excluded n = 21,914       │
┌────────────────────┐      ├──────────▶│ Not relevant to the review│
│ Studies identified │      │           └──────────────────────────┘
│ from searching     │──────┤
│ reference lists    │      │
│    n = 31          │      ▼
└────────────────────┘  ┌──────────────────────────┐
                        │ Full-text articles        │
                        │ retrieved and assessed    │
                        │ for eligibility           │
                        │    n = 276                │
                        └──────────────────────────┘
                                  │            ┌──────────────────────────┐
                                  │            │ Excluded n = 148 (Table 3)│
                                  ├───────────▶│ Not relevant n=30         │
                                  │            │ Review article n=30       │
                                  ▼            │ General population n=20   │
                        ┌──────────────────────────┐ Case study or small case │
                        │ Articles related to       │  series n=14            │
                        │ visual problems following │ <50% stroke diagnosis   │
                        │ stroke                    │  n=26                   │
                        │    n = 128                │ Other non-empirical     │
                        └──────────────────────────┘  articles n=7           │
                                  │            │ Visual defects not        │
                                  ▼            │  discussed n= 4           │
                        ┌──────────────────────────┐ Abstract only n=3       │
                        │ Articles meeting          │ Insufficient information │
                        │ inclusion criteria        │  n=7                    │
                        │ relating to impact        │ Included in Cochrane    │
                        │    n = 11                 │ Systematic review n=5   │
                        └──────────────────────────┘ Duplicate n=2           │
                                               └──────────────────────────┘
```

Fig. 1. Flowchart of the pathway for inclusion of articles

3.3.1 Generic Health-related Instruments

The European Quality of Life Score (EQ-5D), the Medical-Outcome-Study Short-Form-36 Health Survey (SF-36) and the Assessment of Life Habits (LIFE-H) have been used to assess quality of life in individuals with visual impairment post-stroke. More details about these instruments can be viewed in Table 2. They are generic health-related instruments and are not vision specific. Generic instruments include items which are relevant to broad definition of health 'physical, mental and social well-being' (WHO, 1946). This allows comparisons to be made not only within a disease group but across difference disease groups; for example the EQ-5D is currently used in the NHS PROMs programme before and after four common surgeries (hip replacement, knee replacement, hernia repair and varicose vein surgery) [23]. However, they may not be sensitive to specific symptoms caused by visual impairment.

The EQ-5D was reported to show that participants (n=3,859) with visual impairment following stroke had a poorer quality of life at baseline assessment after adjustment for age, thrombolysis treatment, other stroke non-visual related impairment and other medical conditions [20]. Visual impairment was assessed by using the National Institute of Health Stroke Scale (NIHSS), which only tests for homonymous visual field loss and horizontal gaze defects. Therefore, it misses many other forms of visual impairment thus, it is not possible for this study to give an overview of the impact of visual impairment following stroke. It reported that participants with conjugate deviations had reduced scores in all domains with the exception of anxiety/depression. Participants with hemianopia were reported to have reduced scores in self-care and usual activities. If the visual impairment was persistent to 90 days post-stroke onset, those participants had poorer outcomes in all domains for participants with hemianopia and four out of five for participants with gaze palsies with the exception of pain and anxiety/depression [20].

The LIFE-H reported the participants' (n=93) quality of life to be persistently reduced in the presence of perceptual difficulties post-stroke compared to a group (n=96) without visuo-perceptual deficits [22]. This difference was still present when controlling for the use of a walking aid and previous stroke events. The greatest difference was in socialisation rather than activities of daily living. This was shown at all three time points (n=57) of 18-24 days following discharge (baseline), then at three months and six months following baseline [22].

The domains relating to employment and education were not included as part of this study, however, with the increasing number stroke survivors of working age, these areas are critical to examining how a visual defect affects all areas of life.

The SF-36 has been used by three studies in conjunction with the NEI-VFQ and compared against healthy controls [12,16,17]. In each study stroke survivors with visual field defects were reported to have reduced scores in seven out of eight subscales (the exception being role limitation due to emotional problems). Participants with visual field defects were also reported to score better than general stroke survivors one month post-stroke without visual field defects [16]. However, when compared to general stroke survivors six months post-stroke without visual field defects, the participants with visual field defects had a reduced health-related quality of life [12,16]. When the composite scores of participants were compared with stroke survivors with different lesion ages (3, 6 and 12 months post-stroke onset), those with visual field defects scored better in the physical composite score and worse in the mental composite score [12]. Individuals with visual field defects in combination with reduced visual acuity are reported to have a further reduction of scores across four sub-scales: physical functioning, vitality, social functioning and emotional well-being [12]. The comparison groups used by these studies were from previously published data and therefore were not matched.

3.3.2 Vision-specific instruments

The National Eye Institute Visual Function Questionnaire (NEI VFQ-25), the Veterans Low Vision Visual Function Questionnaire (VA LV VFQ-48), the Self-Reported Assessment of Functional Visual Performance (SRAFVP) and the Daily Living Tasks Dependent on Vision (DLTV) have been used to assess quality of life in individuals with visual impairment post-stroke. More details about these instruments can be viewed in Table 2. Vision-specific instruments come under the wider disease-specific instruments umbrella and are tailored to assess quality of life in individuals with visual impairment. They can be more clinically sensitive to changes in visual impairment than generic instruments [24].

Table 1. Quality appraisal of papers using the adapted STROBE checklist

	Intro		Methods							Results					Discussion			
	3 - Objectives	4 - Study design	6 - Participants	7 - Variables	8 - Data source	9 - Bias	10 - Study size	11 - Quantitative variables	12 - Statistical methods	13 - Participants	14 - Descriptive data	15 - Outcome data	16 - Main results	17 - Other analyses	18 - Key results	19 - Limitations	20 - Interpretation	21 - Generalisability
Ali et al. 2013 [20]	+	+	+	+	+	−	+	−	−	?	?	+	+	+	+	+	+	+
Beaudoin et al. 2013 [22]	+	+	+	+	+	+	−	+	−	+	+	−	+	+	+	+	+	+
Chen et al. 2009 [15]	+	+	+	+	+	−	−	+	+	+	+	+	+	n/a	+	−	+	+
Gall et al. 2008 [17]	+	+	+	+	+	+	+	+	+	+	+	+	+	+	+	+	+	+
Gall et al. 2009 [16]	+	+	+	+	+	+	+	+	+	+	+	+	+	n/a	+	−	+	+
Gall et al. 2010 [12]	+	+	+	+	+	+	+	+	+	+	+	+	+	+	+	+	+	+
George et al. 2011 [14]	+	+	+	+	+	+	−	+	+	+	+	+	+	n/a	+	+	+	+
Mennem et al. 2012 [13]	+	+	+	+	+	+	−	+	+	?	+	+	+	+	+	+	+	+
Papageorgiou et al. 2007 [18]	+	+	+	+	+	−	−	+	+	−	+	+	+	n/a	+	+	+	+
Rowe et al. 2013 [19]	+	+	+	+	+	−	+	+	+	−	+	+	+	+	+	+	+	+
Rowe et al. 2013 [21]	+	+	+	+	+	+	+	+	+	+	+	+	+	+	+	+	+	+

+ = Reported ? = Unclear − = Not reported

Table 2. Patient Reported Outcome Measures (PROMs) used with stroke survivors

Questionnaire	Type of instrument	Overview	References
EQ-5D	Generic	5-item instrument, comprising of 5 dimensions: mobility, self-care, usual activities, pain/discomfort and anxiety/depression with an additional health analogue scale.	Ali et al. 2013 [20]
LIFE-H	Generic	77-item instrument comprising of 12 domains split equally between daily activities and social roles.	Beaudoin et al. 2013 [22]
SF-36	Generic	36-item general health instrument consisting of 8 domains. Widely used in health research.	Gall et al. 2010 [12]
NEI-VFQ	Vision-specific	25-item short version instrument, composed of 11 vision-related subscales with an additional question for general health rating. Used to assess many different ocular conditions.	Chen et al. 2009 [15] Gall et al. 2008; 2009; 2010 [12,16,17] George et al. 2011 [14] Papageorgiou et al. 2007 [18]
SRA-FVP	Vision-specific	38 item instrument covering a range of activities of daily living.	Mennem et al. 2012 [13]
VA LV VFQ	Vision-specific	48 item instrument, composed of five domains: visual ability, reading, mobility, visual motor and visual information. Originally developed and validated with patients with ophthalmic pathology such as glaucoma, macular degeneration and diabetic retinopathy	Chen et al. 2009 [15] George et al. 2011 [14]
DLTV	Vision-specific	24-item instrument which are not categorised under named domains, but covers topics such as reading, mobility, self-care and recognition. Originally developed for individuals with macular degeneration.	Rowe et al. 2013 [19,21]

The most commonly used instrument is the NEI VFQ-25, and it is regarded to have good sensitivity to changes in visual impairment [25]. Six studies using the NEI VFQ-25 concentrated on visual field loss post-stroke [12,14-18]. Five studies compared the scores from the NEI VFQ-25 of individuals with visual field loss post stroke and a reference health population and reported a reduced quality of life for those with visual field loss [12,15-18]. Gall et al. [17] also compared the scores of individuals with visual field loss post-stroke to individuals diagnosed with glaucoma and reported the former group to have a poorer quality of life.

The studies reported reduction in several sub-scales in addition to the composite score. The number of affected sub-scales varied from seven up to all 12 sub-scales. Five subscales in common were found to have a significant difference between individuals with visual field loss post-stroke and healthy individuals: General health, general vision, near activities, vision-specific mental health, driving, and peripheral vision [12,15-18]. Chen et al. [15] performed a multivariate analysis, adjusting for visual acuity, reading ability, contrast sensitivity and any pre-existing ocular conditions which changed the sub-scales and were deemed significantly different between the hemianopia and control group. Considering that the study had a very small sample size (n=10), following the multivariate analysis both the NEI VFQ-25 and VA LVQ-48 had a decreased in the number of subscales which were significantly affected, to five and one respectively. The factors adjusted for would not all be considered confounding factors but instead could also be a result of stroke and hemianopia, for example reduced reading ability [21]. The results following this multivariate analysis should be viewed as an assessment of quality of life with an isolated factor of hemianopia rather than visual impairment following stroke.

Five studies used a combination of instruments; two studies used the NEI-VFQ-25 in conjunction with the VA LV VFQ-48 [14,15]. A further three studies used the NEI-VFQ-25 in conjunction with the SF-36 [12,16,17].

Two of the studies investigated the effect of varying degrees of visual field loss post-stroke [12,17]. They reported that those with a greater area of spared central visual field had a better scores in the composite score and the following subscales: distance vision, social functioning and colour vision [12]. Individuals with a quadrantanopia had similar scores to individuals diagnosed with glaucoma, therefore, were less affected than those with hemianopia [17].

Several visual conditions can co-exist post stroke and this has the potential to have a larger impact on quality of life [26]. The presence of visual neglect has been shown to have a negative effect on the general health and mental health domains of the NEI VFQ-25 [16]. However, in the majority of domains participants with combined neglect and visual field loss were reported to have better quality of life than those with visual field loss without neglect. An explanation for this may be that those with visual neglect are less aware of their defect than those with visual field loss alone [21].

Two studies compared and reported the quality of life impact in individuals with visual field loss post-stroke with good visual acuity versus reduced visual acuity [12,16]. Individuals with reduced visual acuity in addition to visual field loss had lower scores (reduced quality of life) in the majority of domains with the exception of ocular pain, the following domains showed a significant reduction; general vision, near vision, distance vision, social functioning, mental health,

role difficulties, and dependency [12]. Furthermore, Gall et al. [16] reported a link between reduced scores for both reduced visual acuity and slower reading speeds.

George et al. [14] reported correlations between the objective assessments of the Behaviour Inattention Test (BIT) and the Mayo-Portland Adaptability Inventory (MPAI) and the subjective NEI VFQ-25 in participants with homonymous hemianopia. The BIT demonstrated the participants did not have attention deficits and it correlated well with eight out of twelve domains of the NEI VFQ-25. The instrument had a good association with both the participation and ability/adjustment scales of the MPAI. The participants (n=24) involved in this study performed well on objective testing, however the details of the patient reported outcome were not discussed [14]. The raw composite score of the NEI VFQ-25 in this study are comparable with those reported by Chen et al. [15], Papageorgiou et al. [18] and Gall et al. [12,16,17], all of these studies investigated participants with homonymous hemianopia.

The Veterans Low Vision Visual Function Questionnaire (VA LV VFQ-48) has been used by two studies investigating quality of life post-stroke in individuals with homonymous hemianopia [14,15]. Chen et al. [15] reported that initially the scores showed that individuals with hemianopia (n=10) had more difficulty with visual ability, mobility and visual motor functioning when compared to healthy controls. The differences for the reading and visual information subscales were found to be much smaller. When visual acuity, contrast sensitivity and the presence of pre-existing ocular conditions were controlled for, the only remaining significant difference was mobility. George et al. [14] reported the correlations between the objective assessments of the Behaviour Inattention Test (BIT) and the Mayo-Portland Adaptability Inventory (MPAI) and the subjective VA LV VFQ-48 for participants with homonymous hemianopia without any attention deficits. The BIT correlated well with four out of five domains of the VA LV VFQ-48. The instrument had a good association with both the participation and ability/adjustment scales of the MPAI [14]. The raw scores for the VA LV VFQ-48 in this study are comparable with those reported by Chen et al. [15].

The Self-Reported Assessment of Functional Visual Performance (SRAFVP) was used in a preliminary prospective observational study with the aim of validating the instrument with individuals with homonymous hemianopia (n=30) [13]. They reported that functional mobility tasks were less difficult to perform than reading and eye-hand co-ordination tasks. Participants without macular sparing had significantly more problems with reading. This study reported good reliability and validity of the SRAFVP [13]. However, the study had several limitations including a small sample size, the majority of the sample were male (29:1) and individuals with inattention, aphasia and other ocular pathology were excluded.

The Daily Living Tasks Dependent on Vision (DLTV) was used in a large cohort study involving individuals with a wide variety of different visual impairments following stroke [21]. Not all patients within the study completed the questionnaire as it was not a compulsory assessment. Two papers relating to visual symptoms and visual field loss report the findings of from the DLTV [21,27]. No significant difference in scores was found between those with visual impairment that reported symptoms and those that did not. Across all the symptom types and an asymptomatic group a wide range of scores was noted. Scores were reported to be reduced in individuals with visual impairment following stroke irrespective if any symptoms were reported [21]. Quality of life was shown to be reduced in individuals with multiple visual impairments when compared to individuals without visual impairment. The reduced score with multiple visual impairments was not significantly different to those diagnosed only with visual field loss [27].

4. CONCLUSION

Issues exist when extracting the specific impact of visual impairment following stroke from the impact of other sequelae of stroke, such as physical and cognitive impairments [8]. The wording of the NEI VFQ aids this task. All questions ask the participant specifically about the impact of vision. However, generic PROMs ask about the impact of their current health state on a particular aspect of health related quality of life. Consequently, the individual's current health state could include any of the sequelae of stroke. This renders it impossible to establish how much of the impact on quality of life is as a result of visual impairment. Studies which adjust for multiple factors have shown that when adjusting for confounders, participants have a poorer

quality of life. This is an important consideration for researchers when choosing PROMs for future studies in this area.

Regardless of the instrument used, all studies similarly report that visual impairment following stroke results in a reduced quality of life. There are some differences in the areas of quality of life affected, relating in part to the range of instruments used and the sub-scales of these.

Eight of the eleven included studies focused on visual field loss following stroke. One of the eleven was found to assess the impact of a specific ocular motility defect (horizontal gaze palsy) occurring following stroke. There is currently no literature reporting the impact of a wider range of ocular motility defects following stroke. Due to this skew towards visual field loss and lack of studies investigating the impact of ocular motility, it was not possible to compare the effects on quality of life due to different visual impairments caused by stroke.

This review highlights the need for further research into the impact of visual impairment following stroke on quality of life using appropriate vision-specific outcome measures.

CONSENT

It is not applicable.

ETHICAL APPROVAL

It is not applicable.

DISCLAIMER

This manuscript was presented in the conference.
Conference name: "Abstracts of the UK Stroke Forum 2015 Conference"
Conference link is "http://onlinelibrary.wiley.com /doi/10.1111/ijs.12634_17/full"
date 1-3 December 2015, Liverpool, UK , Volume 10, Issue Supplement S5

This paper presents independent research funded by the National Institute for Health Research (NIHR). The views expressed are those of the authors and not necessarily those of the NHS, the NIHR or the Department of Health.

ACKNOWLEDGEMENTS

This work was supported by the NIHR Fellowship Award of Dr Fiona Rowe.

COMPETING INTERESTS

Authors have declared that no competing interests exist.

REFERENCES

1. Wang C-W, Chan CLW, Chi I. Overview of quality of life research in older people with visual impairment. Advances in Aging Research. 2014;3(2):79-94.

2. Chia E-M, Wang JJ, Rochtchina E, Smith W, Cumming RR, Mitchell P. Impact of bilateral visual impairment on health-related quality of life: The Blue Mountains eye study. Investigative Ophthalmology & Visual Science. 2004;45(1):71-76.

3. McBain HB, Au CK, Hancox J, MacKenzie KA, Ezra DG, Adams GGW, Newman SP. The impact of strabismus on quality of life in adults with and without diplopia: a systematic review. Survey of Ophthalmology. 2014;59(2):185-191.

4. Tsai SY, Cheng CY, Hsu WM, Su TP, Liu JH, Chou P. Association between visual impairment and depression in the elderly. Journal of the Formosan Medical Association. 2003;102:86-90.

5. World Health Organisation. Preamble to the constitution of the World Health Organisation as adopted by the International Health Conference. in International Health Conference; 1946. New York.

6. Brown MM, Brown GC, Sharma S, Busbee B. Quality of life associated with visual loss: A time tradeoff utility analysis comparison with medical health states. Ophthalmology. 2003;110(6):1076-1081.

7. Finger RP, Fenwick E, Marella M, Dirani M, Holz FG, Chiang PP, Lamoureux EL. The impact of vision impairment on vision-specific quality of life in Germany. Investigative Ophthalmology & Visual Science. 2011;52(6):3613-9.

8. Schenk T, Noble AJ. Better dead than alive? Quality of life after stroke, in The behavioural consequence of stroke. Schweizer TA, MacDonald L, Editors. Springer: New York. 2014;241-255.

9. von Elm E, Altman DG, Egger M, Pocock SJ, Gøtzche PC, Vandenbroucke JP. Strengthening the reporting of observational studies in epidemiology (STROBE): Guidelines for reporting observational studies. PLOS Medicine, 2007;4(10):1623-1627.

10. Vandenbroucke JP, von Elm E, Altman DG, Gøtzche PC, Mulrow CD, Pocock SJ, Poole C, Schlesselman JJ, Egger M. Strengthening the reporting of observational studies in epidemiology (STROBE): Explanation and elaboration. PLOS Medicine. 2007;4(10):1628-1654.

11. Sanderson S, Tatt ID, Higgins JP. Tools for assessing quality and susceptibility to bias in observational studies in epidemiology: A systematic review and annotated bibliography. International Journal of Epidemiology. 2007;36(3):666-676.

12. Gall C, Franke GH, Sabel BA. Vision-related quality of life in first stroke patients with homonymous visual field defects. Health & Quality of Life Outcomes. 2010;8: 33.

13. Mennem TA, Warren M, Yuen HK. Preliminary validation of a vision-dependent activities of daily living instrument on adults with homonymous hemianopia. American Journal of Occupational Therapy. 2012;66(4):478-82.

14. George S, Hayes A, Chen C, Crotty M. Are vision-specific quality of life questionnaires important in assessing rehabilitation for patients with hemianopia post stroke? Topics in Stroke Rehabilitation. 2011; 18(4):394-401.

15. Chen CS, Lee AW, Clarke G, Hayes A, George S, Vincent R, Thompson A, Centrella L, Johnson K, Daly A, Crotty M. Vision-related quality of life in patients with complete homonymous hemianopia post stroke. Topics in Stroke Rehabilitation. 2009;16(6):445-453.

16. Gall C, Lucklum J, Sabel BA, Franke GH. Vision- and health-related quality of life in patients with visual field loss after postchiasmatic lesions. Investigative Ophthalmology and Visual Science. 2009; 50(6):2765-2776.

17. Gall C, Mueller I, Gudlin J, Lindig A, Schlueter D, Jobke S, Franke GH, Sabel BA. Vision- and health-related quality of life before and after vision restoration training in cerebrally damaged patients. Restorative Neurology and Neuroscience. 2008;26(4):341-353.

18. Papageorgiou E, Hardiess G, Schaeffel F, Wiethoelter H, Karnath HO, Mallot H, Schoenfisch B, Schiefer U. Assessment of vision-related quality of life in patients with homonymous visual field defects. Graefe's

Archive for Clinical and Experimental Ophthalmology. 2007;245(12):1749-1758.

19.   Rowe FJ, Wright D, Brand D, Jackson C, Harrison S, Maan T, Scott C, Vogwell L, Peel S, Akerman N, Dodridge C, Howard C, Shipman T, Sperring U, MacDiarmid S, Freeman C. A prospective profile of visual field loss following stroke: Prevalence, type, rehabilitation and outcome. BioMed Research International; 2013.

20.   Ali M, Hazelton C, Lyden P, Pollock A, Brady M, Collaboration V. Recovery from poststroke visual impairment: evidence from a clinical trials resource. Neurorehabilitation & Neural Repair. 2013; 27(2):133-41.

21.   Rowe F, Wright D, Brand D, Vince C, Harrison S, Eccleston C, Maan T, Scott C, Vogwell L, Peel S, Robson L, Akerman N, Dodridge C, Howard C, Shipman T, Sperring U, Yarde S, MacDiarmid S, Freeman C. Symptoms of stroke-related visual impairment. Strabismus. 2013;21(2): 150-154.

22.   Beaudoin AJ, Fournier B, Julien-Caron L, Moleski L, Simard J, Mercier L, Desrosiers J. Visuoperceptual deficits and participation in older adults after stroke. Australian Occupational Therapy Journal. 2013;60(4):260-266.

23.   Health and Social Care Information Centre. Background information about PROMs; 2011. Available:http://www.hscic.gov.uk/article/38 43/Background-information-about-PROMs (13 August 2014)

24.   Hays RD. Generic versus disease-targeted instruments, in Assessing quality of life in clinical trials. Fayers P, Hays R, Editors. Oxford University Press: Oxford. 2005;5-8.

25.   Swamy BN, Chia E-M, Wang JJ, Rochtchina E, Mitchell P. Correlation between vision- and health-related quality of life scores. Acta Ophthalmologica. 2009; 87(3):335-339.

26.   Rowe F, Brand D, Jackson CA, Price A, Walker L, Harrison S, Eccleston C, Scott C, Akerman N, Dodridge C, Howard C, Shipman T, Sperring U, MacDiarmid S, Freeman C. Visual impairment following stroke: do stroke patients require vision assessment? Age & Ageing. 2009;38(2): 188-93.

27.   Rowe F, Wright D, Brand D, Jackson C, Harrison S, Maan T, Scott C, Vogwell L, Peel S, Akerman N, Dodridge C, Howard C, Shipman T, Sperring U, MacDiarmid S, Freeman C. A prospective profile of visual field loss following stroke: prevalence, type, rehabilitation and outcome. BioMed Research International; 2013.

APPENDIX

Appendix 1. Search options and search terms

Databases:

- Cochrane Stroke Group Trials Register
- The Cochrane Eyes and Vision Group Trials Register
- The Cochrane Central Register of Controlled Trials (CENTRAL) (*The Cochrane Library*, latest issue);
- MEDLINE (1950 to May 2014);
- EMBASE (1980 to May 2014);
- CINAHL (1982 to May 2014);
- AMED (1985 to May 2014);
- PsycINFO (1967 to May 2014);
- Dissertations & Theses (PQDT) database (1861 to May 2014);
- British Nursing Index (1985 to May 2014);
- PsycBITE (Psychological Database for Brain Impairment Treatment Efficacy, www.psycbite.com).

Registers:

- ClinicalTrials.gov (http://clinicaltrials.gov/);
- Current Controlled Trials (www.controlledtrials. com);
- Trials Central (www.trialscentral.org);
- Health Service Research Projects in Progress (wwwcf.nlm.nih.gov/hsr_project/home_proj.cfm);
- National Eye Institute Clinical Studies Database (http://clinicalstudies.info.nih.gov/cgi/protinstitute.cgi?NEI.0.html)
- British and Irish Orthoptic Journal, Australian Orthoptic Journal, and proceedings of the European Strabismological Association (ESA), International Strabismological Association (ISA), International Orthoptic Association (IOA) (http://pcwww.liv.ac.uk/~rowef/index_files/Page646.htm)
- Proceedings of Association for Research in Vision and Ophthalmology (www.arvo.org);

Terms:

Cerebrovascular disorders/	Eye Movements/	Quality of Life
Brain ischaemia/	Eye/	Impact
Intracranial Arterial Disease	Eye Disease/	
Intracranial Arteriovenous	Visually Impaired Persons/	
Malformations/	Vision Disorders/	
"Intracranial Embolism and	Blindness/	
Thrombosis*/	Diplopia/	
Stroke/	Vision, Binocular/	
	Vision, Monocular/	
	Visual Acuity/	
	Visual Fields/	
	Vision, Low/	
	Ocular Motility Disorders/	
	Blindness, Cortical/	
	Hemianopsia/	
	Abducens Nerve Diseases/	
	Abducens Nerve/	
	Oculomotor Nerve/	
	Trochlear Nerve/	
	Visual Perception/	

Nystagmus
strabismus
smooth pursuits
saccades
depth perception
stereopsis
gaze disorder
internuclear ophthalmoplegia
Parinaud's syndrome
Weber's syndrome
skew deviation
conjugate deviation
oscillopsia
visual tracking
agnosia
hallucinations

	OR	OR	OR
AND			

Appendix 2. STROBE statement [9,10]

	Item no	Recommendation
Title and abstract	1	(a) Indicate the study's design with a commonly used term in the title or the abstract (b) Provide in the abstract an informative and balanced summary of what was done and what was found
Introduction		
Background/rationale	2	Explain the scientific background and rationale for the investigation being reported
Objectives	3	State specific objectives, including any pre-specified hypotheses
Methods		
Study design	4	Present key elements of study design early in the paper
Setting	5	Describe the setting, locations, and relevant dates, including periods of recruitment, exposure, follow-up, and data collection
Participants	6	(a) Cohort study—Give the eligibility criteria, and the sources and methods of selection of participants. Describe methods of follow-up Case-control study—Give the eligibility criteria, and the sources and methods of case ascertainment and control selection. Give the rationale for the choice of cases and controls Cross-sectional study—Give the eligibility criteria, and the sources and methods of selection of participants (b) Cohort study—For matched studies, give matching criteria and number of exposed and unexposed Case-control study—For matched studies, give matching criteria and the number of controls per case
Variables	7	Clearly define all outcomes, exposures, predictors, potential confounders, and effect modifiers. Give diagnostic criteria, if applicable
Data sources/ measurement	8*	For each variable of interest, give sources of data and details of methods of assessment (measurement). Describe comparability of assessment methods if there is more than one group
Bias	9	Describe any efforts to address potential sources of bias
Study size	10	Explain how the study size was arrived at
Quantitative variables	11	Explain how quantitative variables were handled in the analyses. If applicable, describe which groupings were chosen and why
Statistical methods	12	(a) Describe all statistical methods, including those used to control for confounding (b) Describe any methods used to examine subgroups and interactions (c) Explain how missing data were addressed (d) Cohort study—If applicable, explain how loss to follow-up was addressed Case-control study—If applicable, explain how matching of cases and controls was addressed Cross-sectional study—If applicable, describe analytical methods taking account of sampling strategy (e) Describe any sensitivity analyses
Results		
Participants	13*	(a) Report numbers of individuals at each stage of study—eg numbers potentially eligible, examined for eligibility, confirmed eligible, included in the study, completing follow-up, and analysed (b) Give reasons for non-participation at each stage (c) Consider use of a flow diagram

	Item no	Recommendation
Descriptive data	14*	(a) Give characteristics of study participants (eg demographic, clinical, social) and information on exposures and potential confounders (b) Indicate number of participants with missing data for each variable of interest (c) *Cohort study*—Summarise follow-up time (eg, average and total amount)
Outcome data	15*	*Cohort study*—Report numbers of outcome events or summary measures over time *Case-control study*—Report numbers in each exposure category, or summary measures of exposure *Cross-sectional study*—Report numbers of outcome events or summary measures
Main results	16	(*a*) Give unadjusted estimates and, if applicable, confounder-adjusted estimates and their precision (eg, 95% confidence interval). Make clear which confounders were adjusted for and why they were included (*b*) Report category boundaries when continuous variables were categorized (*c*) If relevant, consider translating estimates of relative risk into absolute risk for a meaningful time period
Other analyses	17	Report other analyses done—eg analyses of subgroups and interactions, and sensitivity analyses
Discussion		
Key results	18	Summarise key results with reference to study objectives
Limitations	19	Discuss limitations of the study, taking into account sources of potential bias or imprecision. Discuss both direction and magnitude of any potential bias
Interpretation	20	Give a cautious overall interpretation of results considering objectives, limitations, multiplicity of analyses, results from similar studies, and other relevant evidence
Generalisability	21	Discuss the generalisability (external validity) of the study results
Other information		
Funding	22	Give the source of funding and the role of the funders for the present study and, if applicable, for the original study on which the present article is based

15

Phenothiazine Group Drug Induced Corneal and Lenticular Deposits in a Patient of Severe Depression – A Case Report

Ojha Sushil[1*], Tandon Anupama[1], Saraswat Neeraj[1] and Shukla Dipendra[1]

[1]*Department of Ophthalmology, UP RIMS and R, Saifai, Etawah, UP, India.*

Authors' contributions

This work was carried out in collaboration between all authors. All authors read and approved the final manuscript.

Editor(s):
(1) Ahmad M. Mansour, Department of Ophthalmology, American University of Beirut, Lebanon.
Reviewers:
(1) Sagili Chandarsekhara Reddy, Department of Ophthlmology, National Defence University of Malaysia, Malaysia.
(2) Italo Giuffre, Ophthalmology Department, University of Rome, Italy.

ABSTRACT

A 50-yr-old man, who had been taking medication for severe depression with psychosis, presented to eye OPD of UPRIMS & R with a chief complaint of visual disturbance of 8 months duration. He was continuously taking chlorpromazine unsupervised in double the dose and doubles the frequency. Slit-lamp examination revealed fine, discrete, and brownish deposits on the posterior cornea. In addition, bilateral star-shaped anterior sub capsular lens opacities, which were dense, dust-like granular deposits, were noted. Best-corrected visual acuity was 6/36 in the right eye and 6/24 in the left eye. Other ocular findings were normal. Dark pigmentation on face was present. The deposition was not reversible even after stopping the drug.

Keywords: Corneal deposits; drug induced lenticular opacity; phenothiazine induced deposits.

Key Message

This case report shows that Phenothiazine group drug, if taken in excess dose and for long duration can lead to visually disabling corneal deposits and star shaped lenticular opacification.

---

*Corresponding author: E-mail: drsushilojha@gmail.com

Phenothiazine group drug must be used with caution and under slit lamp ophthalmic monitoring and strictly under psychiatric monitoring.
The pigmented deposits in cornea are not reversible even after stopping the drug.

1. INTRODUCTION

In 1960s phenothiazine was widely used for the chronic treatment of schizophrenia [1]. However despite its extremely effective antipsychotic action, there is significant decline in the usage of phenothiazine over the last decade due to its tendency to produce ocular complications[1] .In 1964 Greiner and Berry first described the ocular toxicity of phenothiazine over the cornea, conjunctiva and lens [2]. One of the hypothesis for the ocular manifestations of long term phenothiazine therapy is the property of phenothiazine to get deposit in the ocular tissues and to denature the proteins when exposed to light making them opaque [3-4]. Even after the discontinuation of the drug, these ocular changes persists.

Several case reports of chlorpromazine-induced corneal deposits and cataracts have been published till now; however, Chlorpromazine and trifluperazine- induced corneal deposits and cataract are unusual and rare. [1,2] Herein, we report the case of Chlorpromazine and trifluperazine induced corneal deposit and cataract in a case of severe depression. Here we also report severe phototoxic pigmentation of skin in our case which occurs due to binding of phenothiazine to melanin granules [1-4].

2. CASE

A 50-yr-old Indian man, who had been taking medication for severe depression with psychosis, presented to eye OPD with complains of visual disturbance of 8 months duration. He was taking chrorpromazine unsupervised in double the dose and double the frequency. Slit-lamp examination revealed fine, discrete, and brownish deposits on the posterior cornea (Fig. 1). In addition, bilateral star-shaped anterior sub capsular lens opacities, which were dense, dust-like granular deposits, were noted (Fig. 1). Best-corrected visual acuity was 6/36 in the right eye and 6/24 in the left eye. Other ocular findings were normal. No fundal pigmentation noted. Dark pigmentation on forehead, hand and face was present (Fig. 2). Rest systemic examination was within normal limits.

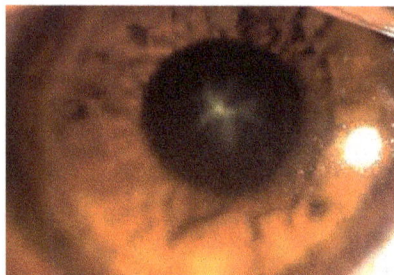

Fig. 1A

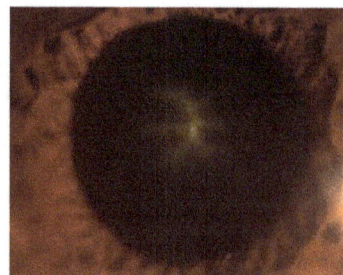

Fig. 1B

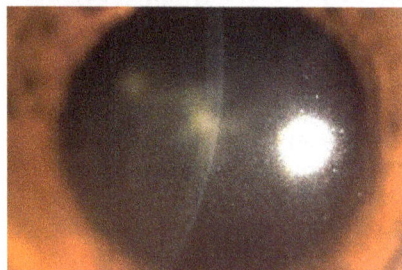

Fig. 1C

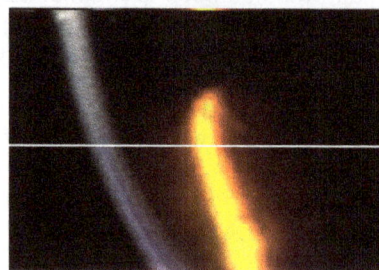

Fig. 1D

Fig. 1A. Right eye showing diffuse brownish coloured deposits in the inferior 2/3 rd of cornea with anterior sub capsular star shaped cataract
Fig. 1B. Left eye showing diffuse brownish coloured deposits in the inferior 2/3 rd of cornea with anterior sub capsular star shaped cataract
Fig. 1C and 1D. showing the level of brownish pigment deposit in right eye and left eye, respectively

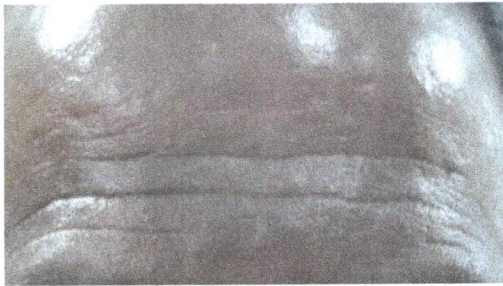

Fig. 2. Shows blackish pigmentation of the forehead of the patient

According to the information provided by his chemist, the patient had received T. Trinicomforte (Trifluperazine 5 mg, Trihexphenidyl 2 mg, T. chlorpromazine 50 mg) and T. Alprex (Alprazolam 0.25 mg). Patient took these drugs for 6 years and now off drugs since 2 months. Psychiatry consultation done which provided information that patient took these drugs in double the dose prescribed and in double the frequency for 6 years without any supervision and suffering from severe depression.

We have done dermatology consultation for pigmentation on face which correlated with Phenothiazine drug induced phototoxicity, causing dark pigmentation.

Patient was counselled and the intake of phenothiazine group drug stopped. Patient is shifted to newer safe anti-psychotic Risperidone after psychiatric consultation.

3. DISCUSSION

Phenothiazines such as chlorpromazine or methotrimeprazine were introduced to the psychiatry clinics in 1953 and have been widely used for the treatment of psychiatric illnesses since then. Multiple studies have been conducted over the phenothiazine for their potential side effects on chronic use and their complications [1,3-5]. On chronic use, phenothiazine were found to have level 50 times higher than blood concentration in the ocular tissues in comparison to that of other tissues of the body [6]. Greiner and Berry were the first to describe the effect of long term medication of chlorpromazine in 70 patients as brownish granular pigmentation in the parenchyma of the cornea and a central star shaped opacity in the centre of anterior capsule of lens [2]. Mc Carty et al reported that the ratio of anterior capsular opacity in cataract patients

not on phenothiazine medication was 0.2%, while the ratio was 26% for the schizophrenics on phenothiazine medication [7]. A study conducted by Ruigomez et al. [8] on the incidence of rate of cataract in Schizophrenics and control group subjects showed that the rate was 8.8 times higher in patients under long term medication of over 300 mg chlorpromazine daily than that of the control group. Many authors have reported that long term medication of phenothiazine increases the risk of cataract. It is believed that the clinical changes in the ocular tissues in patients who received a specific dosage of phenothiazine could be due to an increase in number and melanin content of melanin cells on the exposure of eyes to harmful ultraviolet rays and the accumulation of abnormal metabolites from photosensitization of chlorpromazine which is present in high concentration in the eyes. Still controversy regarding the toxic levels of phenothiazine exists. According to Delong et al. [9] characteristic changes in the eyes were generally observed in patients receiving chlorpromazine dosage of over 1000 mg, and in more than 90% of patients receiving dosage of over 2,500 mg; however these changes were rare when the total dosage was 500 mg. Thaler et al. [10] reported that if daily dosage of chlorpromazine exceeding 800 mg, lenticular pigmentation can begin to occur as early as within 14 to 20 months of treatment. A daily dosage of 2000 mg has caused these changes to appear as early as within 6 months of therapy. As the dosage is increased, the ocular changes became more distinct and remain continued even after stopping the medication. Lal et al. [11] reported the pigmentation i[n the skin and corneal endothelium due to long term usage of phenothiazine and other neuroleptics like haloperidol, trifluoperazine, levomepromazine and thioproperazine. They also reported that skin pigmentation is reversible and might have different mechanism of pigmentation than that of cornea.

Very few cases of corneal and lenticular drug deposits reported so far from use of Phenothiazine group drug and none of them from India. Although corneal and lenticular deposits have been present in literature after Phenothiazine group drug [1-7].

4. CONCLUSION

The purpose of this case study is to highlight the visually disabling corneal and lenticular deposits after the use of Phenothiazine drug which are not reversible after stopping the drug in a patient of severe depression. This case may represent just the tip of the iceberg, and hence calls for establishment of stringent ophthalmic screening protocols for the identification of corneal and lenticular deposits at early stage when patient is on these drugs. This report also re-iterates the fact that ophthalmic manifestations of drugs need to need to discontinue these drugs and to replace them by safer anti-psychotic drugs. Patient will need cataract surgery with intraocular lens implantation to clear lenticular deposits for visual rehabilitation.

CONSENT

It is not applicable.

ETHICAL APPROVAL

Ethical approval was taken from institutional ethical committee.

COMPETING INTERESTS

Authors have declared that no competing interests exist.

REFERENCES

1. Seong Taeck Kim, Jae Woong Koh, Joon Mo Kim, Won Young Kim, Gwang Ju Choi. Methotrimeprazine-induced corneal deposits and cataract revealed by urine drug profiling test J Korean Med Sci. 2010;25:1688-91.
2. Greiner AC, Berry K. Skin pigmentation and corneal and lens opacities with prolonged chlorpromazine therapy. Can Med Assoc J. 1964;90:663-5.
3. Howard RO, McDonald CJ, Dunn B, Creasey WA. Experimental chlorpromazine cataracts. Invest Ophthalmol. 1969;8:413-21.
4. Jung BS, Lee TH, Lee HY. Ocular findings associated with long-term chlorpromazine therapy. J Korean Ophthalmol Soc. 1996;37:1951-7.
5. Kim HS, Choi HJ, Yun YS. Two cases of chlorpromazine-induced corneal and lenticular opacity. J Korean Ophthalmol Soc. 2002;43:2349-53.
6. Potts AM. The concentration of phenothiazines in the eye of experimental animals. Invest Ophthalmol. 1962;1:522-30.
7. McCarty CA, Wood CA, Fu CL, Livingston PM, Mackersey S, Stanislavsky Y, Taylor HR. Schizophrenia, Psychotropic medication and Cataract. Ophthalmology. 1999;106:683-7.
8. Ruigómez A, García Rodríguez LA, Dev VJ, Arellano F, Raniwala J. Are schizophrenia or antipsychotic drugs a risk factor for cataracts? Epidemiology. 2000;11:620-3.
9. DeLong SL, Poley BJ, McFarlane JR Jr. Ocular changes associated with long term chlorpromazine therapy. Arch Ophthalmol. 1965;73:611-7.
10. Thaler JS, Curinga R, Kiracofe G. Relation of graded ocular anterior chamber pigmentation to phenothiazine intake in schizophrenics—quantification procedures. Am J Optom Physiol Opt. 1985;62:600-4.
11. Lal S, Bloom D, Silver B, Desjardins B, Krishnan B, Thavundayil J, Thompson T. Replacement of chlorpromazine with other neuroleptics: effect on abnormal skin pigmentation and ocular changes. J Psychiatry Neurosci. 1993;18:173-7.

16

A Safe, Efficacious and Cost Effective Way of Delivering Sub-Tenon's Anaesthesia during Cataract Surgery

S. Bansal[1], K. Jasani[1*] and K. Taherian[1]

[1]*Department of Ophthalmology, Royal Preston Hospital, Preston PR2 9HT, UK.*

Authors' contributions

This work was carried out in collaboration between all authors. Author SB carried out the study, performed the literature search statistical analysis and wrote the first draft of the manuscript. Author KJ carried out the study, performed statistical analysis and made the final changes to the manuscript prior to submission and author KT designed, supervised and carried out the study. All authors read and approved the final manuscript.

Editor(s):
(1) Ayman Ahmed Alkawas, Department of Ophthalmology, Zagazig University, Egypt.
(2) Mitsuru Nakazawa, Department of Ophthalmology, Hirosaki University, Japan.
Reviewers:
(1) Anonymous, Universidade de São Paulo Medical School, Brazil.
(2) Anonymous, Fourth Military Medical University, China.
(3) Seydi Okumuş, Department of Ophthalmology, University of Gaziantep, Turkey.
(4) Anonymous, Third Military Medical University, Chongqing, China.

ABSTRACT

Aims: There are considerable pressures in various health economies at present to reduce costs whilst maintaining patient safety and clinical efficacy. We report a new simplified regime for the administration of Sub-Tenon's anaesthesia offering a cost saving of up to 95% whilst maintaining to total safety and efficacy.
Study Design: The study compared usage of 2% Xylocaine (2% Lignocaine with 1:200000 Adrenaline) over the more prevalent regime of 2% Bupivacaine + 2% Lignocaine + Hyaluronidase in terms of cost, patient satisfaction, safety and efficacy prior to phacoemulsification surgery.
Place and Duration of Study Sample: Department of Ophthalmology, Royal Preston Hospital, Preston UK between July and November 2010.
Methodology: Following topical anaesthesia with 3 drops of Proxymetacaine 0.5% drops instilled one minute apart and subsequent administration of a drop of 5% Povidone Iodine aqueous solution

into the conjunctival sac, 2ml of 2% Lignocaine with 1:200000 adrenaline was administered as a Sub-Tenon's injection to 100 eyes of consecutive patients undergoing phacoemulsification. Pain levels during the administration of the injection and during surgery were monitored by measuring Visual Analogue Pain (VAP) scores via a prospective questionnaire immediately after the operation.

Results: There were 100 eyes of patients undergoing cataract surgery included in this study. No patient required top up anaesthesia during the surgery and no serious anaesthetic related intra or post-operative complication was noted in any of the patients. The mean VAP score during delivery of anaesthetic and for the duration of surgery were both 0.

Conclusion: Our results show that this regime for administration of Sub-Tenon's anaesthesia meets the standards required in terms of both safety and efficacy whilst delivering considerable cost savings. We recommend its routine use for the reasons cited above.

Keywords: Sub-Tenon's anaesthesia; cataract surgery; local anaesthetic; cost effectiveness.

1. INTRODUCTION

Local anaesthesia for cataract surgery has been shown to be a safe and efficient mode of anaesthesia for routine daycase cataract surgery [1,2] and there is some evidence to suggest that it is preferred by patients [3]. According to a Cochrane review meta-analysis by Davison et al, it is still the anaesthesia of choice with regards to minimising overall pain perception and intraoperative complications [4].

A variety of local anaesthetic agents are employed in the administration of Sub-Tenon's block. The hitherto prevalent regime in our department has been utilising 5ml of a combination of 0.5% Bupivacaine, 2% Lignocaine and Hyalase for the Sub-Tenon's block. Our simplified regime consists of using 2ml of 2% Xylocaine (2% Lignocaine with 1: 200,000 adrenaline).

Our reasons for choosing this preparation were based on our experience that it was an effective and safe method of pain control during surgery and secondly the marked cost advantage over the prevailing regime which amounted to a 95% cost saving per patient. This is highly relevant in the context of a National Health Service that faces considerable pressures to innovate in order to reduce costs whilst maintaining patient safety and clinical efficacy. Cataract surgery is one area in which the high turnover of patients allows for small savings made per person to translate into larger financial gains. Our aim was to assess the effectiveness of our practice in terms of safety, efficacy and meeting the standards required for pain free cataract surgery.

The Royal College of Anaesthesia and Royal College of Ophthalmologists published guidelines in their 2012 paper [5] regarding the administration of local anaesthesia in cataract surgery. In this, the goal of anaesthesia for intraocular surgery is:

- To provide pain-free surgery and to minimise the risk of systemic complications.
- To facilitate the surgical procedure.
- To reduce the risk of surgical complications.

Visual analogue pain (VAP) scores (Fig. 1) have been used in a number of studies to assess pain following Sub-Tenon's anaesthesia [2,6-9]. Stevens was the first to describe a series of 50 patients undergoing Sub-Tenon's anaesthesia and measured pain during both surgery and administration of anaesthesia using a VAP scale [6]. The mean scores were found to be 1 for both of these measurements.

Our aim was to determine if our current practice of administration of Sub-Tenon's local anaesthesia for day case cataract surgery meets the accepted standards required in anaesthesia.

We evaluated the level of pain experienced by the patient during both anaesthesia and surgery. Our standards are:

1. To achieve minimal or no pain during delivery of the Sub-Tenon's block (i.e. VAP score of <2).
2. To achieve pain free surgery (i.e. VAP score of 0).
3. No systemic or serious local adverse effects of anaesthesia.

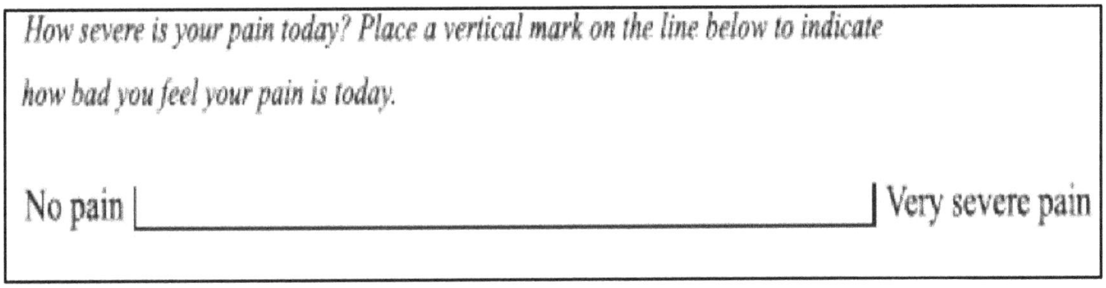

> *How severe is your pain today? Place a vertical mark on the line below to indicate*
>
> *how bad you feel your pain is today.*
>
> No pain | _____ | Very severe pain

Fig. 1. Visual analogue pain (VAP) score scale

2. MATERIALS AND METHODS

This was a prospective longitudinal questionnaire based study where 100 consecutive eyes of all patients undergoing routine cataract surgery as a day-case procedure were included. Exclusion criteria included patients with profound deafness, dementia, learning difficulties, high anxiety or an allergy to any of the compounds being used.

A suitable trained individual as per Royal College recommendations performed patient monitoring of blood pressure, pulse oximetry and heart rate throughout the procedure. In all cases 2ml of Lignocaine and adrenaline 1:200000 was used for injection from a single 20ml bottle. Sterility was maintained by drawing up syringes of anaesthetic for each patient on the list and appropriately labeling them with "anaesthetic" prior to the start of the list.

The Sub-Tenon's anaesthetic was delivered by 1 of 3 surgeons (SB, KJ or KT). Three drops of proxymethacaine were instilled into the inferior fornix at 1-minute intervals. Povidone iodine was given in the conjunctival sac and over the lashes. The patient was asked to look upwards and outwards. The inferonasal bulbar conjunctiva was grabbed using a Moorfields forceps and a small incision was made using curved Wescott scissors. The Sub-Tenon's cannula was inserted along bare sclera and 2 ml of the anaesthetic solution was injected slowly into the Sub-Tenon's space.

The patient was asked to mark their pain score on the visual analogue pain scale immediately after surgery for 1) the delivery of anaesthetic and 2) the duration of surgery.

The patient subsequently underwent cataract surgery using the standard phacoemulsification (Bausch+Lomb Millennium Phaco System) and insertion of intraocular lens technique.

3. RESULTS

There were 100 patients (n=100) included in the study. The mean VAP scores for pain during delivery of the anaesthetic and during the surgery was 0 respectively. 98 patients (98%) gave a VAP score of 0 and 2 patients (2%) recorded a score of 1 for pain during delivery of Sub-Tenon's anaesthesia. This resulted in a mean VAP score of 0.02, or effectively 0 for the purpose of this study. None of the patients (n=100, 100%) felt any pain during the surgery with an average surgical time of 25 minutes. There was no intra or postoperative complications (up to 1 month post surgery) due to anaesthesia recorded in our series.

Our results meet the standards we had defined earlier. Furthermore our findings compare favourably with those in the literature where VAP scores have been used to determine pain during cataract surgery or delivery of anaesthetic.

4. DISCUSSION

Srinavasan et al. [9] report mean VAP scores of 2.42 taken immediately after cataract surgery with Sub-Tenon's anaesthesia in a randomised clinical trial comparing topical and Sub-Tenon's anaesthesia. Similarly Zafirakis et al. [7] report a mean VAP score of 1.53(SD0.63) for delivery of anaesthesia and 0.57(SD1.28) during surgery.

Of note is the study by Rowley et al. [8], in which they used a similar anaesthetic combination to ours, however their group of patients were subdivided into two depending on whether or not hyaluronidase was given. Hyaluronidase was found to improve akinesia however had no significant effect on pain scores. Akinesia was not measured in thisstudy, as many cataract surgeons will nowadays accept a small degree of ocular movement during surgery provided the patient is pain free and cooperative.

Although it has been argued that a limitation with VAP scores is their inter-observer variability, nevertheless as a guide to pain relief, an already subjective modality, they have proved useful in arbitrary comparisons and effectiveness of anaesthesia.

There were no complications from anaesthesia in our series of patients apart from the occasional localized conjunctival chemosis, which is not deemed a significant complication of Sub-Tenon'sanesthesia. Some surgeons may be wary of using adrenaline in the Sub-Tenon's space. Therisks of using dilute adrenaline in Sub-Tenon's anaesthesia are by no means established. Our experience with this study and having used the same preparation in over 800 cases prior to this study has not yielded a single adverse effect of its use in the doses described above. Also, we could not find any reported cases in the English literature of central retinal artery occlusion secondary to the use of adrenaline in the Sub-Tenon's space.

Experiments on rabbits whereby blood flow to ocular structures was analysed using colour Doppler techniques show a reduction in blood flow to certain ocular structures (iris, cilliary body) following retrobulbar injection of adrenaline [10]. In this paper however 2% adrenaline was utilised, approximately 4000 fold more concentrated than our preparation. In addition, we argue that unlike the retrobulbar space, the Sub-Tenon's space is not in direct contact with the optic nerve sheath, which is pierced by the ophthalmic artery and vein. Although some intraconal leakage of anaesthetic might occur, this is perhaps further limited by the relatively smaller volume of anaesthesia administered in our series (2ml) compared with the standard 3-5ml described with Sub-Tenon's techniques.

Krohn et al. [11] report certain distinct advantages of retrobulbar anaesthesia with combined adrenaline in a study involving 75 patients. Compared to patients receiving anaesthetic alone, adrenaline appeared to have a mydriatic as well as an intraocular pressure lowering effect. In addition by virtue of its vasoconstrictor effect it helped increase both the duration of anaesthetic effect and postoperative analgesia by slowing down the absorption of the anaesthetic agent.

Pohjanpelto et al. [12] argue that introduction of epinephrine 5mg/ml into the anaesthetic solution made no difference to the intraocular blood supply over and above that caused by the retro bulbar block alone.

4. CONCLUSION

Our results show that we have met if not surpassed our prescribed standards and the goals set out by the Royal Colleges in terms of providing pain free intraocular surgery. There were also no complications arising as a result of this technique.

The additional cost advantage in the setting of the modern financially constrained NHS can also not be overlooked with the cost of delivery per anaesthetic cocktail per patient being £9.11 per patient for the lignocaine-bupivacaine-hyalase combination regime and only £0.17 per patient with our suggested regime.

We conclude that the use of lignocaine 2% with adrenaline 1:200000 in our current regime of delivery of Sub-Tenon's anaesthesia for cataract surgery is not only safe and effective but also highly cost efficient.

CONSENT

All authors declare that written informed consent was obtained from patients involved in the study as part of their cataract surgery and in line with the Hospitals guidelines.

ETHICAL APPROVAL

No ethical approval was necessary for this study.

ACKNOWLEDGEMENTS

The authors would like to acknowledge patients who participated in the study and thank them for their cooperation and feedback.

COMPETING INTERESTS

Authors have declared that no competing interests exist.

REFERENCES

1. Report of the Joint Working Party on Local Anaesthesia for Intraocular Surgery. London: Royal College of Anaesthetist and College of Ophthalmologists; 2001.
2. Chittenden HB, Meacock WR, Govan JAA. Topical anaesthesia with oxybuprocaine

A Safe, Efficacious and Cost Effective Way of Delivering Sub-Tenon's Anaesthesia...

119

versus subtenon's infiltration with 2% lignocaine for small incision cataract surgery. Br J Ophthalmol. 1997;81:288-290.

3. Desai P, Reidy A, Minassian DC. Profile of patients presenting for cataract surgery:National data collection. Br J Ophthalmol. 1999;83:893-896.

4. Davison M, Padroni S, Bunce C, Rüschen H. Sub-Tenon's anaesthesia versus topical anaesthesia for cataract surgery. The Cochrane Collaboration; 2010.

5. Royal College of Anaesthetists and the Royal College of Ophthalmologists Local anaesthesia for ophthalmic surgery. Joint guidelines from the Royal College of Anaesthetists and the Royal College of Ophthalmologists; 2012. [Online] Available from: http://www.rcoa.ac.uk/docs/la-ophthalmic-surgery-2012.pdf

6. Stevens JD. A new local anesthesia technique for cataract extraction by one quadrant sub-Tenon's infiltration. British Journal of Ophthalmology. 1992;76:670-674.

7. Zafirakis P, Voudouri A, Rowe S, et al. Topical versus sub-tenons anaesthesia without sedation in cataract surgery. Journal of cataract and refractive surgery. 2001;27(6):873-879.

8. Rowley SA, Hale JE, Finlay RD. Sub-Tenon's local anaesthesia: the effect of hyaluronidase Br J Ophthalmol. 2000;84: 435-436.

9. Srinivasan S, Fern AI, Selvaraj S, Hasan S. Randomised double blind clinical trial comparing topical and sub-Tenon's anaesthesia in routine cataract surgery. British J Anaes. 2004;93(5):683-686.

10. Jay WM, Aziz MZ, Green K. Further studies on the effect of retrobulbar epinephrine injection on ocular and optic nerve blood flow. Curr Eye Res. 1986;5:63–7.

11. Krohn J, Høvding G, Seland JH, Aasved H. Retrobulbar anesthesia with and without adrenaline in extracapsular cataract surgery. Acta Ophthalmologica Scandina-vica. 1995;73:56–60.

12. Pohjanpelto P. Pulse induced intraocular pressure variation and retrobulbar anaesthesia with and without adrenaline. Acta Ophthalmologica. 1979;57:136-144.

Child-rated and Parent-rated Quality of Life in Childhood Intermittent Exotropia: Findings from an Observational Cohort Study

Deborah Buck[1][*], Nadeem Ali[2], Peter Tiffin[3], Robert H. Taylor[4], Christine J. Powell[5] and Michael P. Clarke[1,5]

[1]Institute of Neuroscience, Newcastle University, Newcastle Upon Tyne, United Kingdom.
[2]Moorfields Eye Hospital, London, United Kingdom.
[3]Sunderland Eye Infirmary, Sunderland, United Kingdom.
[4]York Hospitals NHS Trust, York, United Kingdom.
[5]Newcastle Eye Centre, Royal Victoria Infirmary, Newcastle upon Tyne Hospitals NHS Foundation Trust, United Kingdom.

Authors' contributions

Author DB contributed to study design, data analysis and interpretation, drafting, revising and approving the manuscript; authors NA, PT and RHT contributed to data interpretation, manuscript revision and approval; author CJP contributed to data acquisition and interpretation, manuscript revision and approval; author MPC contributed to funding acquisition, study design, data interpretation, manuscript revision and approval.

Editor(s):
(1) Tatsuya Mimura, Department of Ophthalmology, Tokyo Women's Medical University Medical Center East, Japan.
Reviewers:
(1) Anonymous, Israel.
(2) Anonymous, Turkey.

ABSTRACT

Purpose: To use the Pediatric Quality of Life Inventory (PedsQL™) to describe generic quality of life (QOL) in children with intermittent exotropia [X(T)], to examine changes in scores, and to compare scores in children with X(T) to those of age-matched healthy cohorts.
Methods: PedsQL™ was administered to children and parents as part of the UK Improving Outcomes in Intermittent Exotropia (IOXT) study. Excluding 27 children with co-morbidity, PedsQL data was available from 365 parents and 152 children. Paired-samples t-tests examined change in PedsQL™ scores over time. One-sample t-tests and mean differences compared scores between

*Corresponding author: E-mail: Deborah.Buck@ncl.ac.uk

children with X(T) and healthy UK samples.

Results: Mean parent-rated PedsQL™ scores from the X(T) cohort at baseline were: 90.6 (Physical Health), 78.2 (Emotional Functioning), 88.8 (Social Functioning), 83.4 (School/Nursery Functioning), 83.6 (Psychosocial Summary), 86.2 (Total). Mean baseline child-rated scores were: 78.1 (Physical Health), 76.5 (Emotional Functioning), 73.6 (Social Functioning), 72.2 (School/Nursery Functioning), 74.2 (Psychosocial Summary), 75.5 (Total). X(T) parents rated their child's QOL similar to healthy children's parents, except for poorer School/Nursery Functioning in 2-4 year olds. X(T) children rated their QOL significantly better than age-matched healthy children. There were no significant changes over time.

Conclusion: Using the PedsQL™ we were unable to detect significant effects of X(T) on generic QOL. However, evidence for PedsQL's utility in this condition remains limited without further investigation in larger samples and concurrent control groups. Further qualitative work and consideration of condition-specific measures in UK cohorts are needed before practitioners can better inform parents about psychosocial impacts of X(T).

Keywords: Intermittent exotropia; divergent strabismus; quality of life; surgery; child; parent; proxy.

1. INTRODUCTION

Intermittent exotropia [X(T)] is one of the commonest forms of childhood strabismus. In X(T), one eye intermittently drifts outwards when the child is looking at distant objects, or is tired or inattentive. Potential functional consequences include loss of stereovision and amblyopia. Parents often have concerns relating to social exclusion and bullying because of the appearance of the strabismus [1].

Childhood X(T) has been associated with subsequent poor psychological well-being into young adulthood [2,3]. There may also be more immediate implications for the child's quality of life (QOL) yet relatively little exists in the literature about this [4-8]. One group of researchers, from the Mayo Clinic in North America, has studied parental and children's concerns regarding the effect of X(T) on QOL, leading to the recent development of their Intermittent Exotropia Questionnaire (IXTQ) [6-10]. As far as we are aware, there have been no other reports of paediatric QOL in this specific condition and the relevance of this group's work to a different population and healthcare system in the UK is unestablished.

QOL estimates of patients, including those with ophthalmologic conditions, often differ significantly from those of physicians [11]. Capturing child and parental perspectives is important since parental insight may not correspond with that of their children [12] and there is growing recognition that each needs to be taken into consideration. Parent-child agreement on QOL ratings in X(T) has been found to be poor [13].

A widely-used and accepted generic QOL instrument is the Pediatric Quality of Life Inventory (PedsQL™), which has strong evidence of reliability and validity in healthy children and those with a range of acute and chronic illnesses [14]. However, evidence of its usefulness in assessing generic QOL in children with X(T) is very limited. Here we describe parent- and child-rated PedsQL™ scores from a UK observational study of X(T) (the Improving Outcomes in Intermittent Exotropia (IOXT) study) [15-17]. The primary aim of this paper is to examine change over time in self- and parent-rated PedsQL™ scores. A secondary aim is to compare baseline PedsQL™ scores to those of unaffected age-matched cohorts.

2. METHODS

2.1 Participants

The IOXT study involved 26 children's eye clinics /orthoptic departments [15]. Between May 2005 and December 2006, collaborating departments approached parents/carers of children under 12 years, diagnosed with X(T) within the previous 12 months, without significant coexisting ocular pathology (e.g. cataract). In addition to clinical assessment, demographic details were recorded at enrolment including age, gender, and general health. Treatment status was documented (observation only, conservative treatment for squint such as glasses/patching, eye muscle surgery, or treatment for visual acuity only). Clinical and QOL follow-up ended in December 2008 (December 2009 for surgery patients). As this was an observational study, clinicians managed children according to their usual clinical criteria. Informed consent was obtained from parents/guardians. The study received a favourable opinion from UK North West Multi-Centre Research Ethics Committee.

2.2 Outcome Measures

Generic QOL data were collected from parents and children using the PedsQL[TM] 4.0 Generic Core Scales (http://www.pedsql.org/index.html). We used the age-appropriate 'proxy' (parent/carer) version for those with children aged 2-4 years (toddler version), 5-7 years and 8 years or older, and the child's self-rated version for those aged 5-7 and 8 years or older. The PedsQL assesses QOL on four individual scales: Physical Health (8 items), Emotional Functioning (5 items), Social Functioning (5 items) and School Functioning (5 items, or 'Nursery/Day Care Functioning' for the toddler version which has 3 items). These four scales can be amalgamated to form a Total score (23 or 21 items) and 2 summary scores: Physical Health summary and Psychosocial Health summary. We followed developers' scoring instructions by reversing and linearly transforming scores to a 0-100 scale (higher scores indicating better QOL), and, for missing data, imputation of the mean of completed items in a scale when 50% or more are completed.

PedsQL[TM] questionnaires were administered in the clinic setting as part of the IOXT study assessment in all except 2 cases. In accordance with PedsQL[TM] administration guidelines, child versions were self-completed by those aged 8 or older. If the child was 5-7 years, instructions and questions were read to the child word for word by an orthoptist who then circled his/her response. Parent versions were self-completed. A written protocol and training video were produced for use by study orthoptists to ensure PedsQLs were administered in a standardised way. This generic instrument has been widely validated in numerous conditions and in healthy groups, and we found that its psychometric properties specifically in children with X(T) were generally good [13].

Baseline PedsQL[TM] data were scheduled to be collected within 12 weeks of enrolment. Follow-up appointments were arranged on a 3-monthly basis during the first year of the study and 6-monthly thereafter for an average period of 2 years. These visits involved both clinical and QOL review. Outcome QOL is the latest PedsQL[TM] completed, but at least 6 months after the initial QOL assessment.

2.3 Data Analysis

Data were analysed using SPSS version 19.0. Summary statistics (mean scores, standard deviations (SD)) are reported for each PedsQL[TM] scale. Analyses are performed across the whole cohort of children with X(T), i.e. for all age groups combined, and (see Supplemental Material) repeated for age-specific versions of the PedsQL[TM]. Paired-samples t-tests were performed to examine change over time.

Baseline scores are compared with age-matched published scores [18,19] from healthy UK samples: mean differences and one-sample t-tests were used. Comparisons with healthy UK samples are possible for those aged between 2 years and 4 years 11 months [18] and for those aged between 5.5 and 8.5 years [19]. All scales/sub-scales are available for use in the 2-4 year old comparison. Only the Total, Physical Health and Psychosocial Summary scores can be used in the older age-group comparison, as individual scores for Emotional, Social and School/Nursery Functioning were not published for the 5.5 to 8.5 year-old healthy group.

One-way analysis of variance was used to examine whether severity of X(T) at baseline was associated with QOL at initial assessment. Severity was determined by scores on the Newcastle Control Score (NCS) [20] with a score of 1 to 3 denoting mild, 4 to 6 moderate, and 7 to 9 severe X(T). One-way analysis of variance was used to explore any association between treatment and PedsQL[TM] scores (see Supplemental Material). Given the scarcity of reports of QOL in X(T), and to place this study in context, further descriptive comparison was made of PedsQL[TM] scores in this sample and those reported in the American study [8].

Co-morbidity was present in 27 children, the most common co-existing health issues being asthma and developmental delay. We have excluded those with co-morbidity from our analyses as they had significantly poorer QOL compared to those without other health conditions (see Supplemental Material).

2.4 Statement of Ethics

We certify that all applicable institutional and governmental regulations concerning the ethical use of human volunteers were followed during this research.

3. RESULTS

3.1 Participant Characteristics

Baseline PedsQL[TM] data were available from 365 parents and 152 children (excluding 27 children with comorbidity). Mean (SD) age at time of initial parent PedsQL[TM] was 52 (22) months. Mean (SD) age at time of initial child PedsQL[TM] was 74 (16) months. 57% of the children were female.

3.2 Baseline PedsQL[TM] Scores

Mean (SD) baseline parent-rated scores for all 365 parents were 86.2 (12.8) on Total score, 90.6 (12.8) on Physical Health, 78.2 (18.8) on Emotional Functioning, 88.8 (15.5) on Social, 83.4 (17.6) on School and 83.6 (14.7) on Psychosocial Summary. Mean (SD) baseline scores for all 152 children with QOL data were 75.5 (14.7) on Total score, 78.1 (17.4) on Physical Health, 76.5 (19.5) on Emotional Functioning, 73.6 (23.2) on Social, 72.2 (19.6) on School and 74.2 (16.2) on Psychosocial Summary. Age-specific PedsQL[TM] scores are provided in the Supplemental Material.

3.3 Paired Data

Mean interval between baseline and outcome PedsQL[TM] was 24 months (range 6 to 48) for parents and 20 months (6 to 48) for children. Paired data (baseline and outcome scores) were available from 301 parents and 128 children: Fig. 1 shows their baseline and corresponding outcome scores. For parent-ratings there was a small, statistically significant deterioration over time on Total (mean difference 1.5, 95% CIs 0.1 to 2.9, p=0.036), School/Nursery (mean difference 2.5, 95% CIs 0.3 to 4.8, p=0.025), and Psychosocial Summary (mean difference 1.9, 95% CIs 0.3 to 3.5, p=0.023) scales. Paired data within age-specific versions are provided in the Supplemental Material. For child-ratings (Fig. 1) there were no significant changes in self-rated scores.

Treatment received was not significantly associated with PedsQL[TM] scores in any of the parent- or child-rated PedsQL[TM] scales at baseline or outcome (see Supplemental Material). Mean parental PedsQL[TM] scores were higher at outcome on each scale (except Physical Health) for those with a better surgical outcome, defined as a NCS of between 0 and 2. However, this was not statistically significant (see Supplemental Material).

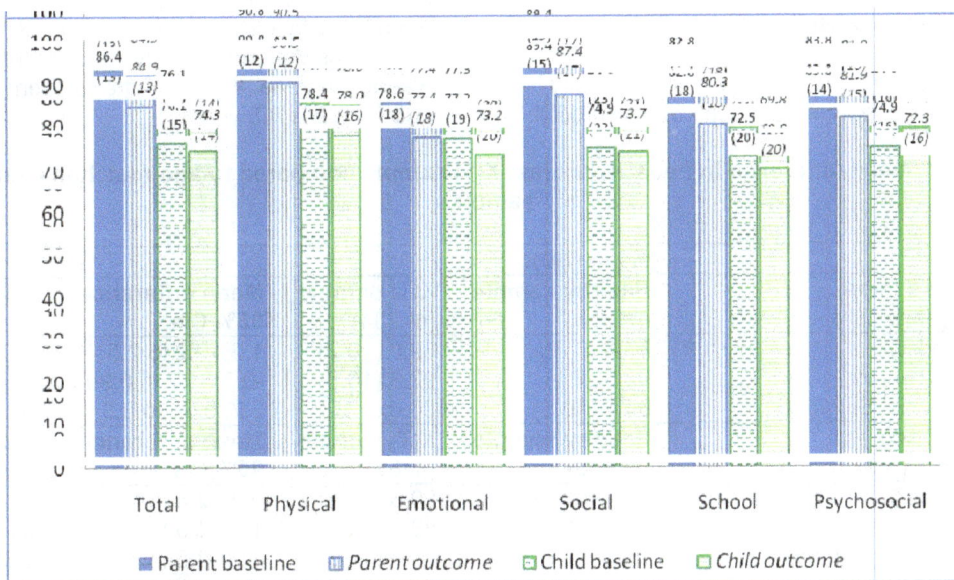

Fig. 1. Mean (SD) parent and child PedsQL scores at baseline and outcome

3.4 Comparisons with Unaffected Children (UK Sample)

3.4.1 2-4 year olds

Parents of 2 to 4 year-old children with X(T) rated their child's QOL similarly to those of age-matched healthy children in terms of Total and summary (Physical Health and Psychosocial) scores (Table 1). Further details are provided in the Supplemental Material.

3.4.2 5.5 to 8.5 year olds

In the 5.5 to 8.5 year-old group, there were no significant differences between X(T) parents' and healthy parents' ratings on Total or summary scores (Table 1). Children with X(T) rated their own QOL as significantly better than the age-matched healthy sample on the Total, Physical and Psychosocial Summary scales (Table 1).

3.5 Cross-cultural Comparisons

Fig. 2 shows that baseline parental PedsQL[TM] scores were very similar to those in a recent North American study of QOL in X(T).[7] In contrast, child-rated scores were significantly lower amongst our sample compared to their American counterparts with X(T) (one-sample t tests, p=0.005 to p<0.001).

3.6 Squint Severity

Although children with severe X(T) generally had poorer mean parent- and self-rated PedsQL[TM]

scores than those with mild or moderate X(T), this was not statistically significant. Details are reported in the Supplemental Material.

4. DISCUSSION

Drawing on data from a large UK multicentre observational study of children with X(T), we have described child-rated and parent-rated generic QOL using the widely-used and validated PedsQL[TM]. We found that parent-rated PedsQL[TM] scores for children with X(T) were similar to those of unaffected cohorts in the UK, while the self-rated scores of the children themselves were better than those of unaffected children. While this finding is of interest, it is important to keep in mind that, as a generic measure, the PedsQL[TM] may not be detecting QOL issues that are especially pertinent to X(T). Our findings differ from those of a research group from the Mayo Clinic in North America (the only other group to have used the PedsQL[TM] specifically in this condition) [8]. In their study of 51 children with X(T) and 47 controls, they found that parent-rated scores were poorer in children with X(T) than in controls, while child-rated scores were similar between affected and unaffected children [8]. The differences between the UK and North American studies are most likely due to variations in the way the healthy samples were recruited given that the latter benefitted from a concurrent control group. Age is also a likely factor, since the age of the healthy sample in the American study ranged from 5 to 16 years whereas those in the present study ranged from 2 to 8.5 years.

Table 1. Mean difference in PedsQL scores: X(T) sample compared to age-matched healthy samples

	Mean (SD):			
Parental scores 2 to 4 years	**Healthy sample (n=256)**	**X(T) sample (n=234)**	**Mean difference; 95% CIs**	**p value**
Total PedsQL	87.8 (8.7)	89.0 (10.2)	1.2; -0.2 to 2.5	0.083
Physical Health	92.6 (9.1)	92.3 (10.3)	-0.3; -1.7 to 0.99	0.62
Psychosocial Summary	84.6 (10.5)	86.8 (12.2)	2.2; 0.63 to 3.8	0.006
Parental scores 5.5 to 8.5 years	**Healthy sample (n=149)**	**X(T) sample (n=82)**	**Mean difference; 95% CIs**	**p value**
Total PedsQL	79.9 (11.7)	80.8 (15.2)	0.9; -2.4 to 4.3	0.58
Physical Health	86.1 (11.4)	88.0 (15.9)	1.9; -1.6 to 5.4	0.28
Psychosocial Summary	76.7 (13.0)	76.9 (17.0)	0.2; -3.5 to 3.9	0.89
Child scores 5.5 to 8.5 years	**Healthy sample (n=149)**	**X(T) sample (n=92)**	**Mean difference; 95% CIs**	**p value**
Total PedsQL	71.8 (14.4)	77.8 (13.9)	6.0; 3.1 to 8.9	<0.001
Physical Health	76.4 (14.0)	80.8 (15.7)	4.4; 1.1 to 7.6	<0.001
Psychosocial Summary	68.9 (16.2)	76.3 (15.2)	7.4; 4.2 to 10.5	<0.001

*one-sample t-test

a) Parental scores

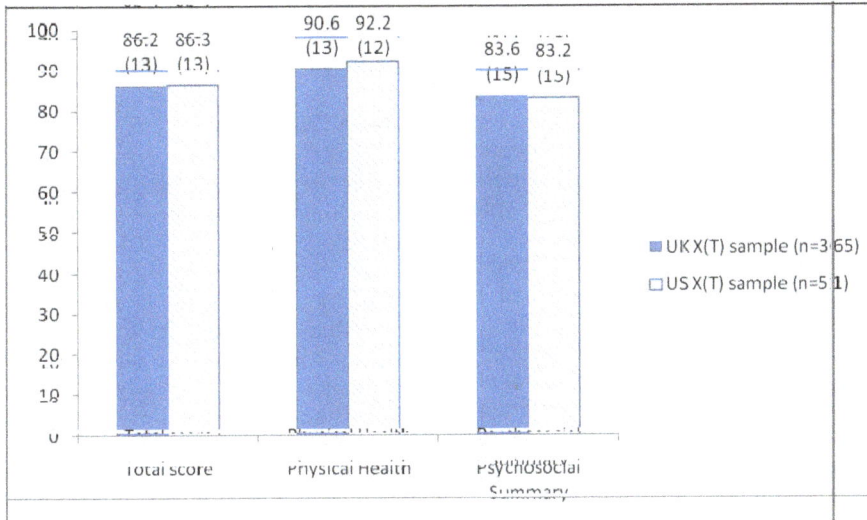

b) Child-rated scores

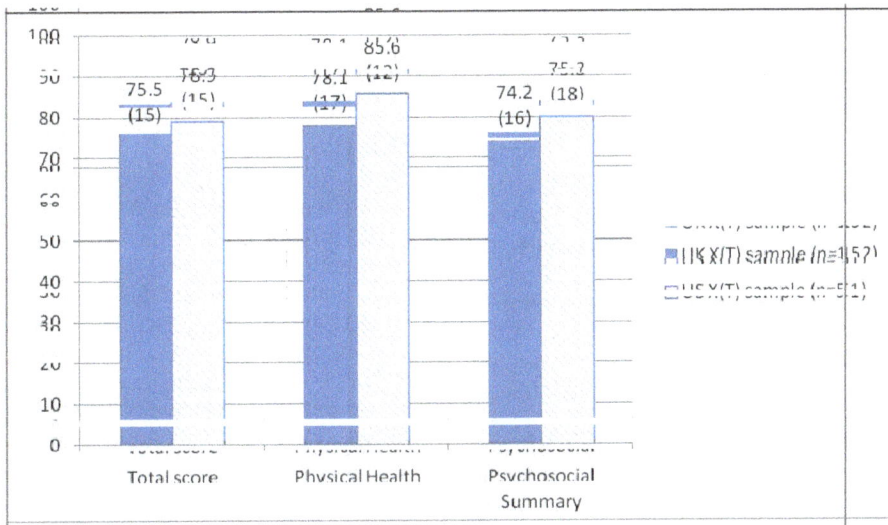

Fig. 2. Comparison of IOXT study PedsQL^{TM} scores with those from a recent study of X(T) in North America

We found no effects of treatment on PedsQL^{TM} scores, and no significant deterioration in self-rated PedsQL^{TM} scores over an average follow-up period two years. While some parent-rated PedsQL^{TM} scores did worsen slightly over time within the youngest age group, the size of these changes is unlikely to be meaningful [21].

Generic measures such as the PedsQL^{TM} are important because of their applicability to a diverse range of conditions, enabling comparisons between various groups including healthy populations and thereby placing scores into context. However, they may not be sensitive enough to demonstrate effects associated with strabismus generally or X(T) in particular, or its treatment. A particularly informative way to determine any effect of X(T) on QOL is through qualitative methods. Indeed qualitative research, also by the Mayo Group in North America, reveals the most frequently mentioned QOL 'concerns' of children with X(T) was worry [6]. From the parents' perspective, "comments from other people" was the most frequently mentioned concern.

Although no paediatric strabismus-specific measures were available at the start of our study, the qualitative findings in America have recently informed the development of the Intermittent Exotropia Questionnaire (IXTQ) [7]. The advantage of such condition-specific measures is that they should be responsive to any change over time, for example in those who undergo treatment for their condition, while the main disadvantage is that they can not be used across different conditions or to compare with unaffected populations. Thus there will remain a need for both condition-specific and generic patient-reported outcome measures, depending on the context of the study. A popular solution is the use of a 'battery' of outcome measures incorporating both specific and generic components, although this can be more time-consuming and may result in respondent burden.

An important limitation of this paper is that we did not have a concurrent control group with which to compare the PedsQL^{TM} scores of children with X(T) and we therefore used published, age-matched scores from unaffected UK children. The published data for the older control group were collected from one region of the UK. Consequently, there may have been geographical and socio-economic differences between this group and our national IOXT cohort. The data for unaffected toddlers were collected from a wider geographical area and from a variety of sources. Another important limitation is that, due to the young age of the children in the IOXT study, there were less baseline child-rated PedsQL^{TM} data with which to evaluate change over time from their own perspective.

The findings from the IOXT study show that UK children with X(T) did not appear to fare any worse than unaffected peers in terms of PedsQL^{TM} scores, and that there was no detrimental effect on their PedsQL^{TM} scores over time. These findings do not necessarily imply a lack of effect of X(T) on QOL. However, they do add to the sparse literature on the condition itself and on the utility of the universally-accepted PedsQL^{TM} as an outcome measure specifically in ophthalmology. While the PedsQL^{TM} has demonstrated reasonable psychometric properties in X(T),[13] the evidence regarding its direct relevance to children with eye conditions remains limited. The implications for the management of this condition in the UK are difficult to establish, although the lack of any significant difference between children with X(T) and those without it should be reassuring to worried parents. Further investigation of the comparison of generic and condition-specific instruments in larger cohorts will further help clinicians.

5. CONCLUSION

In conclusion, parent- and child-rated PedsQL^{TM} scores were similar to or better than those of unaffected cohorts in the UK. Scores were not altered by treatment or time. Local and international evidence about the impact of intermittent exotropia on a child's quality of life remains limited. Further qualitative work should be pursued together with further investigation of established QOL measures in larger samples, and with concurrent control groups, in order to inform researchers, practitioners and parents about the specific effects of childhood X(T) and in turn how to evaluate its treatment.

COMPETING INTERESTS

Authors have declared that no competing interests exist.

REFERENCES

1. Horwood J, Waylen A, Herrick D, Williams C, Wolke D. Common visual defects and peer victimisation in children. Invest Ophthalmol Vis Sci. 2005;46:1177-1181.

2. McKenzie JA, Capo JA, Nusz KJ, Diehl NN, Mohney BG. Prevalence and sex differences of psychiatric disorders in young adults who had intermittent exotropia as children. Arch Ophthalmol. 2009;127:743-747.

3. Mohney BG, McKenzie JA, Capo JA, Nusz KJ, Mrazek D, Diehl NN. Mental illness in young adults who had strabismus as children. Pediatr. 2008;122:1033-1038.

4. Wen G, McKean-Cowdin R, Varma R, Tarczy-Hornoch K, Cotter SA, Borchert M, et al. General health-related quality of life in preschool children with strabismus or amblyopia. Ophthalmol. 2011;118:574-80.

5. Archer SM, Musch DC, Wren PA, Guire KE, Del Monte MA. Social and emotional impact of strabismus surgery on quality of life in children. J AAPOS. 2005;9:148-151.

6. Hatt SR, Leske DA, Adams WE, Kirgis PA, Bradley EA, Holmes JM. Quality of life in intermittent exotropia: child and parent concerns. Arch Ophthalmol. 2008;126:1525-1529.

7. Hatt SR, Leske DA, Yamada T, Bradley EA, Cole SR, Holmes JM. Development and initial validation of quality-of-life questionnaires for intermittent exotropia. Ophthalmol. 2010;117:163-168.

8. Hatt SR, Leske DA, Holmes JM. Comparison of quality-of-life instruments in childhood intermittent exotropia. J AAPOS. 2010;14:221-226.

9. Yamada T, Hatt SR, Leske DA, Holmes JM. Spectacle wear in children reduces parental health-related quality of life. J AAPOS. 2011;15:24-28.

10. Yamada T, Hatt SR, Leske DA, Holmes JM. Specific health-related quality of life concerns in children with intermittent exotropia. Strabismus. 2012;20:145-151.

11. Stein JD. Disparities between ophthalmologists and their patients in estimating quality of life. Curr Opin Ophthalmol. 2004;15:238-243.

12. Upton P, Lawford J, Eiser C. Parent–child agreement across child health-related quality of life instruments: a review of the literature. Qual Life Res. 2008;17:895-913.

13. Buck D, Clarke MP, Powell C, Tiffin P, Drewett RF. Use of the PedsQL in childhood intermittent exotropia: estimates of feasibility, internal consistency reliability and parent-child agreement. Qual Life Res. 2012; 21: 727-736.

14. Varni JW, Seid M, Kurtin PS. PedsQL 4.0: Reliability and validity of the Pediatric Quality of Life Inventory version 4.0 generic core scales in healthy and patient populations. Med Care. 2001; 39: 800-812.

15. Buck D, Powell C, Cumberland P, Davis H, Dawson E, Rahi J, et al. Presenting features and early management of childhood intermittent exotropia in the UK: inception cohort study. Br J Ophthalmol. 2009;93:1620-1624.

16. Buck D, Powell CJ, Rahi J, Cumberland P, Tiffin P, Sloper J, et al. The improving outcomes in intermittent exotropia study: outcomes at 2 years after diagnosis in an observational cohort. BMC Ophthalmol. 2012;12:1.

17. Buck D, Powell CJ, Sloper JJ, Taylor R, Tiffin P, Clarke MP. Surgical intervention in childhood intermittent exotropia: Current practice and clinical outcomes from an observational cohort study. Br J Ophthalmol. 2012;96: 1291-1295.

18. Buck D. The PedsQL™ as a measure of parent-rated quality of life in healthy UK toddlers: psychometric properties and cross-cultural comparisons. J Child Health Care. 2012;16:331-338.

19. Cremeens J, Eiser C, Blades M. Factors influencing agreement between child self-report and parent proxy-reports on the Pediatric Quality of Life Inventory 4.0 (PedsQL) generic core scales. Health Qual Life Outcomes. 2006;4:58.

20. Buck D, Clarke MP, Haggerty H, Hrisos S, Powell C, Sloper J, et al. Grading the severity of intermittent distance exotropia: the revised Newcastle Control Score. Br J Ophthalmol. 2008;92:577.

21. Varni JW, Burwinkle TM, Seid M, Skarr D.The PedsQL 4.0 as a pediatric population health measure: feasibility, reliability, and validity. Ambul Pediatr. 2003;3:329-341.

18

Fashioned 25G Cannula for Injection of Heavy Liquid during 23G Vitrectomy for Primary Simple Rhegmatogenous Retinal Detachment

Wael A. Ewais[1], Malak I. El Shazly[1*] and Ashraf A. Nossair[1]

[1]*Department of Ophthalmology, Cairo University, Egypt.*

Authors' contributions

This work was carried out in collaboration between all authors. The three authors designed altogether the study, Author AAN wrote the protocol, and wrote the first draft of the manuscript. Author MIES managed the literature searches, and author WAE carried out the surgeries with the assistance of the other two authors AAN and MIES. All three authors read and approved the final manuscript.

<u>Editor(s):</u>
(1) Stephen G Schwartz, Department of Clinical Ophthalmology, Bascom Palmer Eye Institute, University of Miami Miller School of Medicine, USA.
<u>Reviewers:</u>
(1) Otzem chassid, Ophthalmology Bar Ilan University, Israel.
(2) Anonymous, Mayo Clinic Florida, USA.
(3) Jose D Luna, Chief Vitreoretinal Department, Centro Privado de Ojos Romagosa, Argentina.
(4) Sameh Mohamed Elgouhary, Menoufia College of Medicine, Egypt.
(5) Anonymous, Venezuela.

ABSTRACT

Purpose: To evaluate ease of fashioning of 25G cannula, safety and efficacy of injection of heavy liquid using this fashioned cannula during Vitrectomy for simple Rhegmatogenous Retinal Detachment.

Methods: This is a prospective non-comparative case series including 28 cases of simple Rhegmatogenous Retinal Detachment (without PVR, with PVR A, B, and C1). A 25G cannula was fashioned by unbending of a 25G Healon cannula. This cannula was applied on the nozzle of a 5 cc syringe filled with perfluorocarbon liquid, and then the heavy liquid was injected inside the vitreous cavity to reattach a detached retina. The outcome measures were: ease of fashioning of the cannula (no cutting off of the shaft), ease of injection (no resistance), need to replace by a back flush needle, iatrogenic retinal breaks / hemorrhage, retinal reattachment.

Results: The cannula was fashioned easily without cutting off of the shaft in all cases (100%). There was no resistance or interruption of the stream of heavy liquid through the cannula during

---

Corresponding author: E-mail: Melshazly75@hotmail.com

injection in all cases, and thus no need to replace by an industrialized back flush needle in any case (100%). No iatrogenic retinal breaks or hemorrhages in any case. Complete intraoperative retinal reattachment in all cases (100%).

Conclusion: Fashioned 25G cannula is safe and effective for injection of heavy liquids for reattachment of the retina during Vitrectomy for Rhegmatogenous Retinal Detachment. However, further studies are required to evaluate suction function using this fashioned cannula.

Keywords: RRD; PVR; perfluorodecalin; healon; 23G; 25G cannula.

1. INTRODUCTION

Heavy liquids are used during Vitrectomy for several purposes. For reattachment of detached retina from posterior to anterior, thus allowing for peripheral laser Retinopexy and avoiding the hazards of a posterior drainage retinotomy [1-6]. They are also used for stabilizing the posterior retina to allow for peripheral shaving of vitreous base and addressing peripheral proliferative vitreoretinopathy (PVR). They are used to protect the macula during retrieval of dropped nuclear fragments and in intraocular foreign bodies. They may also be used as hemostatic agents in diabetic Vitrectomy [5-12].

Heavy liquids are usually injected during 23G Vitrectomy using a manufactured 23G back flush needle. It is a homogenous straight blunt tipped metal cannula 22.2 mm long, with 0.75 mm diameter. It is fitted to the nozzle of a 5cc syringe, which is filled with heavy liquid. Then it is introduced through the trocar cannula to the mid-vitreous. The injection process is always safe on retina.it is smooth and sustained enough to reattach the retina during Rhegmatogenous Retinal Detachment [1-10].

Heavy liquids include: Perfluorodecalin (C10F18), perfluorooctane (C8F18), perfluorotributyla mine, and perfluoroethylcyclohexane. The most commonly used is Perfluorodecalin.

In this study, we are looking for a credible, cheap, safe, and efficient alternative to the back flush needle, which can help whenever the back flush needle is not available for use. This alternative is achieved by fashioning a 25G cannula from Healon cannula used in cataract surgery.

2. MATERIALS AND METHODS

This is a prospective non-comparative study that was done for 28 eyes of 28 patients with simple Rhegmatogenous Retinal Detachment (RRD). It was carried out at the period from April 2012 to December 2012 at Kasr El Ainy Hospital, Cairo University.

The study and data collection conformed to all local laws and were compliant with the principles of the Declaration of Helsinki. Detailed informed consent was taken from all patients.

Inclusion criteria included: RRD without proliferative vitreoretinopathy (PVR), RRD with PVR A, B, and C1.

2.1 Exclusion Criteria Included

RRD with PVR C2-12, RRD due to Trauma or intraocular foreign body (IOFB), Hypotony (intraocular pressure (IOP) < 6 mmHg), Tractional Retinal Detachment (Diabetic or other causes), Exudative Retinal Detachment.

All patients underwent slit lamp examination, IOP measurement using an Applanation Tonometer. Fundus examination was performed using a +90.0 D non-contact lens, and a 3-mirror contact lens.

All patients underwent a 4-port 23G pars plana Vitrectomy. The 4th port was used for chandelier illumination. Additional phacoemulsification was performed for phakic eyes. The 25G cannula was fashioned from a Healon cannula (BIOCORNEAL II, 0.5 mm diameter, 22.2 mm long shaft with a bending angle 35°, CROMA, Leobendorf, Austria). A 10/0 suture needle holder was used to fashion the cannula by straightening (unbending) of the shaft. This was done at the bending angle point then at the distal part of the shaft (Fig. 1). This was done gently to avoid cutting - off of the shaft. Then the cannula was fitted to the nozzle of a 5cc syringe filled with heavy liquid. The heavy liquid, which was used, was Perfluorodecalin (Eftiar Decalin, 5 ml vial, DORC, Netherlands). It was injected into the vitreous cavity to reattach the detached retina in all cases. The infusion cannula was closed during the perfluorodecalin injection, and the surgeon. They were done in the period between April 2012 and December 2012.

The analyzed variables were intraoperative, and they included: ease of fashioning (No cut off), resistance to injection, need to replace by back flush needle, iatrogenic retinal breaks/ hemorrhages, and retinal reattachment.

Statistical analysis was done mainly for the baseline characteristics for the mean, range, and standard deviation, and also paired t-test was done to correlate age and baseline IOP to sex. SPSS package 20 was used.

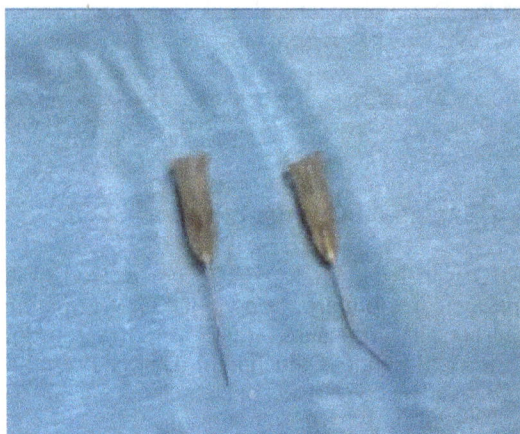

Fig. 1. 25G Healon cannula before and after unbending

3. RESULTS

The study was done on 28 eyes of 28 cases, of which 13 eyes were right (46.4%), and 15 eyes were left (53.6%). Fourteen cases (14) were females, and 14 cases were males (F: M = 1:1). The mean age of patients was 35 (range, 17-65 years, standard deviation: 15.17). The lens status was as follows: 15 phakic eyes (53.6%), 10 pseudophakic eyes (35.7%), and 3 aphakic eyes (10.7%). The mean preoperative intraocular pressure was 12 (range, 8-16 mmHg, SD: 1.97). All the cases were simple RRD, of which 8 cases had no PVR (28.6%), 14 cases had PVR A-B (50%) and 6 cases had PVR C1 (21.4%).

Fashioning of 25G cannula was easy and not time consuming (mean 23 seconds, range 15-27 seconds), the shaft of the cannula wasn't cut off in all cases (100%), however, the shaft was not perfectly straight, and there was a minimal

optic nerve head was observed for pallor and pulsations. All surgeries were done by the same residual bending angle in all cases (100%). The residual bending impeded entry via the trocar at 1 case, and it was further straightened and introduced easily.

The injection of perfluorodecalin went on smooth, and non-pulsatile in all cases (100%). There was no undue gush of perfluorodecalin during the injection, no iatrogenic retinal breaks or retinal hemorrhage in any case (100%). There was no need to replace the cannula by a manufactured back flush needle in any case. Retina was smoothly and properly reattached, from posterior pole to periphery, with the perfluorodecalin in all cases (100%). There was no optic nerve head pulsation or pallor in any case. (Fig. 2).

4. DISCUSSION

Although scleral buckle was the standard treatment for most of Rhegmatogenous retinal detachment without significant PVR, [11,12] primary pars plana Vitrectomy became more commonly used [1-6]. Heavy liquids are now a substantial tool for 23G Vitrectomy in cases of Rhegmatogenous retinal detachment. They are injected to flatten the posterior pole, allow for proper shaving of vitreous base, prevent retinal incarceration, and thus retina can be flattened and lasered accurately. The instrument, that is usually adopted for heavy liquid injection, is a manufactured back flush needle [5-12].

In our study, we fashioned a blunt cannula for the injection of the heavy liquid. We used a 25G healon cannula, not a 23G cannula (Hydroxy propyl methyl cellulose). This is because the unbending of the Healon cannula is never 100% perfect, and thus the straight shaft of the fashioned cannula is never homogenously straight. There is always a residual bending angle. This makes the overall diameter of the cannula 0.75 mm (23G) rather than the 0.5 mm (25G). This prevents getting locked at entry or exit through the 23G trocar cannula system.

The fashioning of 25G cannula was easy without cutting off in any case, because it was done very gently, using a blunt 10/0 needle holder, it was done on a relatively resilient cannula (Healon), and the unbending process was mainly at the distal part of the shaft, and not on the point of bending which may be the weakest point of the shaft (Fig. 3).

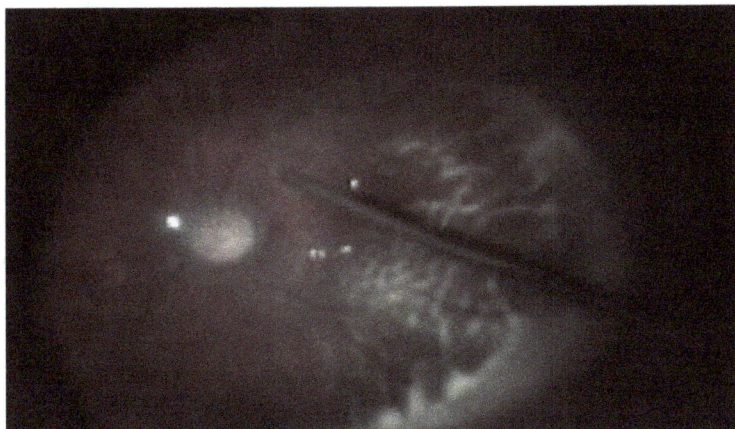

Fig. 2. Perfluorodecalin injection using fashioned 25G cannula

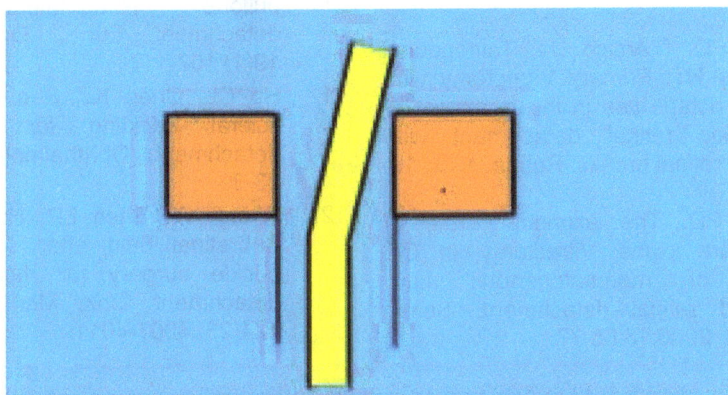

Fig. 3. Residual bending of 25G cannula

The injection process went on smoothly because it was an active step, and in the direction of gravity. Despite the residual bending, the injection was non-pulsatile. This is because the residual bending didn't occlude the lumen of the shaft.

Retina was properly and smoothly reattached from posterior to peripheral because of the smooth heavy liquid injection, proper removal of peripheral vitreous, in addition to the absence of significant PVR C2-5.

However, the fashioned 25 cannula was not efficient for passive aspiration of PFC. we had to use the 23G back flush needle (passive aspiration) or the 23G vitreous cutter (active aspiration) for PFC aspiration.

5. CONCLUSION

The fashioned 25-gauge cannula is safe and efficient for injection of heavy liquid during vitrectomy for retinal detachment. On the other hand, it isn't efficient for suction purpose. Further studies are needed for proper evaluation of all possible use of this fashioned cannula. Further studies are also needed for cheap efficient manufactured instruments (like the Dual Bore cannula) for proper comparison.

ETHICAL APPROVAL

All authors hereby declare that all the study have been approved by the appropriate ethical committee and have therefore been performed in accordance with the ethical standards laid down in the 1964 Declaration Of Helsinki

COMPETING INTERESTS

Authors have declared that no competing interests exist.

REFERENCES

1.   Escoffery RF, Olk RJ, Grand MG, Boniuk I. Vitrectomy   without   scleral   buckling

for primary Rhegmatogenous retinal detachment. Am J Ophthalmol. 1985;99: 275-281.

2. Hakin KN, Lavin MJ, Leaver PK. Primary vitrectomy for rhegmatogenous retinal detachment. Graefes Arch Clin Exp Ophthalmol. 1993;231:344-346.

3. Gartry DS, Chignell AH, Franks WA, Wong D. pars plana Vitrectomy for the treatment of Rhegmatogenous retinal detachment uncomplicated by advanced proliferative vitreoretinopathy. Br J Ophthalmol. 1993;77: 199-203.

4. Heinmann H, Bornfeld N, Friedrichs W. Primary vitrectomy without scleral buckling for rhegmatogenous retinal detachment. Graefes Arch Clin Exp Ophthalmol. 1996; 234:561-568.

5. Brazitikos PD, D'Amico DJ, Tsinopoulos IT, Stangos NT. Primary Vitrectomy with perfluoro-n-octane use in the treatment of pseudophakic retinal detachment with undetected retinal breaks. Retina. 1999;19: 103-109.

6. Brazitikos PD. The expanding role of primary pars plana Vitrectomy in the treatment of rhegmatogenous non-complicated retinal detachment. Semin Ophthalmol. 2000;15:65-77.

7. Larrison WI, Frederick AR, Peterson TJ, Topping TM. Posterior retinal folds following vitreoretinal surgery. Am J Ophthalmol. 1994;111:621-625.

8. Thompson JT. Use of perfluorocarbon liquids in vitreoretinal surgery. Ryan SJ ed. Retina. St. Louis: CV Mosby. 1994;21-97.

9. Brazitikos PD, Androudi S, D'Amico DJ, Papadopoulos N, Dimitrakos MD, Dereklis DL, Alexandridis A, Lake S, Stangos NT. Perfluorocarbon liquid utilization in primary vitrectomy repair of retinal detachment with multiple breaks. Retina. 2003;23:615-621.

10. Abu El Asrar AM, El Kwikbi HF, Kangave D. Prognostic factors after primary Vitrectomy and perfluorocarbon liquids for bullous Rhegmatogenous retinal detachment. Eur J Ophthalmol. 2009; 19(1):107-117.

11. Ho CL, Chen KJ, See LC. Selection of scleral buckling for primary retinal detachment. Ophthalmologica. 2002;216: 33-39.

12. Wang XY, Shen LP, Hu RR. Persistent Subretinal fluid after successful scleral buckle surgery for macula- off retinal detachment. Chin Med J (Eng). 2011; 124(23):4007-4011.

19

Isolated Medial Orbital Wall Fracture: A Rare Presentation

Raşit Kılıç[1*], Abdi Bahadır Çetin[1] and Gülay Çetin[2]

[1]Department of Ophthalmology, Numune Hospital, Sivas, Turkey.
[2]Department of Radiology, Numune Hospital, Sivas, Turkey.

Authors' contributions

This work was carried out in collaboration between all authors. All authors read and approved the final manuscript.

Editor(s):
(1) Jimmy S. M. Lai, Department of Ophthalmology, The University of Hong Kong, Hong Kong and Honorary Consultant Ophthalmologist, Queen Mary Hospital, Hong Kong.
Reviewers:
(1) Gabor Nemeth, Department of Ophthalmology, University of Debrecen, Debrecen, Hungary.
(2) Anonymous, Catholic University of Campinas, Brazil.

ABSTRACT

Aim: The aim of this study was to evaluate the clinical course and treatment of a case that developed right orbital medial wall fracture following the rare etiological factor of nose blowing.

Presentation of Case: A 20-year-old male patient presented with suddenly developing swelling of the right eye following strong nose blowing the same day. The examination revealed swelling of the right eye and mild pain with eye movements. The visual acuity was full with normal anterior and posterior segments in both eyes. Computed tomography revealed an ethmoid bone fracture and medial rectus muscle and orbital contents had prolapsed inside the sinus. The eyelid swelling had decreased and the pain with eye movements had disappeared at the 2-week follow-up. Complete recovery without any sequel was seen in the 3-month follow-up.

Discussion: Considering the complications that may develop after surgical treatment, the cases should be thoroughly evaluated at presentation with surgery only being considered in appropriate cases. Small fractures with no or minor herniation, or cases with diplopia recovering quickly can be monitored without treatment. Our patient was followed-up without treatment as the bone defect was small, and there was no enophtalmus, eye movement limitation or diplopia. Full recovery was seen without sequel at the end of the short-term follow-up of our patient.

*Corresponding author: E-mail: kilicrasit@gmail.com

> **Conclusion:** Small fractures with no enophtalmus, eye movement limitation or diplopia can be followed-up without treatment, as in the presented case.

Keywords: Diplopia; enophtalmus; orbital blowout fracture; orbital surgery.

1. INTRODUCTION

Orbital blowout fractures are usually the result of blunt orbital or maxillofacial trauma and most commonly develop in the medial and inferior walls [1]. Orbital floor fractures may less commonly be accompanied by intracranial trauma such as epidural hematoma [2]. Other potential findings are subcutaneous emphysema in the periorbital region, ecchymosis, enophthalmus, limited ocular movement, diplopia, hyphema, traumatic uveitis and corneal perforation [1,3]. The gold standard diagnostic method is computerized tomography (CT) [4]. CT enables evaluation of the fracture's location and size and the prolapse of the extraocular muscles and orbital content into the fracture. Small fractures are monitored while large ones require surgical treatment. The aim of surgical treatment is to repair to defect and preserve ocular functions and the cosmetic structure.

The etiology of orbital blowout fractures includes accidents, assault and falls [1]. The aim of this study was to evaluate the clinical course and treatment of a case that developed right orbital medial wall fracture following the rare etiological factor of nose blowing.

2. PRESENTATİON OF CASE

A 20-year-old male patient presented with suddenly developing swelling of the right eye following strong nose blowing the same day. The examination revealed swelling of the right eye and mild pain with eye movements. Eye movements were full and there was no diplopia or enophtalmus. The visual acuity was full with normal anterior and posterior segments in both eyes. Computed tomography revealed an ethmoid bone fracture approximately 1x1.5 cm in size that was depressed towards the sinus in the right medial orbital wall. The medial rectus muscle and orbital contents had prolapsed inside the sinus with increased hemorrhagic density secondary to the fracture together with air in the orbit and anterior periorbital region (Fig. 1). Systemic antibiotic therapy that oral ampicillin sulbactam 750 mg two times a day was given the patient for one week long period. The eyelid swelling had decreased and the pain with eye

movements had disappeared at the 2-week follow-up. Visual acuity and other eye findings were normal. Complete recovery without any sequel was seen in the 3-month follow-up.

3. DISCUSSION

Orbital blowout fractures occur in the weakest part of the bone structure due to increased intraorbital pressure after trauma. Çağatay et al. [1] reported that medial wall fracture (39 cases, 51.3%) was the most common isolated orbital wall fracture and all their cases were the result of trauma. Isolated medial wall fractures can occur at the ethmoid bone when the patient blows his nose [5]. Most untreated orbital blowout fractures can heal by themselves. The patients should avoid nose blowing due to the possibility of sending infected sinus content towards the orbit in such cases. However, complications such as diplopia and enophtalmus can be seen in some untreated cases. Bone defects can be surgically repaired with transconjunctival and transnasal procedures, among others [3]. Bone tissues are frequently divided into small pieces during orbital blowout fractures and it is not possible to return them to their original anatomic position. Grafts and implants are therefore used in defect repair [6-9]. Autogenous grafts such as bone and cartilage and allogeneic implants such as silicone or hydroxyapatite are used in such surgical procedures. Early period complications such as infection, implant expulsion or valve malposition and late period complications such as diplopia and proptosis can develop due to the use of orbital implants [10]. Autogenous grafts may cause volume reduction followed by recurrence of the corrected enophtalmus [9].

Considering the complications that may develop after surgical treatment, the cases should be thoroughly evaluated at presentation with surgery only being considered in appropriate cases. Small fractures with no or minor herniation, or cases with diplopia recovering quickly can be monitored without treatment. Our patient was followed-up without treatment as the bone defect was small, and there was no enophtalmus, eye movement limitation or diplopia. Full recovery was seen without sequel at the end of the short-term follow-up of our patient.

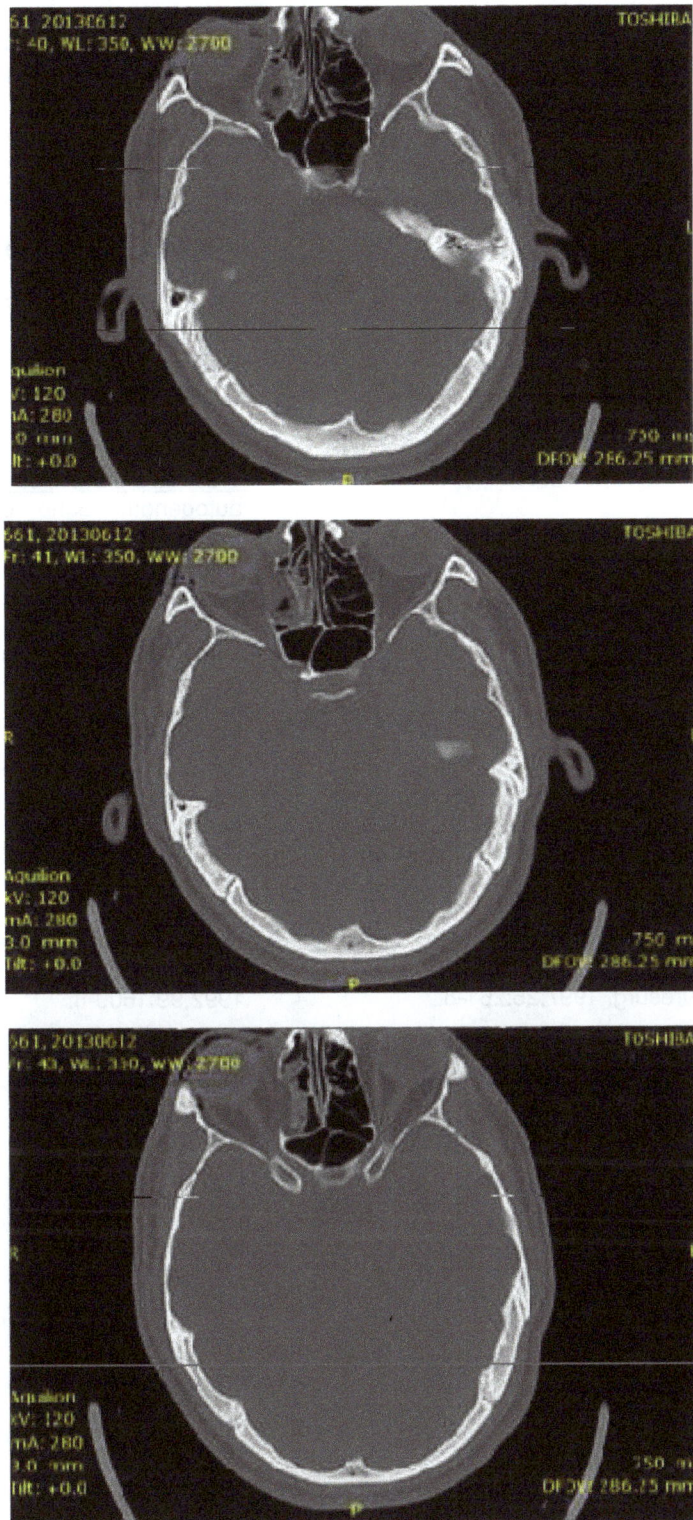

Fig. 1. Fracture of the right orbital medial wall. The medial rectus muscle and orbital content have prolapsed inside the sinus

4. CONCLUSION

In conclusion, fractures can occur at the ethmoid bone with strong nose blowing as it is one of the thinner bones of the orbit. Small fractures with no enophtalmus, eye movement limitation or diplopia can be followed-up without treatment, as in the presented case.

CONSENT

A written informed consent was obtained from the patient.

ETHICAL APPROVAL

It is not applicable.

COMPETING INTERESTS

Authors have declared that no competing interests exist.

REFERENCES

1. Çağatay HH, Ekinci M, Pamukcu C, Oba ME, Özcan AA, Karşıdağ S. Retrospective analysis of 132 patients with orbital fracture. Ulus Travma Acil Cerr Derg. 2013;19:449-55.

2. Donahue DJ, Smith K, Church E, Chadduck WM. Intracranial neurological injuries associated with orbital fracture. Pediatr Neurosurg. 1997;26:261-8.

3. Lim NK, Kang DH, Oh SA, Gu JH. Orbital Wall Restoring Surgery in Pure Blowout Fractures. Arch Plast Surg. 2014;41:686-92.

4. Courtney DJ, Thomas S, Whitfield PH. Isolated orbital blowout fractures: survey and review. Br J Oral Maxillofac Surg. 2000;38:496-504.

5. Watanabe T, Kawano T, Kodama S, Suzuki M. Orbital blowout fracture caused by nose blowing. Ear Nose Throat J. 2012;91:24-5.

6. Bratton EM, Durairaj VD. Orbital implants for fracture repair. Curr Opin Ophthalmol. 2011;22:400-6.

7. Zunz E, Blanc O, Leibovitch I. Traumatic orbital floor fractures: repair with autogenous bone grafts in a tertiary trauma center. J Oral Maxillofac Surg. 2012;70:584-92.

8. Talesh KT, Babaee S, Vahdati SA, Tabeshfar Sh. Effectiveness of a nasoseptal cartilaginous graft for repairin g traumatic fractures of theinferior orbital Wall. Br J Oral Maxillofac Surg. 2009;47:10-3.

9. Kraus M, Gatot A, Fliss DM. Repair of traumatic inferior orbital wall defects with nasoseptal cartilage. J Oral Maxillofac Surg. 2001;59:1397-400.

10. Jordan DR, St Onge P, Anderson RL, Patrinely JR, Nerad JA. Complications associated with alloplastic implants used in orbital fracture repair. Ophthalmology 1992;99:1600-8.

20

Bilateral Endogenous Endophthalmitis as an Initial Presentation of *Klebsiella pneumoniae* Bacteremia in Advanced Hepatocellular Carcinoma

Rhuen Chiou Chow[1,2*] and Tengku Ain Kamalden[1,2]

[1]*University of Malaya Eye Research Center (UMERC), Malaysia.*
[2]*Department of Ophthalmology, Faculty of Medicine, University of Malaya, Kuala Lumpur, Malaysia.*

Authors' contributions

This work was carried out in collaboration between both authors. Author RCC wrote the first draft of the manuscript. Authors RCC and TAK managed the literature searches and author TAK revised it critically for important intellectual content. Both authors read and approved the final manuscript.

Editor(s):
(1) Ahmad M. Mansour, Department of Ophthalmology, American University of Beirut, Lebanon.
Reviewers:
(1) Anonymous, Mansoura Uinversity, Egypt.
(2) Mitzy E. Torres Soriano, Retina Department, Centro Medico Cagua, Cagua, Venezuela.

ABSTRACT

Aims: To report a case of *Klebsiella pneumoniae* bacteremia presenting as bilateral endogenous endophthalmitis in a patient with advanced hepatocellular carcinoma and liver failure.
Presentation of Case: We describe a 55 year-old man with diabetes, Hepatitis B, metastatic hepatocellular carcinoma with liver failure who presented with sudden, painful, bilateral rapid loss of vision accompanied with hypopyon, intense anterior chamber fibrinous reaction and vitritis. Systematic workup revealed bilateral endogenous *K. pneumonia* endophthalmitis secondary to hepatobiliary sepsis. Conservative management with systemic piperacillin/tazobactam, intravitreal and topical ceftazidime and vancomycin led to successful sepsis control, however visual outcome was dismal.
Discussion: *Klebsiella* endogenous endophthalmitis has become extremely prevalent in southeast Asia, most commonly occurring as a metastatic complication of pyogenic liver abscess. Early systemic and intravitreal antibiotics remain the cornerstone of its management. Despite adequate treatment, visual prognosis is grave.
Conclusion: This highlights the rapidly destructive nature of this virulent organism. Clinicians must

*Corresponding author: E-mail: rhuen_chiou@yahoo.com

be mindful that endophthalmitis can be the initial presenting sign of *Klebsiella* bacteremia and the search for a primary infective source is paramount. Identification of prognostic factors for poor vision following an attack allows early intervention, in hope to improve patient outcomes.

Keywords: Klebsiella pneumoniae; bilateral; endogenous endophthalmitis; bacteremia.

1. INTRODUCTION

Endogenous endophthalmitis, also termed metastatic endophthalmitis results from hematogenous spread of pathogens from a remote primary site across the blood ocular barrier to affect the internal structures of the eye. *Klebsiella pneumoniae* is now recognized as the leading cause of endogenous endophthalmitis in Southeast Asia, accounting for up to 60% of cases in this region, especially in the presence of pyogenic liver disease [1-3]. This is in vast contrast to western countries like Europe, United States and Australia where *K. pneumoniae* is the causative organism in only 3-5% of endogenous endophthalmitis cases [4]. This case report highlights the rising prevalence of invasive *Klebsiella* infection in Asia and its known risk factors.

2. PRESENTATION OF CASE

A 55 year-old Malay gentleman, presented to the emergency department of a tertiary hospital in the city he lived in, complaining of bilateral, painful sudden reduced vision and sticky discharge for two days, worse on the left compared to the right eye. There was associated fever and lethargy for a week. He had a background of type 2 diabetes mellitus, Hepatitis B infection, newly diagnosed advanced hepatocellular carcinoma with liver failure (Child-Pugh class B) and lung base metastasis. The past medical history and family history was negative for autoimmune conditions nor thyroid dysfunction. Prior to this episode, he denied similar episodes of painful red eye in the past and there was no history of any eye trauma, contact lens use or eye surgery. Premorbidly, our patient did not have any vision problems and has never undergone treatment for diabetic retinopathy either.

The right vision on presentation was light perception in all quadrants and there was no light perception in the left eye. An initial ophthalmic examination revealed bilaterally injected conjunctivas, with chemosis on the left. Both corneas were edematous and there was no

evidence of infiltrates or gross keratic precipitates. He had severe anterior uveitis bilaterally with dense fibrin and hypopyon. There was no view of iris details nor of the fundus in either eyes due to the cloudy corneas and dense inflammation in the anterior chambers. The intraocular pressures in the right and left eyes were 22 mmHg and 23 mmHg respectively. The lids in both eyes, however, were not swollen and there was no proptosis. An ultrasound scan (B-scan) of both eyes revealed dense vitritis, with no evidence of retinal detachment or traction.

Our patient was treated empirically for sepsis with bilateral endogenous endophthalmitis. He received intravenous piperacillin/tazobactam (Tazosin) 4.5 g tds, alongside intravitreal ceftazidime 2.25 mg/0.1 ml and vancomycin 1 mg/0.1 ml. Intensive hourly topical ceftazidime and vancomycin was also commenced.

Laboratory parameters showed marked neutrophilic leukocytosis (53.6×10^9) and elevated C-reactive protein 21.5 µg/dl. Blood and bilateral vitreous tap cultures yielded *Klebsiella pneumoniae*, sensitive to piperacillin/ tazobactam, ceftazidime, cefuroxime and amoxycillin/clauvulanate. A computerized tomography (CT) scan of the abdomen showed multiple hypodense necrotic areas and air pockets within the large, multinodular tumour mass occupying the entire left lobe of the liver (Fig. 1).

He showed good response to treatment and was afebrile after 48 hours. Leukocytosis reduced to 21.8×10^9 after five days. Surgical option of bilateral vitrectomy was offered to the patient however was declined due to the high risk from general anaesthesia and the patient's unwillingness to undergo the surgery under local anaesthesia. A total of six doses of intravitreal ceftazidime and vancomycin were given at 72-hour intervals, after which our patient refused any further injections. Topical steroids 4-hourly were also commenced. By two weeks, there was clinical improvement noted as evidenced by gradual resolution of the conjunctival inflammation, hypopyon and fibrin

(Fig. 2a and 2b). Our patient also reported drastic reduction in eye pain. Vision in both eyes, however, remained the same i.e. light perception in the right and no light perception in the left.

Systemic antibiotics were continued for three weeks and subsequently downgraded to oral cefuroxime, as he remained afebrile and blood cultures twice repeated were negative.

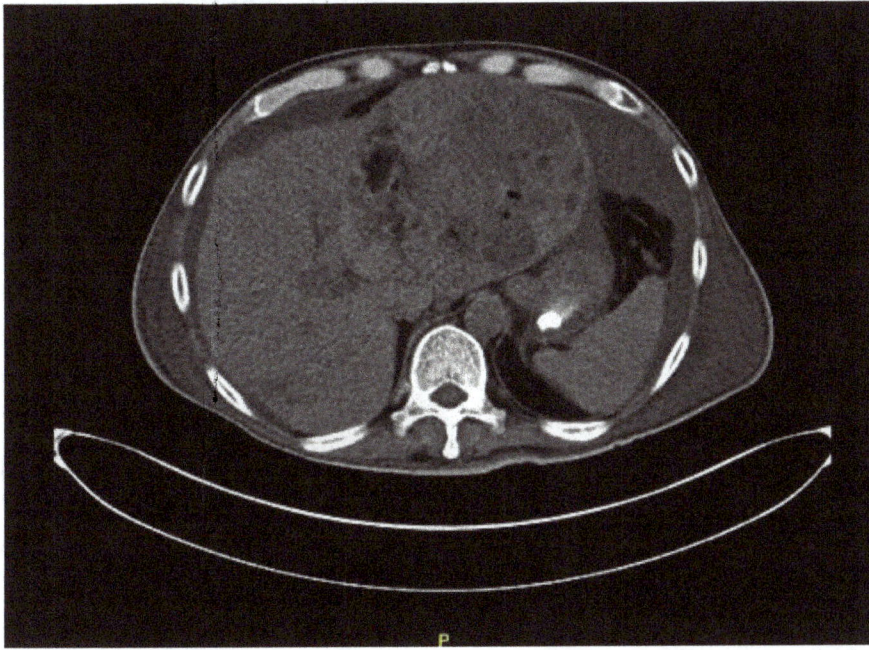

Fig. 1. Large multinodular heterogeneously enhancing mass occupying the entire left lobe of liver with multiple necrotic areas and air pockets within, suggestive of infected tumour

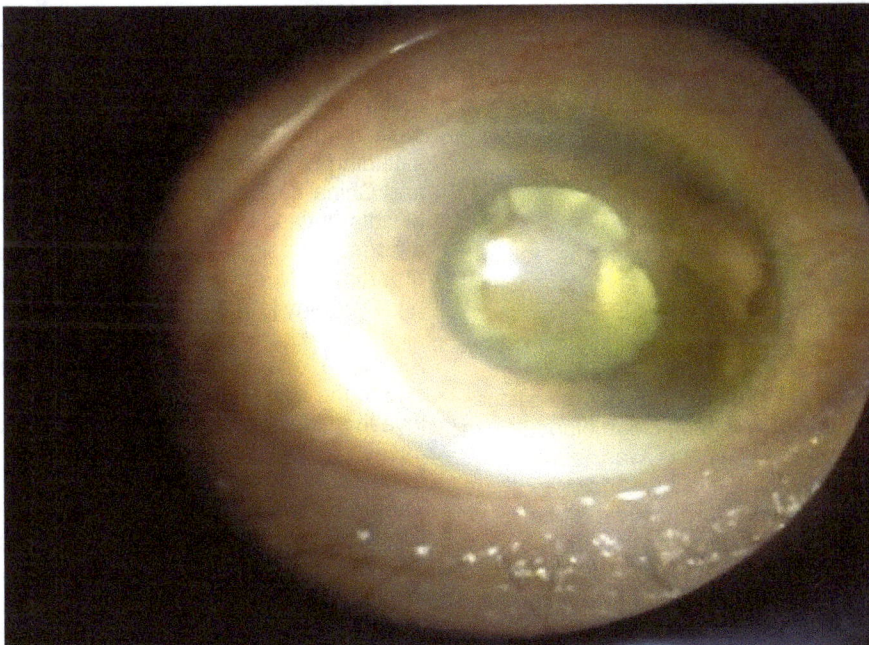

Fig. 2a. Right eye showing contracting pupillary fibrin and hypopyon

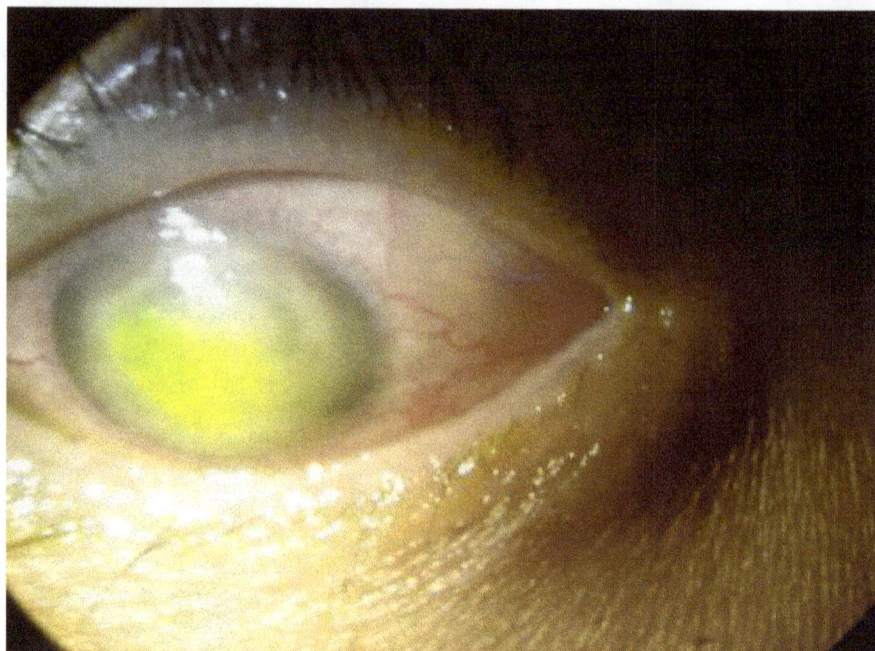

Fig. 2b. Left eye conjunctiva is less injected with resolved chemosis. Anterior chamber fibrinous material reduced, revealing superior pupillary margins. Central large corneal epithelial defect present

Topical antibiotics were also tapered to two hourly since ocular infection appeared to be under control, prior to discharge home for palliative care after one month of hospitalization. Our patient eventually succumbed to liver failure secondary to advanced hepatocellular carcinoma three weeks after discharge. He had no evidence of worsening ocular infection within this period however.

3. DISCUSSION

Klebsiella pneumoniae is the second leading cause of community acquired and nosocomial Gram-negative bacteremia, after Escherichia coli [5].

Ko et al. [6] reports significant global differences in clinical patterns of K. pneumoniae bloodstream infection. Although pneumonia was found to be the commonest infection site worldwide, there was a distinctive syndrome of liver abscess in conjunction with Klebsiella bacteremia almost exclusive to cases in Taiwan. This is resonated by more than 900 case reports of K. pneumoniae liver abscesses in Taiwan over the past decade. Specific organism virulence factors such as K1 and K2 capsular serotype, mucoid phenotype and aerobactin production have been implicated

to account for this geographic difference in disease spectrum [4,7,8].

First described in Taiwan during the 1980s, Klebsiella invasive syndrome is defined as K. pneumoniae liver abscess with extrahepatic complications including endophthalmitis, meningitis and necrotizing fasciitis. Subsequent case reports in other Southeast Asian countries including Singapore, Hong Kong, Korea, Vietnam and China have highlighted the rapid emergence of this invasive entity. Outside Asia, isolated reports on similar presentations have been reported in North and South America [8] Europe [9], Germany [10] and Qatar [11].

Klebsiella endogenous endophthalmitis (EE) is one of the most feared metastatic complication in invasive Klebsiella syndrome. In up to 4.9% of cases, ocular symptoms may precede diagnosis of hepatobiliary sepsis [2,12,13], like in our case. The reported risk of developing EE in the presence of Klebsiella liver abscess ranges from 3-7.8%. A review by Sheu et al. [14] found 42 individuals (53 eyes) out of 602 patients (6.9%) with pyogenic Klebsiella liver disease had developed EE, of which 11 patients (26.1%) experienced bilateral involvement.

Diabetes mellitus has been consistently implicated as a major risk factor for the development of EE in *Klebsiella* bacteremia, especially in cases with poor glycaemic control. This is due to impaired chemotactic and phagocytosis mechanisms by polymorphonuclear leukocytes [14-16]. Sng et al. [2] however had previously reported that diabetes and other comorbid pathologies were not risk factors for endophthalmitis in *K. pneumoniae* bacteraemia.

In a case-control study of 133 patients, definite risk factors for *Klebsiella* EE were hepatic abscess and disseminated intravascular coagulation. Additional risk factors included a lower white cell count at presentation and a longer interval between onset of symptoms and administration of systemic antibiotics [2]. In our patient, significant associations for development of metastatic endophthalmitis are underlying diabetes, hepatobiliary sepsis and delayed presentation of 2 days between onset of ocular symptoms and administration of intravenous antibiotics.

The management of *Klebsiella* EE is challenging for a variety of reasons. Currently, there are no guidelines available, specifically on the role of vitrectomy. In contrast to post-operative endophthalmitis, prompt administration of intravenous antibiotics is key to address the primary source of infection, which in Southeast Asia is of hepatobiliary origin in up to 77.5% of cases [1,3,13,14,17].

The choice of antimicrobial should be guided according to in-vitro sensitivity results and clinical response. Successfully treated cases in the literature employed first to third generation cephalosporins, aminoglycosides and anti-pseudomonal penicillins [8]. Antibiotics need to be continued for at least 2-3 weeks until systemic infection has been eradicated for certain. In conjunction to this, intravitreal antibiotics such as amikacin 400 μg/0.1 ml, gentamicin 0.05 mg/0.1 ml, ceftazidime 2.25 mg/0.1 ml and vancomycin 1 mg/0.1 ml have been used [14,15].

Pars plana vitrectomy in endogenous *Klebsiella* endophthalmitis can reduce the bacterial load and inflammatory mediators within the vitreous cavity, as well as enhance ocular penetration of antibiotics [4,14]. In some cases series, early vitrectomy was shown to save eyes from enucleation or evisceration [14,18]. However, due to poor systemic conditions these patients present with, combined with high risk for general anesthesia, early vitrectomy is not always feasible [1,17]. The shift towards 23-gauge and 25-gauge transconjunctival sutureless vitrectomy offers increased patient comfort, shorter operation duration and performance under local anaesthesia. Hence, small gauge vitrectomy may be a solution for ill and high-risk patients who are not fit for general anaesthesia and long operations [17]. Perhaps early posterior vitrectomy under local anaesthesia could have improved visual outcome in our patient. To date, most studies have concluded no significant difference in visual outcome between conservative management and vitrectomy [13-15].

Over the years, despite improved recognition and aggressive treatment of endogenous *Klebsiella* endophthalmitis, the final visual outcome remains grim. In a case series of 71 eyes, 41 patients (57.6%) had a final vision of no light perception [13]. Experimental animal models have demonstrated rapid and irreversible destruction of retinal photoreceptors occurred as early as 48 hours of infection, due to the extremely virulent nature of *K. pneumoniae* [14]. Ang et al. [13] revealed the prognostic factors for poor visual outcomes to be presence of hypopyon, unilateral involvement, short time interval from onset of sepsis to ocular symptoms (4 days or less) and panophthalmitis. Identification of these poor prognostic factors allows clinicians to intervene early, in hope to improve outcomes in such patients.

4. CONCLUSION

In summary, this case highlights the well-known risk factors for *K. pneumoniae* bacteremia including diabetes, liver failure and malignancy. Ophthalmologists faced with endophthalmitis in a patient of Asian decent with the mentioned risk factors must actively search for a primary infective focus, most commonly *Klebsiella* hepatobiliary sepsis, as ocular disturbances may be the first presenting sign. Although drainage of pyogenic liver abscesses is advocated to control *Klebsiella* bacteremia, not all patients will be suitable candidates. This is particularly so in our case of advanced hepatocellular carcinoma with superimposed necrotic areas within the tumour. Despite this, our patient recovered from sepsis with intensive and prolonged systemic antibiotics. With conservative management of the bilateral endophthalmitis, he did not require evisceration or enucleation either. However, final visual outcome was poor, further emphasizing the grave prognosis of this increasingly prevalent entity. Further research on the exact virulence factors in *K. pneumoniae* strains in Southeast Asia is crucial and vaccination in high-risk groups could potentially be achieved in the near future.

CONSENT

All authors declare that written informed consent was obtained from the patient and his wife for publication of this case report and accompanying images.

ETHICAL APPROVAL

It is not applicable.

COMPETING INTERESTS

Authors have declared that no competing interests exist.

REFERENCES

1. Wong JS, Chan TK, Lee HM, Chee SP. Endogenous bacterial endophthalmitis-An east asian experience and a reappraisal of a severe ocular affliction. Ophthalmology. 2000;107(8):1483-1491.

2. Sng CCA, Jap A, Chan YH, Chee SP. Risk factors for endogenous *Klebsiella* endophthalmitis in patients With *Klebsiella* Bacteremia: A Case-control Study. Br J. Ophthalmol. 2008;92:673-677.

    DOI: 10.1136/bjo.2007.132522.

3. Chen YJ, Kuo HK, Wu PC, Kuo ML, Tsai HH, Liu CC, et al. A 10-Year Comparison of Endogenous Endophthalmitis Outcomes: An East Asian Experience with *Klebsiella pneumoniae* Infection. Retina. 2004;24(3):383-390.

4. Sridhar J, Flynn HW, Kuriyan AE, Dubovy S, Miller D. Endophthalmitis caused by *Klebsiella* species. Retina. 2014; 34(9):1875-1881.

5. Meatherall BL, Gregson D, Ross T, Pitout J, Laupland K. Incidene, risk factors and outcomes of *Klebsiella pneumoniae* bacteremia. The American Journal of Medicine. 2009;122:866-873.

    DOI: 10.1016/j.amjmed.2009.03.034.

6. Ko WC, Paterson DL, Sagnimeni AJ, Hansen DS, Gottberg AV, Mohapatra S, et al. Community-acquired *Klebsiella*

7. Yu VL, Hansen DS, Ko WC, Sagnimeni A, Klugman FP, Gottberg AV, et al. Virulence characteristics of *Klebsiella* and clinical manifestations of *K. pneumoniae* bloodstream infections. Emerging Infectious Diseases. 2007;13(7):986-993.

8. Siu LK, Yeh KM, Lin JC, Fung CP, Chang FY. *Klebsiella pneumoniae* liver abscess: A new invasive syndrome. Lancet Infect Dis. 2012;12:881-887.

9. Sobirk SK, Struve C, Jacobsson SG. Primary *Klebsiella pneumoniae* liver abscess with metastatic spread to lung and eye, a North-European case report of an emerging syndrome. Open Microbiol J. 2010;4:5-7.

10. Bilal S, Volz MS, Fiedler T, Podschun R, Schneider T. *Klebsiella pneumoniae*-induced liver abscesses, Germany. Emerg Infect Dis. 2014;20(11):1939-1940. DOI: 10.3201/eid2011.140149.

11. Al Ani AARM, Elzouki AN, Rahil A, Al-Ani F. Endogenous endophthalmitis and liver abscess syndrome secondary to *Klebsiella pneumoniae*: Report of Three Cases from Qatar. Asian Pacific Journal of Tropical Biomedicine. 2015;5:930-935.

12. Iglesias APB, Cabeza MIP, Pardo MJR, Castano M. Endogenous endophthalmitis as a first clinical manifestation of *Klebsiella* sepsis. The Importance of an Early Diagnosis. Arch Soc Esp Oftalmol. 2011;86(12):412-414.

13. Ang M, Jap A, Chee SP. Prognostic factors and outcomes in endogenous *Klebsiella pneumoniae* endophthalmitis. Am J. Ophthalmol. 2011;151:338-344.

14. Sheu SJ, Kung YH, Wu TT, Chang FP, Horng YH. Risk factors for endogenous endophthalmitis secondary to *Klebsiella pneumoniae* liver abscess-20 year experience in Southern Taiwan. Retina. 2011;31(10):2026-2031.

15. Chen KJ, Hwang YS, Chen YP, Lai CC, Chen TL, Wang NK. Endogenous *Klebsiella* endophthalmitis associated with *Klebsiella pneumoniae* pneumonia. Ocular Immunology and Inflammation. 2009; 17:153-159.

    DOI: 10.1080/09273940902752250.

16. Lin YT, Wang FD, Wu PF, Fung CP. *Klebsiella pneumoniae* liver abscess in

pneumoniae bacteremia: Global differences in clinical patterns. Emerging Infectious Disease. 2002;8(2):160-166.

diabetic patients: Association of glycaemic control with the clinical characteristics. BMC Infectious Diseases. 2013;13:56.

DOI: 10.1186/1471-2334-13-56.

17. Lee SH, Um TW, Joe SG, Hwang JU, Kim JG, Yoon YH, et al. Changes in the clincial features and prognostic factors of endogenous endophthalmitis-fifteen years of clinical experience in Korea. Retina. 2012;32:977-984.

18. Yoon YH, Lee SU, Sohn JH, Lee SE. Result of early vitrectomy for endogenous *Klebsiella pneumoniae* endophthalmitis. Retina. 2003;23:366-370.

21

A Clinical Sign for Aiding the Diagnosis of Unilateral Subconjunctival Orbital Fat Herniation

Saul N. Rajak[1,2*] and Geoffrey E. Rose[3]

[1]*The Sussex Eye Hospital, Brighton, United Kingdom.*
[2]*The London School of Hygiene and Tropical Medicine, United Kingdom.*
[3]*Moorfields Eye Hospital, London, United Kingdom.*

Authors' contributions

This work was carried out in collaboration between both authors. Both authors read and approved the final manuscript.

<u>Editor(s):</u>
(1) Rachid Tahiri Joutei Hassani, Ophthalmology Department III, XV – XX National Ophthalmologic Hospital, France.
<u>Reviewers:</u>
(1) Anonymous, USA.
(2) Anonymous, Egypt.
(3) C. O. Adeoti, Ophthalmology Department, Ladoke Akintola University of Technology Teaching Hospital, Osogbo, Nigeria.
(4) Gabor Nemeth, Department of Ophthalmology, University of Debrecen, Debrecen, Hungary.
(5) José Francisco de Sales Chagas, Department of Surgery, Head and Neck Service, Medical School, Catholic University of Campinas, Brazil.
(6) Rahmi Duman, Department of Ophthalmology, Dr. Abdurrahman Yurtaslan Oncology Training and Research Hospital, 06105, Yenimahalle, Ankara, Turkey.

ABSTRACT

Subconjunctival orbital fat herniation is a rare occurrence. These masses can be easily mis-diagnosed as more sinister lesions. We present a unilateral case of this condition and a useful, previously undescribed clinical sign, which obviated the need for orbital imaging.

Keywords: Orbital; fat; herniation; prolapsed; subconjunctival.

1. INTRODUCTION

Subconjunctival orbital fat herniation (SOFH) is a rare finding [1-6]. Intraconal orbital fat herniates through a dehiscence in Tenon's capsule to form a mass, usually under the supero-temporal bulbar conjunctiva. SOFH has been mistaken for choristomas (dermoid cysts and dermolipomas),

*Corresponding author: E-mail: saul.rajak@lshtm.ac.uk

lymphomas, pleomorphic lipomas and lacrimal gland tumours or cysts [4].

A more common finding is protuberances of the lateral area of the lower lid an upper cheek from orbital fat herniation through the inferior orbital septum. This is particularly common in elderly, obese males. It has been referred to as 'steatoblepharon' or 'palpebral bags' [1].

SOFH is frequently misdiagnosed. We report a previously unreported, useful clinical sign that helped confirm the clinical diagnosis.

2. CASE REPORT

A 76-year-old man was referred to the orbital clinic with an asymptomatic right, supero-temporal anterior orbital mass, which had been present for five years. The patient had diabetes mellitus, hypertension, high cholesterol and had had a cardiac bypass for which he took multiple medications. There was no history of ophthalmic disease or trauma. On examination there was a large, soft, yellow, mobile, subconjunctival mass in the supero-temporal orbit, directly inferior to the palpebral lobe of the lacrimal gland (Fig. 1). The posterior edge of the mass was not visible. The mass did not have dermis, glands, keratin or hair on it. There was also bilateral infero-temporal preseptal fat prolapse, with the left prolapse being markedly larger than the right (Figs. 2a and b). There was no proptosis, diplopia, acuity/colour vision reduction, pupillary abnormalities, tenderness or conjunctival inflammation. The mass was diagnosed clinically as SOFH and no imaging or investigations were performed. The patient declined surgical intervention.

3. DISCUSSION

Supero-temporal subconjunctival masses may be intraorbital fat herniation, dermoid cyst, dermolipoma, lymphoma, pleomorphic lipoma and dacryops [4]. Unlike the present case, dermoid cysts and dermolipomas usually present in childhood. They are typically firm and white and their surface can contain sebaceous glands and hair follicles. Lymphomas are usually flat and 'salmon pink' in colour. Orbital pleomorphic lipomas are extremely rare, with only a few cases in the literature [7]. Although similar in appearance to SOFH they gradually increase in size. SOFH should not be confused with the lacrimal gland, which is located superiorly to the fatty mass. The present case was suspected as being an SOFH as the lesion was soft, yellow and mobile. The finding of bilateral, but asymmetrical inferior fat pads supported the diagnosis. The inferior fat pad on the side with the subconjunctival fatty mass was markedly smaller than the fellow side. There appears to have been a similar degree overall of fat herniation on each side, but on one side all the herniated fat was located in the inferior fat pad but on the other side it was split between the inferior fat pad and the superior subconjunctival fatty mass. This useful clinical sign, which has not been previously reported, obviated the need for CT scanning.

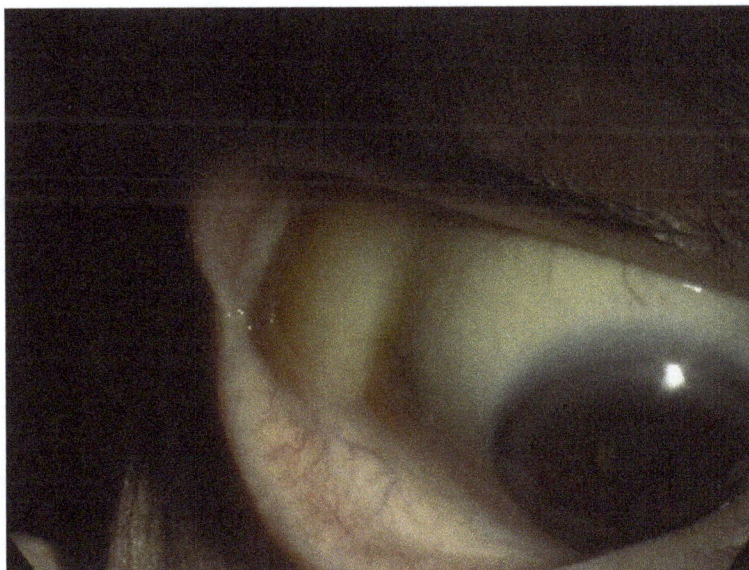

Fig. 1. Supero-temporal subconjunctival orbital fat herniation

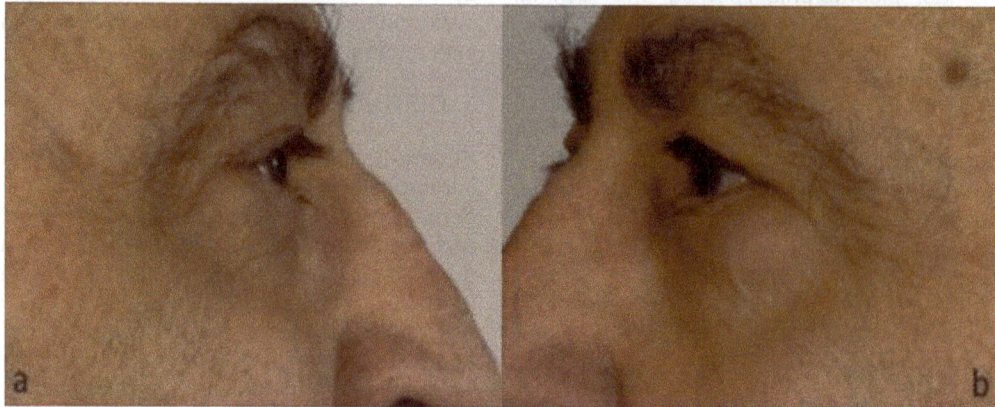

Fig. 2. Asymmetrical infero-temporal pre-septal fat pads: right smaller than left

The orbit contains both intraconal fat (within Tenon's capsule) and extra-conal fat (outside Tenon's capsule). CT scanning from other case series of SOFH showed extrusion of intra-conal fat.1, 4 Inferior fat pads are usually thought to derive from extra-conal fat. However, in the present cases, the clear splitting of fat between the superior conjunctival area and the inferior lid indicates a common source. It is likely that inferiorly, intra-conal fat herniated through both tenons and orbital septum – both of which atrophy with age - to form the lower lid fat pad.

SOFH is usually unilateral and supero-temporal, but has been described to occur bilaterally and nasally and inferiorly [4]. The reported case series are all small, but age, male sex and obesity all seem to be risk factors [2,4]. There are two reports of SOFH in children, one of which was thought to be congenital and the other probably caused by penetration with a wire [4,6].

The patient in the present report was asymptomatic and elected for conservative management. Surgical excision has been conducted in other case series for both diagnostic and cosmetic reasons [4]. The lesions have been clamped, cut and the base diathermied prior to releasing the clamp. No recurrences or complications have been reported, but there is a risk of retrobulbar haemorrhage.

4. CONCLUSION

SOFH is frequently misdiagnosed. Assessment of the inferior fat pads may facilitate a clinical diagnosis avoiding the need for further investigations, referrals or excision.

CONSENT

The patient gave written consent for his photographs to be taken and for these photographs to be used for publication.

ETHICAL APPROVAL

It is not applicable.

COMPETING INTERESTS

The authors report no conflicts of interest. The authors alone are responsible for the content and writing of the paper.

REFERENCES

1.   Viana GA, Osaki MH, Filho VT, Sant'Anna AE. Prolapsed orbital fat: 15 consecutive cases. Scand J Plast Reconstr Surg Hand Surg. 2009;43(6):330-4.

2.   Schmack I, Patel RM, Folpe AL, et al. Subconjunctival herniated orbital fat: A benign adipocytic lesion that may mimic pleomorphic lipoma and atypical lipomatous tumor. Am J Surg Pathol. 2007;31(2):193-8.

3.   Stangos AN, Hamedani M. Spontaneous subconjunctival orbital fat prolapse: presentation of four cases. Klin Monbl Augenheilkd. 2006;223(5):415-7.

4.   McNab AA. Subconjunctival fat prolapse. Aust N Z J Ophthalmol. 1999;27(1):33-6.

5.   Skorin L Jr, Rink C. Diagnosis and excision of subconjunctival herniation of orbital fat. Optom Vis Sci. 2014;91(9):e236-40.

6. Bernhard MK, Starke S, Hirsch W. A yellowish subconjunctival lesion in an infant-congenital orbital fat herniation. Eur J Pediatr. 2010;169(11):1427-8.

7. Daniel CS, Beaconsfield M, Rose GE, et al. Pleomorphic lipoma of the orbit: a case series and review of literature. Ophthalmology. 2003;110(1):101-5.

22

Laser-Assisted Opening of Gold Micro Shunt's Windows in Glaucoma: Efficacy and Safety

Nicolas Cadet[1] and Paul Harasymowycz[1,2*]

[1]*Department of Ophthalmology, Université de Montréal, Montreal, Canada.*
[2]*Montreal Glaucoma Institute, Montreal, Canada.*

Authors' contributions

This work was carried out in collaboration between the two authors. Author PH designed the study and edited the manuscript. Author NC wrote the protocol and the first draft of the manuscript. Both authors read and approved the final manuscript.

Editor(s):
(1) Tatsuya Mimura, Department of Ophthalmology, Tokyo Women's Medical University Medical Center East, Japan.
Reviewers:
(1) S. K. Prabhakar, Ophthalmology, JSS University, India.
(2) Barbara Giambene, SOD Oculistica, University of Firenze, Italy.

ABSTRACT

Objective: To determine the intraocular pressure-lowering effect and safety of opening the Gold Micro Shunt Plus' (GMS+) windows with a titanium-sapphire laser.
Design: Retrospective case series.
Participants: The charts of 5 patients were reviewed. Diagnoses included primary open-angle glaucoma (n=3), aphakic glaucoma (n=1) and neovascular glaucoma (n=1). There were 4 males and 1 female, aged between 56 and 81 (mean age 70±11). They had undergone a mean of 2±1.6 surgeries (range: 0-4) before GMS implantation.
Methods: IOP and number of glaucoma medications were recorded before and after the implantation of the GMS in 5 patients, as well as before and after the opening of the GMS' windows with a titanium-sapphire (Ti-Sap) laser. Patients were assessed for complications arising from implanting the GMS and opening its windows. Follow-up lasted 17 to 42 months.
Results: The GMS+ had 8 closed windows and one open flow port upon implantation. Four of these windows were opened in all five patients. Mean IOP before GMS implantation was 29.9±8.5 mmHg and it was 18.6±6.5 mmHg after implantation. Hence, implantation of the GMS was associated with an average decrease in IOP of 11.3±4.2 mmHg or 37.0% (p=0.076). The mean IOP before window-opening was 24.9±5.8 mmHg and after window opening, it was 17.6±5.7 mmHg. The IOP thus dropped 7.3±4.6 mmHg or 29.3% (p=0.055) on average after opening the

*Corresponding author: E-mail: pavloh@igmtl.com, nicolas.cadet2@gmail.com

GMS' windows. The windows were opened an average 6.4±4.5 months after GMS implantation. IOP at follow-ups remained lower than pre-GMS levels in all patients. The IOP reduction post window opening lasted throughout follow-up, i.e. from 17 to 42 months (average 30±10 months). The number of glaucoma drops for each patient did not decrease after opening the GMS' windows. One patient developed transitory cystoid macular edema after GMS implantation that resolved with a course of NSAID drops. No complications arose from the opening of the GMS' windows.
Conclusions: In our small case series, opening the GMS' windows was safe and was associated with a substantial and sustained reduction in IOP.

Keywords: Glaucoma; gold micro shunt (GMS); gold micro-shunt window opening; glaucoma shunt; suprachoroidal glaucoma shunt.

1. INTRODUCTION

Several surgical treatments exist for glaucoma. Conventional surgical approaches such as trabeculectomy and glaucoma drainage devices connect the anterior chamber (AC) to the subconjunctival space, and form a filtering bleb. These procedures have been effective in many cases but are associated with potential complications, including bleb leaks with hypotony, tube erosions and endophthalmitis [1].

A surgical technique that allows drainage of aqueous humour from the anterior chamber to the suprachoroidal space, while avoiding the complications linked to bleb formation, has been previously described [2]. The Gold Micro Shunt (GMS) (SOLX Inc, Waltham, MA) is a newer suprachoroidal shunt that also lowers IOP without bleb formation [3] and has been proven to reduce IOP from 32.6 to 45.3% [4,5].

It has been noted that both traditional shunts as well as suprachoroidal shunts, may fail due to marked encapsulation secondary to the high degree of scarring [1,2,6]. This may be due to the initial high flow through the implant, which induces fibrosis [7]. It is thus hypothesized that using a shunt in which the windows are initially closed like the GMS, and opening the windows after a few months, May lead to a slower egress of fluid and thus decrease the incidence of fibrosis and the pressure elevations associated with it.

The goal of this study was to determine the IOP-lowering effect and safety of opening the GMS' windows.

2. METHODS

2.1 Shunt Design

The Gold Micro Shunt Plus is a sterile, flat drainage device made from 24-K medical-grade (99.95%) gold. The device used in this study is approximately 6 mm long, 3 mm wide and 80 μm thick. The proximal or "head" end of the device has 8 closed ports and 1 open flow port which directs aqueous flow into the device. The 8 closed ports have a width of 100 micron and a height of 60 micron. The 1 open port is 50 micron wide by 60 micron height. The distal or "tail" end terminates in the suprachoroidal space with openings that allow aqueous to flow out through that end of the device. Larger reinforced openings aligned along the centerline of the device are designed to help in positioning the device. A protective, sterile insertion tool is supplied to aid with handling and insertion of the implant.

The GMS+ used in this study had eight closed windows. Four of these windows were opened all at once in all our patients when IOP was above target. The windows were opened with a Latina lens and Ti-Sap laser after an average of 6.4±4.5 months [range: 1-9].

2.2 Clinical Study

All cases that have undergone GMS insertion between December 2008 and March 2010 were included in this study. These five cases were retrospectively analysed from July to September 2012. The main outcomes were the complications and IOP associated with opening the GMS windows. The study was accepted by the IRB of Maisonneuve-Rosemont Hospital, and followed the tenets of the Helsinki Agreement. All patients signed an informed consent form to participate in the study.

After an initial fornix based conjunctival flap was made, a square-shaped scleral flap measuring 3.5 x 3.5 mm was dissected. Mitomycin C (500 mcg per mL) was then applied to the scleral bed for one minute, and washed with BSS. A full thickness incision into the suprachoroidal space was made posteriorly, and then the anterior chamber was penetrated using a 2.75 keratome and enlarged. The GMS was implanted into the AC and the tail end in the suprachoroidal space. The superficial scleral flap was closed with a single 10.0 Nylon suture and the conjunctiva was closed with a 10.0 Vicryl suture using a modified Wise technique.

IOP was monitored regularly and if it was judged to be above target, the patient was scheduled for laser assisted window opening. The windows were opened after an average of 6.4±4.5 months [range: 1-9]. The Titanium-Sapphire laser procedure was performed with a 200 micron spot size, 790 nm wavelength, and 7 msec exposure time using 1-2 shots per window of 30-40 mJ. Topical Nepafenac (Nevanac, Alcon) drops were applied qid for four days after window ablation. The IOP (using a Goldmann tonometer) and number of glaucoma medications were recorded immediately after laser, as well as one, three, six and twelve months after laser. Follow-up was organized every 4-6 months thereafter.

2.3 Statistical Analysis

The paired student t-test was used to calculate differences between pre- and post-GMS implantation IOP, as well as between pre- and post-window opening IOP. The Friedman p-value was calculated to compare the pre-GMS and last follow-up's IOP (see Fig. 1), as an average of the five patients. A paired student t-test was also used to compare the number of glaucoma drops pre-GMS and at the most recent follow-up.

3. RESULTS

Among the research subjects, there were 4 males and 1 female, with a mean age of 70±11 year (range: 56-81). Three patients had primary open-angle glaucoma, one had aphakic glaucoma and one had neovascular glaucoma (Table 1). Four of the patients were Caucasian and one was Hispanic. They had undergone a mean of 2±1.6 surgeries (range: 0-4) before GMS implantation. Three patients were pseudophakic, one was phakic and one was aphakic. In terms of previous glaucoma surgeries, three had undergone a trabeculectomy, two had undergone a laser trabeculoplasty and three had other glaucoma drainage devices.

The GMS had 8 closed windows and one open port upon implantation. Four of these windows were opened in all five patients. Average follow-up post GMS implantation was 30±10 months.

Mean IOP before GMS implantation was 29.9±8.5 mmHg and it was 18.6±6.5 mmHg after implantation. Hence, implantation of the GMS was associated with an average decrease in IOP of 11.3±4.2 mmHg or 37.0% (p=0.076) (Fig. 1). The mean IOP before window-opening was 24.9±5.8 mmHg and after window opening, it was 17.6±5.7 mmHg. The IOP thus dropped 7.3±4.6 mmHg or 29.3% (p=0.055) on average after opening the GMS' windows (Fig. 1). The windows were opened an average 6.4±4.5 months after GMS implantation. IOP dropped 2.3 to 10.7% per window opened (mean 7.3%). Mean IOP at the last follow-up was 18.4±5.0 mmHg. Mean IOP reduction from pre-GMS to most recent follow-up is 38.5%.

Long-term IOP at follow-ups remained lower than pre-GMS levels in all patients. The IOP reduction post window opening lasted throughout follow-up, i.e. from 17 to 42 months (average 30 months).

The mean number of glaucoma drops was 2.6±1.1 before GMS implantation and 2.8±1.1 afterwards. The pre-operative glaucoma drops were continued as is after GMS implantation. Before opening the GMS' windows, the average number of drops was 2.4±0.9 and remained identical after opening the GMS' windows (Fig. 2). At the last follow-up, the average number of drops was 3.0±0.7 (p=0.26, student t-test). One patient developed transitory cystoid macular edema after GMS implantation that resolved with a course of Nepafenac (Nevanac, Alcon) drops four times per day during a month. No complication arose from opening of the GMS' windows.

4. DISCUSSION

Molteno et al. [7] suggested that a rapid egress of aqueous humour from the anterior chamber into the subconjuctival space after implanting a glaucoma shunt can lead to conjunctival fibrosis and subsequent elevation in IOP. In order to minimize this effect, the current study analyzed the effect of implanting a GMS with 8 closed windows and only one small open channel to limit the initial egress of fluid from the anterior chamber to the suprachoroidal space. In opening the GMS' windows a few months after implantation to decrease IOP further, it was postulated that this would limit the conjunctival fibrosis and subsequent IOP spikes described by Molteno et al. [7].

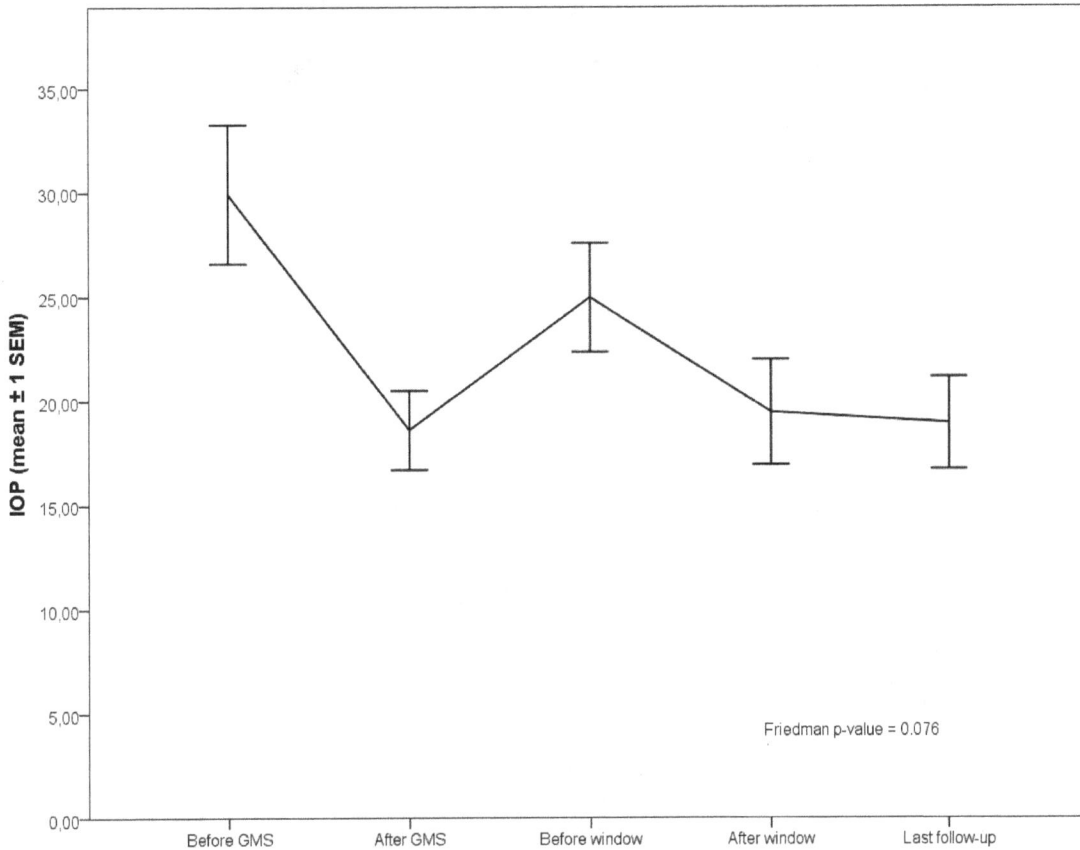

Fig. 1. IOP vs time, as an average of the five patients. IOP was measured before and after GMS implantation, before and after window opening and at the most recent follow-up

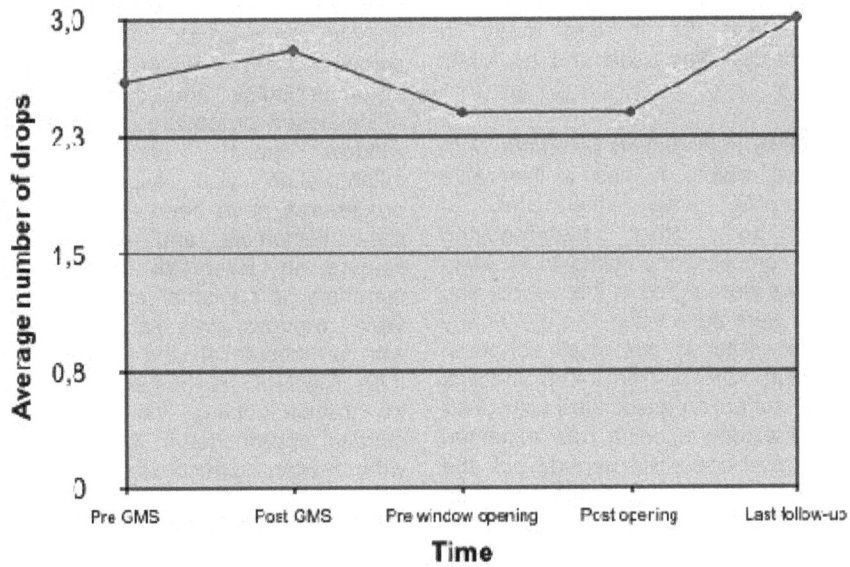

Fig. 2. Average number of drops versus time. The number of drops averaged between the 5 Patients was measured before and after GMS implantation, before and after window opening and at the most recent follow-up

Table 1. Clinical characteristics of patients enrolled in the study

	Patient 1	Patient 2	Patient 3	Patient 4	Patient 5
Type of glaucoma	Neovascular	Aphakic	POAG	POAG	POAG
Lens status	Pseudophakic	Aphakic	Pseudophakic	Pseudiphakic	Phakic
Pre-GMS filtration procedures	Trabeculectomy	Trabeculectomy Ahmed valve	Trabectome	none	Trabeculectomy with ex-press shunt
Maximal IOP recorded	34 OS	30 OD	34 OD	33 OD	26 OS
Central corneal thickness (in microns)	540 OS (Normal)	620 OD (High)	501 OD (Low)	535 OD (Normal)	567 OS (Slightly high)
Number of medications before GMS implantation	4	3	1	3	2

In this study, IOP decreased significantly after GMS implantation. There was still a moderate increase in IOP post-operatively, suggesting some healing response, however after opening the GMS' windows, the IOP decreased below the post-implantation level. In our small case series, this lowered IOP was sustained until the end of our patients' follow-up, without further pressure elevations. This is in contrast to a recent study that noted failure in almost all of their GMS cases [8]. This series is different not only in shunt design but in the use of MMC in our series as well. We postulate that the use of MMC diminishes fibrosis around the GMS and helps prevent late pressure spikes seen in other studies. Another recent study found that failure was associated with inflammatory cells in the suprachoroidal space [9]. In that study, a different shunt design was used and no MMC was deployed.

In this series, GMS implantation was safe, with no post-operative blebs. It has a favorable complication profile when compared to trabeculectomy and other bleb-requiring procedures. No complications linked to opening the GMS' windows were noted in this series, and no gold particles were seen within the eye at any of the post laser visits. In this small cohort of patients with high IOP on maximum medical therapy, the IOP reduction associated with GMS implantation and window opening was sustained throughout the post-operative period, but the average number of hypotensive drops remained largely constant throughout follow-up. One potential reason why the number of hypotensive drops was not decreased after laser opening of the GMS windows was that a lower target IOP was required. It has to be noted that the pre- vs post-GMS implantation (p=0.07) and pre- vs

post-window opening (p=0.055) IOP reduction was not statistically significant. However, we consider that the IOP reduction was definitely significant from a clinical standpoint. The small sample size accounts for the lack of statistical significance in this study. It is also possible that had the remaining four windows also been opened, further IOP lowering may occur.

5. CONCLUSION

One of the current study's strengths is its follow-up duration (averaging 30 months and up to 42 months in one patient). However, the obvious limitation is its small sample size. Larger cohorts of patients with suprachoroidal implants that initially limit flow, used concomitantly with anti-fibrotics are needed. Future shunt designs may consider using a similar strategy that limit initial aqueous outflow, and permit future increase with office based procedures such as laser-assisted window opening, once the post-operative inflammation has subsided. Similar laser procedures have been used for suture lysis in trabeculectomies and removal of the tube ligature in Baerveldt drainage devices. In summary, in our small case series, opening the GMS' windows was safe and was associated with a substantial and sustained reduction in IOP. The GMS is thus an interesting alternative to trabeculectomy and other conventional surgical approaches in the treatment of patients with refractory glaucoma.

ETHICAL APPROVAL

All authors hereby declare that all experiments have been examined and approved by the appropriate ethics committee and have therefore been performed in accordance with the ethical standards laid down in the 1964 Declaration of Helsinki.

COMPETING INTERESTS

Authors have declared that no competing interests exist.

REFERENCES

1. Gedde SJ. Postoperative complications in the Tube Versus Trabeculectomy (TVT) study during five years of follow-up. Am J Ophthalmol. 2012;153(5):804-814.
2. Jordan JF, et al. A novel approach to suprachoroidal drainage for the surgical treatment of intractable glaucoma. J Glaucoma. 2006;15:200-205.
3. Mastropasqua, et al. *In vivo* analysis of conjunctiva in GMS implantation for glaucoma. Br J Ophthalmol. 2010;94:1592-96.
4. Melamed, et al. Efficacy and safety of GMS implantation in supraciliary space of patients with glaucoma. Arch Ophthalmol. 2009;127:264-9.
5. Figus, et al. Supraciliary shunt in refractory glaucoma. Br J Ophthalmol. 2012;95:1537-44.
6. Agnifili, et al. Histological findings of failed gold micro shunts in POAG. Graefes Arch Oph. 2012;250(1):143-9.
7. Molteno, et al. Otago Glaucoma Surgery Outcome Study: Factors controlling capsule fibrosis around molteno implants with histopathological correlation. Ophthalmol. 2003;110(11):2198-206.
8. Hueber A, Roters S, Jordan JF, Konen W. Retrospective analysis of the success and safety of Gold Micro Shunt Implantation in glaucoma. BMC Ophthalmol. 2013;18; 13(1):35.
9. Rękas M, Pawlik B, Grala B, et al, Clinical and morphological evaluation of gold micro shunt after unsuccessful surgical treatment of patients with primary open-angle glaucoma. Eye (Lond). 2013;27(10): 1214-17.

23

Ishihara Electronic Color Blindness Test: An Evaluation Study

Hatem M. Marey[1*], Noura A. Semary[2] and Sameh S. Mandour[1]

[1]*Ophthalmology Department, Faculty of Medicine Menofia University, Shebin El-Kom, Egypt.*
[2]*Faculty of Computers and Information Menofia University, Shebin El-Kom, Egypt.*

Authors' contributions

This work was carried out in collaboration between all authors. All authors read and approved the final manuscript.

Editor(s):
(1) Jimmy S.M. Lai, Department of Ophthalmology, The University of Hong Kong, Hong Kong and Honorary Consultant Ophthalmologist, Queen Mary Hospital, Hong Kong.
(2) Li Wang, Department of Ophthalmology, Cullen Eye Institute, Baylor College of Medicine, USA.
Reviewers:
(1) Anonymous, India.
(2) Anonymous, Canada.
(3) Ricardo Franco de Lima, Department of Neurology, State University of Campinas (UNICAMP), Brazil.
(4) Anonymous, Turkey.

ABSTRACT

Purpose: Evaluation of computer based color deficiency test.
Materials and Methods: Two hundred and sixty seven volunteers have been checked using both traditional Ishihara plates and a computer diagnosis program using LCD monitors.
Results: The prevalence of red green color vision deficiency (RG-CVD) was 8.75% of male participants, no female participants were diagnosed, both in the paper based test, and in the computer based test. Computer based test gave 100% sensitivity and 98.78% specificity.
Conclusion: Presenting the computer based color deficiency test software on LCD screen can be used for screening of color vision deficiency with nearly similar sensitivity and specificity to the Ishihara test with the advantage reducing the cost through decreasing required resources over time, and decreasing the time to analyze the results.

Keywords: Color blindness; color vision deficiency; color vision screening.

---

*Corresponding author: E-mail: hatemmarey@yahoo.com

1. INTRODUCTION

Color vision is provided by three types of photoreceptors; sensitive to blue, green, and red wavelengths of the visible spectrum [1]. Color vision deficiency (CVD) could be congenital or acquired; the acquired form reflects a problem that occurred anywhere along the visual pathway from the photoreceptors to the cortex [2]. While congenital color deficiency is due to a genetic disorder where the color deficient person could miss one, some pigments, where anomalous trichromats are the most common, and they have an anomalous pigment in either the red or green cone [3].

Up to 8% of the world's male population exhibits a type of CVD. This is made up of 1% red-blind (protanope) and 1.1% green-blind (deuteranope) dichromats and of 1% red-insensitive (protanomolous) and 4.9% green-insensitive (deuteranomolous) trichromats. Only 0.4% of women have any sort of color vision deficiency. More than 80% of CVD subjects have one form of anomalous trichromacy, which demonstrates a milder and variable severity than those with dichromacy [4].

Due to abnormal cone characteristics, people with CVD may have great difficulty with color discrimination that affects their social life and careers [5].

Different methods are used for diagnosing color vision deficiency including; Anomaloscope, arrangement tests, and Pseudoisochromatic plates which are the most popular and easy applicable screening test [4]. Different test books have significant variations, and the pigment technology, and age of the test could affect the result of the test [6].

Ishihara color test is most often used to screen for congenital and acquired red green deficiencies, and the characteristics of the responses may change with the severity of the defect [7].

Computer software programs had been previously used to test different visual functions such as; visual acuity, stereo vision, visual field, and color vision [8-12].

This study was conducted to evaluate the use of computer software for CVD screening as compared to the results of Ishihara test.

2. METHODOLOGY AND VOLUNTEERS

A prospective non randomized controlled study was conducted in the period from January 2012 to June 2013, where 267 volunteers from the Menofia University Campus students were examined for red green color vision deficiency (RG-CVD). Announcements were made using posters in different places of the campus besides electronic announcement in different internet social groups. The announcements highlight the aim of this screening test, how, and where the volunteer would be examined.

2.1 Collection of Volunteers' Data

The Volunteers were asked to fill a registration form containing personal information; age, gender, residence, telephone number. Volunteers with vision disorders, other than requiring spectacles or contact lenses to correct refractive errors, were excluded. This study was approved by the clinical research committee of the Menoufia University Hospital and it followed the tenets of the Declaration of Helsinki. An informed consent were signed by all volunteers. These data with the results of examination of volunteers on the first 21 plates of the 36 Ishihara test and the computer based test were documented in a spread sheet of SPSS software program version 16.

2.2 Paper-Based Ishihara Test

To get the best results on color vision testing, the examined person should wear his/her vision correction whether spectacles or contact lenses. Any add-on materials in the vision correction aid that could alter color perception should be prohibited. The examiner (who was previously assessed and classified as having normal color vision) has to check these points carefully before starting the test.

Brand new Ishihara 38 plates were used for screening. A full CVD test has been performed using the first 21 numerical plates. As noted in the instruction sheet of this brand [13], examinations were done in ordinary day light (opened windows in the examination room in a non cloudy morning in the middle east area, with a sufficient white fluorescent lambs for room lighting), with no direct sun exposure, plates were held 75 cm from the volunteer and tilted so that the plane of the paper is at right angle to the line of vision, the numerals seen on the plates were stated within 3 seconds, and recorded by the examiner.

2.3 Computer-Based Ishihara Test

The first 21 plates of a brand new Ishihara color vision deficiency examination plates were scanned using HP Deskjet 1050 J410 all in one scanner with 600 dpi resolution, no adjustments or modifications of the scanned images were made. The test program has been written in Matlab code and converted to an executable program. The test has been performed on Acer Veriton M 290 PC (Intel Core i3 Processor, 4GB-Ram).

The test starts when the volunteer pushes the Start button of the first screen, where the first plate appears to the volunteer with the instructions of using the test. After submitting the first answer (all cases should answer it correctly), next plate is displayed one after another for 3 seconds only after which the image disappears and he records the numeral in the specified place, then he switches to the next plate. Fig. 1 shows a screenshot of the program. At the end of the 21 plates, the program summarizes the test presenting which answer is correct and which is not, final score and the final diagnosis decision according to the instructions sheet.

2.4 Screen Adjustment

The test has been performed on Acer Professional 24" Widescreen LCD Monitor with 1920 x 1080 Full HD resolution. To achieve an approximate accurate color reproduction, the following screen adjustments were made; the monitor was kept half an hour in operation. Monitor resolution was set to max. Color calibration process has been performed to insure the quality of the presented colors on the screen. The sufficient specs for this test were: Color temperature 6500° K, Color intensities of red, green, and blue respectively to 50%. Set in the "Control Panel" mode "true color" and "16 million colors".

2.5 Statistical Analysis

Validation of screening tests for CVD had been approached [12], which was guided by simplicity, acceptance, and reliability of the procedure; this validation was mainly focused on analysis of sensitivity, and specificity of the test [11].

Sensitivity is defined as the proportion of volunteers classified as having CVD among those with Ishihara plates proven CVD. While specificity is the proportion of volunteers classified as not having CVD among those in whom the disease was excluded by Ishihara plates.

Sensitivity and Specificity were calculated to the results of the computer based test using the paper based test results as a reference.

Screening inefficiency (SI) for each plate was used by Crone, which measures the quality of the discriminating ability of the each plate [11],

$$SI = \sum \text{(false positive answers)} + \sum \text{(false negative answers) divided by} \sum \text{(answers)} \quad \text{Eq. (1)}$$

Student t test was used to calculate the statistical difference between numerical variables, while the *Chi* square test was used for categorical variables.

3. RESULTS

The study included 267 volunteer, 240 males (89.9%), and 27 females (10.1%) with an age range from 19 to 23 years, with a mean 20.7 years, and standard deviation 1.34 years.

Using the paper based test, twenty one volunteers were diagnosed as having RG-CVD, all were males, with a percent 8.75% of male participants, and 246 volunteers were diagnosed as normal, no female volunteers were diagnosed as RG-CVD as shown in Table 1.

Table 1. Results of the paper based test

Diagnosis	Number of plates answered correctly	Number of volunteers	Total number of volunteers
RG-CVD	4	3	21
	6	3	
	8	3	
	10	9	
	13	3	
Normal	19	3	246
	20	18	
	21	225	

Volunteers were diagnosed as normal if they were able to read 17 or more plates correctly, and diagnosed as RG-CVD if they were able to read 13 or less plates only correctly.

Using the computer based test, also 21 volunteers were diagnosed as RG-CVD, and all were males, with a percent 8.75% of male participants, and 243 volunteers were diagnosed as normal, and three volunteers answered 16 plates correctly, so they were not classified as RG-CVD nor normal, no female volunteers were diagnosed as having RG-CVD as shown in Table 2.

The same number of volunteers were diagnosed as red green CVD by both tests, with 100% sensitivity of the computer based test compared to the paper based test, and 243 volunteers were diagnosed as normal in computer based test, when compared to the 246 volunteers diagnosed as normal by the paper based test gave a 98.78% specificity for the computer based test. Table 3 shows that the results of the computer based test was the same as that of the paper based test in 150 volunteers, where all volunteers answered the same number of plates in a correct way.

Table 2. Results of computer based test

Diagnosis	Number of plates answered correctly	Number of volunteers	Total number of volunteers
RD-CVD	6	3	21
	8	3	
	12	3	
	13	12	
Not diagnosed	16	3	3
Normal	17	15	243
	18	6	
	19	24	
	20	57	
	21	141	

In 102 volunteers the numbers of correct plates answered by the volunteers were more in paper based test than in computer based test, where; in

54 volunteers there were one more correct answer, in 24 volunteers there were 2 more correct answers, in 6 volunteers there were 3 more correct answers, in 12 volunteer there were 4 more correct answers, and in 6 volunteer there were 5 more correct answers, however these differences in the number of correct answers did not affect the end result of the computer based test whether the volunteer is a RG-CVD or not (Table 3).

In 15 volunteers, the number of correct plates answered were more in computer based test, out of them; twelve participants answered 1 more correct plate, and 3 participants answered 2 more correct plates, these differences in the number of correct answers did not affect the end result of the computer based test whether the volunteer is a RG-CVD or not (Table 3).

The mean and the standard deviation of the screening inefficiency for the paper and the computer based test were 0.04 ± 0.02, and 0.05 ± 0.02 respectively with no significant difference between both tests (P=0.092) (Table 4).

On comparing the results of both tests according to categorization into normal, and RG-CVD, we found that the same number of volunteers were diagnosed as RG-CVD, and 247 volunteer were diagnosed as normal by the paper test and only 243 were diagnosed as normal with the computer based test, without significant difference between both tests (P=0.0912) as shown in Table 4.

Comparing all answers to the whole set of plates, the paper based test resulted in 5376 correct answers , and 231 false answers , and in the computer based test there were 5310 correct answers, and 297 wrong answers with a significant difference between both tests (P=0.004) (Table 4).

Table 3. Difference between both tests regarding the number of correct answers in each test

Two test difference	Number of difference	Number of volunteers	Total number of volunteers
Number of correct answers more in the computer based test	1	12	15
	2	3	
Number of correct answers more in the paper based test	1	84	102
	2	24	
	3	6	
	4	12	
	5	6	
No difference			150

Table 4. Difference between both tests regarding the screening inefficiency, the categorization into normal or RG-CVD, and the total number of answers in each test

Variable		Paper based test	Computer based test	P value
Screening inefficiency	Mean	0.04	0.05	0.092
	STD	0.02	0.02	
Categorization into	Normal	247	243	0.0912
	RG-CVD	21	21	
Total number of answers	Correct	5376	5310	0.004
	Wrong	231	297	

4. DISCUSSION

Different tests had been used for screening of color vision deficiency; Cavanagh et al. [10] mentioned that at least two approaches are accepted to detect color anomaly, Ishihara plates and the American optical pseudoisochromatic plates. Long and Tuck mentioned that other methods can be used, such as Nagel anomaloscope or the Fransworth-Munsell 100-Hue test [14].

Pseudoisochromatic plates are the most popular and easily applicable for screening of color vision deficiency [4]. Several experiments have shown a high reliability of Ishihara test to detect RG-CVD [15-18]; however the printing technology, and the age of the test could affect the end result of the test [6].

Integration of tests of human sensory functions to computer can improve the quality of the results, reduces the required resources, and decrease the time to analyze the results [19,20].

There have been a number of attempts to develop methods of color testing based on computer software; Pardo et al. [21,22] have presented a system of characterizing red–green color vision anomalies by simulating the Pickford–Nicholson type anomaloscope on a cathode ray tubes (CRT) monitor. Toufeeq in 2004 has described an inexpensive computer based test for detection of color defect [23], also, Miyahara et al., developed a computerized system to diagnose red green color defects using Cathode Ray Tube (CRT) screen [24].

In 2007, Kuchenbecker et al. [25] has developed a German-language web-based color vision test with 25 pseudoisochromatic color plates based on the color plates of Velhagen and Broschmann and of Ishihara.

These entire computer based tests for examination of color vision deficiency used CRT screens, with some technical restrictions, that not all perceivable colors can be adequately presented on a CRT monitor [26].

Derefeldt and Hedin [27] investigated the spectral emission of colors on CRT monitors, and showed that certain shades of orange yellow and blue green colors cannot be represented on a monitor using CRT technology, this lead to the assumption that the spectral emission of Ishihara plates on a CRT monitor will be different from the spectral emission of the reflected day light on the paper plates.

In 2004; Pardo et al. [28] conducted a comparative study of the color gamuts that can be generated by three of the TFT-LCD, as well as of their variations in the chromaticity of the primary stimuli and of the white point as a function of viewing angle, and came to a conclusion that these monitors are valid for color vision research and diagnosis.

In this study, all participants were examined using the paper based test, and the computer based test with plates presented on LCD monitor, the prevalence of RG-CVD was 8.75% of male participants, no female participants were diagnosed, both in the paper based test, and in the computer based test, which is similar to that of Modarres et al. [29] (8.18% of male participants), and Buckalew et al. [30] (8% of male participants).

Computer based test gave 100% sensitivity and 98.78% specificity, which makes the use of computer based test convenient for screening RG-CVD without losing any positive cases, or misdiagnosing negative cases as RG-CVD, there were three cases that fall in the zone between normal, and RG-CVD, where volunteers did not fulfill the criteria to be normal, or RG-CVD with the computer based test.

Comparing the number of volunteers diagnosed as normal or RG-CVD by both tests, resulted in statistically insignificant difference, so, the computer based test could be used in screening of RG-CVD.

Comparing the total correct and wrong answers in both tests resulted in a significant difference, however this did not affect the reliability of the computer based test, as the total number of correct and wrong answers did not diagnose RG-CVD from normal, where it depends on the number of correct and wrong answers in all plates for each, not all participants.

Some plates are better detectable than others, this assumption was confirmed by Haskett and Hovis [31] where they found that plate number 7 is the one most misread by participants, also in this study, plates number 9, and 10 were the most misread (21 mistake in each test), for that, screening inefficiency was calculated for each plate independently, and the mean and the standard deviation values for all plates were calculated, and compared, which resulted in statistically insignificant difference between both tests, so both tests can be used for screening of RG-CVD without significant difference in the mean result of the discriminating ability of these plates.

5. CONCLUSION

Presenting the computer based color deficiency test software on LCD screen can be used for screening of color vision deficiency with nearly similar sensitivity and specificity to the Ishihara test with the advantage reducing the cost through decreasing required resources over time, and decreasing the time to analyze the results.

COMPETING INTERESTS

Authors have declared that no competing interests exist.

REFERENCES

1. Stockman A, Sharpe LT. Spectral Sensitivities of the Middle- and Long-wavelength sensitive cones derived from measurements in observers of known genotype. Vision Research. 2000;40:1711–1737.

2. Marre M. Investigation of acquired color vision deficiencies. Colour.1973;73:99-136.

3. Neitz M, Neitz J. Molecular genetics of color vision and color vision defects. Arch Ophthalm. 2000;118:691–700.

4. McIntyre D. Color blindness: Causes and effects, Dalton Publishing, Chester, UK; 2002.

5. Cole BL. Assessment of inherited colour vision defects in clinical practice. Clinical and experimental optometry. 2007;90(3).

6. Lee DY, Honson M. Chromatic variation of ishihara diagnostic plates. Color Research and Application Supplement. 2003;28(4):267–276.

7. Birch J. Diagnosis of defective color vision. Butterworth-Heinemann, Edinburgh; 2003.

8. Arden G, Gunduz K, Perry S. Color vision testing with a computer graphics system: Preliminary results. Doc Ophthalmol. 1988;69:167–174.

9. Bach M, Schmitt C, Kromeier M, Kommerell G. The freiburg stereoacuity test: Automatic measurement of stereo threshold. Graefes Arch Clin Exp Ophthalmol. 2001;239:562–566.

10. Cavanagh P, Maurer D, Lewis T, MacLoad DAI, Mather G. Computer-generated screening test for color blindness. Color Res. 1986;11:63-66.

11. Crone R. Qunatitative diagnosis of defictive color vision Am J Ophthalmol. 1961;51:298–305.

12. Cochrane AL, Holland WW. Validation of screening procedures. Br. Med. Bull. 1971;27(1):3-8.

13. Ishihara S. The series of plates designed for colour deficiency. Instruction sheet; 1917.

14. Long ML, Tuck JP. Colour vision screening and viewing conditions: The problem of diagnosis. Nars Res. 1986;35(1):52-55.

15. Birch J. Efficiency of the Ishihara test for identifying red–green colour deficiency. Opthal Physiol Opt. 1997;17(5):403–408.

16. Perales J, Hita E. Influence of some factors on non-typical responces to three tests of colour vision in children. Documenta Ophthalmologica Proceedings Series.1984;39:211-219.

17. Chapanis A. A comparative study of five tests of colour vision. J Optom Soc Am. 1984;38:626-649.

18. Mäntyjäri M, Karppa T, Karvonen P, Markkanen H, Myöhänen T. Comparison of six color vision tests for occupational screening. Int Arch Occup Environ Health. 1986;58:53–59.

19. Krueger H. Der betriebsarzt im spannumgsfeld zwischen arbeitsplatz begehumgund spezieller arbeitsmedizinischer vorsorgeuntersuchung aus der sicht eines arbeitsphysiologen. Zbl. Arbeitsmedizin. 1991;41:361–368.

20. Menozzi M. Der personal computer im einsatz beim screening visueller funktionen. Klin. Monatsbl. Augenheillkd.1995;206(5):405–407.

21. Pardo PJ, Pérez AL, Suero MI. A new colour vision test in a PC-based screening system. Displays. 2000;21:203–206.

22. Pardo PJ, Pérez AL, Suero MI. Characterization of dichromat and trichromat observers using a PC-based anomaloscope. Displays. 2001;22(5):165-168.

23. Toufeeq A. Specifying colours for color vision testing using computer graphics. Eye. 2004;18:1001-1005.

24. Miyahara E, Pokorny J, Smith VC. et al. Computerized color vision test based upon postreceptoral channel sensitivities. Vis Neurosci. 2004;1(3):465-469.

25. Kuchenbecker J, Röhl FW, Wesselburg A, Bernarding J, Behrens-Baumann W. Validity of a web-based color vision test for screening examinations of color vision. Ophthalmologe. 2007;104(1);47–53.

26. Walraven J. Color basics for the display designer, color in electronic displays, Plenum Press, New York. 1992;3–38.

27. Derefeldt G0, Hedin CE. Visualisation of VDU colors by means of the CIELUV color space. Displays.1989;10(3):125–128.

28. Pardo PJ, Pérez AL, Suero MI. Validity of TFT-LCD displays for colour vision deficiency research and diagnosis. Displays. 2004;25(4):159-163.

29. Modarres M, Mirsamadi M, Peyman GA. Prevalence of congenital color deficiencies in secondary-school students in Tehran. Int Ophthalmol. 1996;20:221-222.

30. Buckalew LW, Buckalew NM, Ross S. Note on color preference and color vision test performance. Percept Mot Skills. 1989;69:1039-1042.

31. Haskett MK, Hovis JK. Comparison of the standard pseudoisochromatic plates to the Ishihara color vision test. Am J Optorm Physiol Opt.1987;64(3):211-216.

APPENDICES

A. Figures

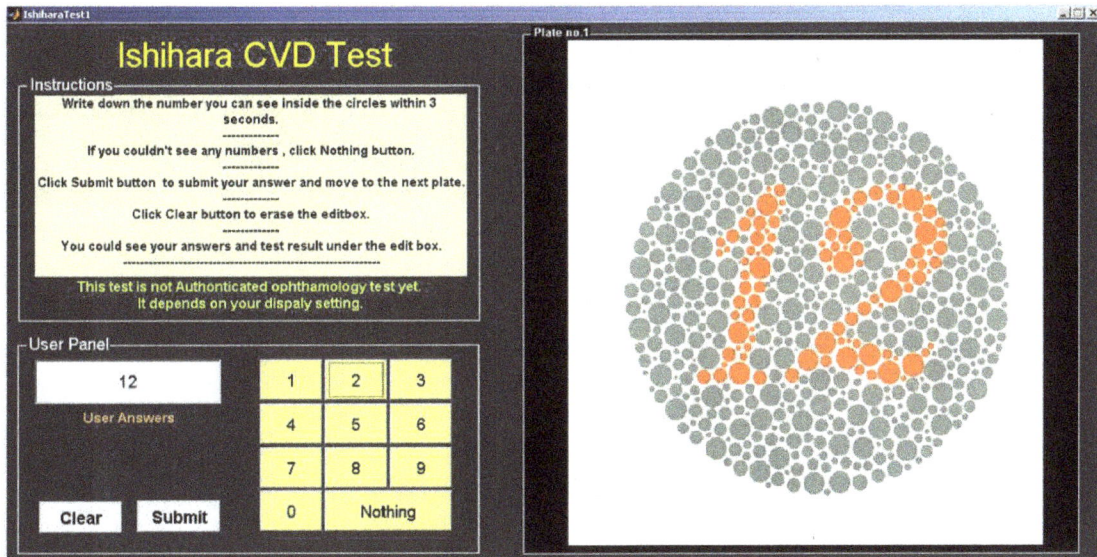

Fig. 1. Computer-based ishihara test

2a

2b

Fig. 2a and b. Contrast / brigtness screen adjustment test

Fig. 3. Color screen adjustment test.

B. Equations

Equation (1): Screening inefficiency.

C- Appendix

For actual reproduction of the test, the following target could be used to judge whether the monitor used is adjusted for best viewing. Set contrast to maximum and the brightness so that you can identify by black 11 degrees in the graphics in Fig. 2.a and 7 degrees (2 of white, 3 for gray and 2 for black) as in Fig. 2.b. Also, you should see red, green and blue graphics in Fig. 3 each of 2 different colors. If this is not the case, your settings are not correct, or your monitor is not suitable for accurate color reproduction.

24

Applications of Thin Films in Ophthalmology

L. Lamprogiannis[1,2*], A. Karamitsos[1,2], V. Karagkiozaki[1], I. Tsinopoulos[2], S. Dimitrakos[2] and S. Logothetidis[1]

[1]*Department of Physics, Laboratory for Thin Films Nanosystems and Nanometrology- LTFN, Aristotle University of Thessaloniki, Thessaloniki, Greece.*
[2]*Department of Ophthalmology, School of Medicine, Aristotle University of Thessaloniki, "Papageorgiou" General Hospital, Thessaloniki, Greece.*

Authors' contributions

This work was carried out in collaboration between all authors. Authors LL and AK collected the literature and prepared the manuscript. Authors VK and IT organized the structure of the review and contributed to the bibliographic search. Authors SL and SD revised it critically. All authors read and approved the final manuscript.

Editor(s):
(1) Rachid Tahiri Joutei Hassani, Ophthalmology Department III, XV – XX National Ophthalmologic Hospital, France.
Reviewers:
(1) Rahmi Duman, Bursa Sevket Yilmaz Training and Research Hospital, Department of Ophthalmology, 16800, Bursa, Turkey.
(2) Anonymous, Finland.

ABSTRACT

Nanotechnology provides a revolutionary approach to therapeutic challenges. Drug delivery, gene therapy, novel diagnostic methods and tissue engineering rank among the main fields of current nanomedical research. Thin films, with their unique optical and mechanical properties, are regarded as valuable biomedical tools and research is conducted to incorporate them in a variety of nanomedical devices. Main applications of thin films in ophthalmology include intraocular drug delivery, coatings for intraocular implants, scaffolds for retinal and corneal tissue engineering, novel diagnostic methods and modified intraocular lenses. A variety of chemical substances and nanotechnology techniques are used to fabricate thin films for ophthalmic use and it is clear that this burgeoning field may overcome hurdles and produce significant results that will revolutionize our approach to ocular diseases.

Keywords: Thin films; nanotechnology; ophthalmology; diagnosis; drug delivery; therapy.

*Corresponding author: E-mail: lamproslamprogiannis@hotmail.com

1. INTRODUCTION

Nanomedicine represents a multidisciplinary scientific field with promising perspectives in the fields of diagnosis and treatment of a broad variety of diseases [1]. Tissue engineering [2], drug delivery [3], novel imaging and diagnostic methods [4] and gene therapy [5] rank among the most important applications of Nanomedicine and commercialization efforts are expected to increase rapidly within the following years.

Ophthalmology is viewed as one of the medical specialties with the greatest potential to incorporate Nanotechnology advancements [6]. Relatively small size of the eye, the blood-ocular barrier and low permeability of drugs through the cornea, the conjunctiva and the sclera render ocular diseases excellent candidates for research at the nanolevel. Significant progress has been recorded during the last decades and development of revolutionary treatments for a number of ocular diseases is currently under way. Intraocular drug delivery nanosystems [7], corneal and retinal tissue regeneration [8], noninvasive diagnostic techniques [9] and gene therapies [10] with the use of nanoparticles lie at the epicenter of current research. It is reasonable to expect that Nanotechnology will enable us to address sight-threatening diseases such as age-related macular degeneration (AMD) and glaucoma in the future.

Thin films, developed and characterized with Nanotechnology methods, are commonly used as biomaterials because of their unique interfacial and mechanical properties. Application of thin films in medical specialties such as cardiology [11-13], orthopedics [14] and urology [15,16] leads to new approaches to therapeutic challenges. Obstacles related to safety and cost-effectiveness of nanotechnology research remain, however those are not insurmountable and thin films are expected to contribute significantly to biomedical research.

Primary aim of this review is to summarize and discuss applications of thin films in diagnosis, monitoring and treatment of ophthalmic diseases.

2. DRUG-ELUTING CONTACT LENSES

Low efficiency of ophthalmic drops is a common problem in Ophthalmology. Although they account for the vast majority of ophthalmic medications, they do not achieve a steady and uniform therapeutic concentration. Their absorbance is relatively low, they cause side effects related to the ocular surface and patient compliance tends to be insufficient.

Ciolino et al. [17] have suggested a drug eluting contact lens as an alternative drug delivery system. They have fabricated a prototype lens consisting of a thin film of poly (lactic-co-glycolic) acid (PLGA) that contained the drugs, coated by poly (hydroxyethylmethacrylate) (pHEMA). This dual polymer system provided zero-order kinetic drug release of ciprofloxacin and fluoroscein over a period of four weeks and therapeutical concentrations were achieved. It is underlined that storage of the prototype lenses is an issue that remains to be addressed.

3. COATINGS FOR INTRAOCULAR IMPLANTABLE DEVICES

Retinal photoreceptors degeneration ranks among the main causes of irreversible blindness. Retinal implants are viewed as a possible solution to this sight-threatening situation and great progress has been recorded in the design and fabrication of implantable stimulating devices. Li et al. [18] have developed biocompatible ultrananocrystalline diamond thin films to encapsulate intraocular implants, enabling ophthalmic surgeons to place them inside the eye without the risk of damaging interaction with the tissues. They have also fabricated bioinert materials with high dielectric constant based on Al_2O_3 and TiO_2 nanolaminate structures and they have produced high-capacitance capacitors which are necessary to allow intraocular implantation of the artificial retina. It is noteworthy that these advances may also be applied in other implantable biomedical devices.

Glaucoma is also a major cause of blindness worldwide. It refers to a group of ocular disorders that may lead to peripheral vision loss and eventually to loss of central vision. Although in most cases eye drops, if administered properly, provide a sufficient treatment, surgical treatment is often necessary. Implantation of glaucoma drainage devices (GDD), such as Ahmed glaucoma valve, may lead to satisfactory results, but fibrosis represents a common complication that reduces their success rate. Ponnusamy et al [19] have designed and manufactured porous mitomycin C (MMC) and 5-fluorouracil (5-FU) releasing thin films of PLGA, using a spin-coating technique. The double-layered biodegradable films provided a continuous release of antifibrotic drugs for a period of 28 days and may be used as coating for GDD implants.

4. DIAGNOSTICS

Optical coherence tomography (OCT) is a valuable tool that allows diagnosis and monitoring of a number of ophthalmic diseases, such as AMD, diabetic retinopathy and glaucoma. The growing impact of OCT on management of ocular diseases underlines the necessity of standardized assessment of OCT devices. According to Baxi et al. [20], thin films may contribute to the standardization process. Their research has led to the development of a retina-simulating phantom, consisting of thin scattering films of polydimethylsiloxane (PDMS), that mimics the optical properties and structure of retinal layers. Spin coating and laser etching were the methods that were applied in the fabrication of the phantom, which displayed promising results.

5. CORNEAL TISSUE ENGINEERING

The cornea is the outermost layer of the eye and it serves as a protective barrier for the eye, providing also over two thirds of its refractive power. Corneal disease may lead to blindness, with corneal transplant being the only therapeutic method in many cases. Corneal transplants' relatively high rate of rejection and failure and shortage of donors are obstacles that could be overcome with the development of an artificial cornea.

Young et al. [21,22] have conducted extensive research on cornea bioengineering. They have developed membranes consisting of chitosan and polycaprolactone (PCL) which may serve as a biocompatible scaffold for corneal endothelium. Endothelial cells demonstrated a satisfactory proliferation and they formed a continuous layer. Lawrence et al. [23] prepared optically transparent thin silk films and investigated their suitability for culture of corneal fibroblasts. While further research is deemed necessary, silk film biomaterials demonstrated promising results as scaffolding for corneal tissue.

Collagen has also been used to prepare corneal scaffolds. As Crabb et al. [24] have demonstrated, collagen films displayed suitable mechanical properties and may be used to produce bioengineered corneal stroma. Ozcelik et al. [25] developed poly(ethylene glycol) (PEG)-based hydrogel films with satisfactory optical and mechanical properties. These biocompatible, biodegradable films allow proliferation of corneal endothelial cells on their surface.

6. INTRAOCULAR DRUG DELIVERY SYSTEMS

Intraocular drug delivery represents a major challenge to scientists because of the unique anatomical and physiological characteristics of the eye. Nanomedicine advancements have been used to overcome obstacles such as the blood-ocular barrier and low permeability of ophthalmic tissues and to lead to more effective and convenient treatment of ophthalmic diseases. PCL thin films are often used in intraocular drug delivery applications and it has been demonstrated by Bernards et al. [26] that they are safe, structurally stable and well-tolerated.

Thin films have also been applied in novel methods of glaucoma pharmaceutical treatment. Huang et al. [27] prepared PLGA films loaded with timolol and observed a satisfactory intraocular pressure (IOP) lowering effect. Okuda et al. [28,29] developed a honeycomb- patterned thin film that can be used in filtration surgery in glaucoma patients that fail to respond to medication. In vivo experiments in rabbits illustrated that the poly (L-lactide-co-epsilon-caprolactone) thin film successfully protected the conjunctiva from MMc and reduced bleb avascularity.

Posterior capsule opacification (PCO) or secondary cataract, as it is also known, is a common complication of cataract surgery and it has been suggested that modified intraocular lenses (IOLs) may contribute to its prevention. Liu et al. [30,31] designed and fabricated PLGA thin films that were loaded with rapamycin and were developed on the surface of IOLS. In vivo experiments demonstrated satisfactory anti-inflammatory and anti-proliferative results.

7. RETINAL SCAFFOLDS

Retina is a unique tissue and it is involved in the vision process. Retina contains neural cells that are very sensitive if changes occur to the retinal environment. Therefore, the presence of the physiological barrier structure, the blood-retinal barrier (BRB), is of imperative importance in order to maintain optimal retinal homeostasis [32].

The BRB consists of the inner and the outer BRB. The tight junctions of the retinal endothelial cells that are covered by pericytes and glial cells form the inner BRB, while the outer BRB is formed by the tight junctions of retinal pigment epithelial cells (RPE) and the choriocapillaries that are fenestrated. [33] More specific, the retinal endothelial cells of the inner BRB form a tightly sealed monolayer, separating the retinal from blood side of the endothelium, and thus prevent paracellular transport of materials between the retina and the circulating blood. This paracellular impermeability of hydrophilic molecules is governed by the tight junctions in the healthy retinal capillary endothelium and the desirable molecules are transported to the retinal cells by a transcellular route. [34] These unique anatomical and physiological features of the retina impart the difficulties of a drug to reach and act through the circulating blood to the retinal cells. For these reasons, in the majority of the retinal diseases the drug is injected in the eye via pars plana, in the vitreous cavity.

AMD is the leading cause of blindness in patients over the age of sixty in United States of America. [35] Patients suffering from AMD have 10-15% risk of severe central vision loss. The majority of the these patients (75%) lose their vision due exudative AMD, which is characterized by choroidal neovascularization that invades Bruch's membrane and causes intraretinal hemorrhage and damage to the RPE. [36] Exudative AMD could be effectively treated with anti-vascular endothelial growth factors (anti-VEGF), which are injected in the vitreous cavity.

Bruch's membrane and RPE cells compose the outer retinal layer and perform a crucial role in maintaining photoreceptor viability. Degeneration of RPE cells and Bruch's membrane may lead to accumulation of metabolic cell products and decreased level of nutrient transport to the photoreceptors. [37] These alterations have impact on photoreceptor function and may affect visual acuity. A potential treatment of non-exudative AMD should prevent the degeneration of RPE cells and prevent also the alterations of Bruch's membrane. Potentially, replacing the outer retina with healthy RPE cells could prevent the damage to the photoreceptors.

Thomson et al tried to manufacture thin films of poly (L-lactic acid) (PLLA) and PLGA 75:25 and 50:50 biocompatible and biodegradable materials. [38] These materials were shown to be non-toxic when employed intraocularly for drug delivery purposes. [39] Furthermore, their degradation products are removed from the body through either the respiratory or the urinary systems. [40] PLLA and PLGA are approved for specific human clinical uses by the Food and Drug Administration. [41] The investigators manufactured the thin films using solvent casting technique. PLLA thin films could not be removed from the glass surface and they were not suitable for further experiments. PLGA films were easily removed. Despite the films were non-porus, RPE cells were found to attach on these substrates when cultured in vitro [38].

Other researchers design a synthetic biodegradable polymer substrate with specific chemical micropattern from PLGA and diblock copolymers of poly (ethylene glycol) and poly (DL-lactic acid) (PEG/PLA). [42] Previous experiments demonstrated that RPE cells cultured on PLGA films formed cell monolayers. [43] In order to improve RPE function, a microcontact printing technique was used to obtain thin films chemically micropatterned surfaces. The model thin films contained organized arrays of unmodified glass domains of micrometer scale separated by regions modified with octadecyltrichlorosilane (OTS) self-assembled monolayers. The investigators observed that the RPE cells cultured on these thin films retained their characteristic cuboidal morphology [42].

Tezcaner et al. [44] manufactured thin films from poly (hydroxybutyrate-co-hydroxyvalerate) (PHBV) in order to culture RPE cells. PHBV has been found to exhibit low toxicity and well tolerated by the tissue when implanted subcutaneously. No inflammation, abscess formation or tissue necrosis was observed in tissues adjacent to this material. The researchers manufactured thin films using solvent casting technique and functionalized the surface by oxygen plasma treatment. The investigators observed that RPE cells grown to confluency as an organized monolayer in treated PHBV thin films [44].

Lu et al. [45] tried to design a scaffold that mimic the Bruch's membrane in order to culture RPE cells. The film was made of cross-linked collagen fibers and exhibited diffusion properties, which allow the flow of nutrients and waste of RPE cells. The researchers also observed that the attached on the collagen film RPE cells formed an epithelial phenotype capable to phagocytize photoreceptor outer segments.

Other investigators designed thin films as scaffolds for RPE cells from polyurethanes. [46] Biodegradable polyurethanes, derived from poly (caprolactone), poly (ethylene glycol), isophorone diisocyanate and hydrazine have been developed by producing water dispersion of the polymers, following by a drying step and thus the usage of organic solvent is avoiding. [47] Also, these polymers displayed high elasticity and biocompatibility and they can be manufactured with the desirable thickness. [48] The researchers manufactured the thin films by casting the polymer dispersions in a Teflon mold and allowing them to dry in room temperature for one week. Culture experiments using RPE cells demonstrated the formation of an organized monolayer of cells, which exhibited polygonal appearance and the establishment of cell-cell interaction. Also, these thin films display the desirable mechanical properties for an easy transcleral-driven subretinal implantation [46].

8. CONCLUSION

Nanotechnology advancements play an increasingly significant role in ophthalmic research. It is safe to predict that nanodevices will contribute to the development of new diagnostic and therapeutic strategies in the future. Thin films technology is a valuable tool in the fabrication of nanomedical devices and it is likely to offer solutions to otherwise intractable problems. It is clear that issues such as safety and cost-effectiveness still need to be addressed. However, applications of thin films with their unique properties in Ophthalmology are expected to lead to revolutionary changes.

CONSENT

It is not applicable.

ETHICAL ISSUE

There are no ethical issues in this review.

COMPETING INTERESTS

Authors have declared that no competing interests exist.

REFERENCES

1. Thorley AJ, Tetley TD. New perspectives in nanomedicine. Pharmacol Ther. 2013;140(2):176-85.

2. Walmsley GG, McArdle A, Tevlin R, Momeni A, Atashroo D, Hu MS, et al. Nanotechnology in bone tissue engineering. Nanomedicine; 2015.

3. Park W, Na K. Advances in the synthesis and application of nanoparticles for drug delivery. Wiley Interdiscip Rev Nanomed Nanobiotechnol; 2015.

4. Ahmed MU, Saaem I, Wu PC, Brown AS. Personalized diagnostics and biosensors: a review of the biology and technology needed for personalized medicine. Crit Rev Biotechnol. 2014;34(2):180-96.

5. Krishnamurthy S, Ke X, Yang YY. Delivery of therapeutics using nanocarriers for targeting cancer cells and cancer stem cells. Nanomedicine (Lond). 2015;10(1): 143-60.

6. Zarbin MA, Montemagno C, Leary JF, Ritch R. Nanotechnology in ophthalmology. Can J Ophthalmol. 2010; 45(5):457-76.

7. Kim SJ. Novel Approaches for Retinal Drug and Gene Delivery. Transl Vis Sci Technol. 2014;3(5):7.

8. Kopsachilis N, Tsinopoulos I, Tsaousis KT, Meiller R, Dimitrakos SA, Kruse FE, et al. Cross-linking in an artificial human cornea via induction of tissue transglutaminases. Ophthalmologe. 2012;109(6):583-90.

9. Zarbin MA, Montemagno C, Leary JF, Ritch R. Nanomedicine for the treatment of retinal and optic nerve diseases. Curr Opin Pharmacol. 2013;13(1):134-48.

10. Zarbin MA, Montemagno C, Leary JF, Ritch R. Regenerative nanomedicine and the treatment of degenerative retinal diseases. Wiley Interdiscip Rev Nanomed Nanobiotechnol. 2012;4(1):113-37.

11. Karagkiozaki V, Logothetidis S, Lousinian S, Giannoglou G. Impact of surface electric properties of carbon-based thin films on platelets activation for nano-medical and nano-sensing applications. Int J Nanomedicine. 2008;3(4):461-9.

12. Karagkiozaki VC, Logothetidis SD, Kassavetis SN, Giannoglou GD. Nanomedicine for the reduction of the thrombogenicity of stent coatings. Int J Nanomedicine. 2010;5:239-48.

13. Karagkiozaki V, Karagiannidis PG, Kalfagiannis N, Kavatzikidou P, Patsalas P, Georgiou D, Logothetidis S. Novel nanostructured biomaterials: implications for coronary stent thrombosis. Int J Nanomedicine. 2012;7:6063-76.

14. Pleshko N, Grande DA, Myers KR. Nanotechnology in orthopaedics. J Am Acad Orthop Surg. 2012;20(1):60-2.

15. Maddox M, Liu J, Mandava SH, Callaghan C, John V, Lee BR. Nanotechnology applications in urology: a review. BJU Int. 2014 ;114(5):653-60.

16. Jin S, Labhasetwar V. Nanotechnology in urology. Urol Clin North Am. 2009;36(2): 179-88.

17. Ciolino JB, Hoare TR, Iwata NG, Behlau I, Dohlman CH, Langer R, et al. A drug-eluting contact lens.Invest Ophthalmol Vis Sci. 2009;50(7):3346-52.

18. Wei Li, Bernd Kabius, Orlando Auciello. Science and technology of biocompatible thin films for implantable biomedical devices. Conf Proc IEEE Eng Med Biol Soc. 2010;2010:6237-42.

19. Ponnusamy T, Yu H, John VT, Ayyala RS, Blake DA. A novel antiproliferative drug coating for glaucoma drainage devices. J Glaucoma. 2014;23(8):526-34.

20. Baxi J, Calhoun W, Sepah YJ, Hammer DX, Ilev I, Pfefer TJ, et al. Retina-simulating phantom for optical coherence tomography. J Biomed Opt. 2014;19(2): 21106.

21. Tsung-Jen Wang, I-Jong Wang, Jui-Nan Lu, Tai-Horng Young. Novel chitosan-polycaprolactone blends as potential scaffold and carrier for corneal endothelial transplantation. Mol Vis. 2012;31(18):255-64.

22. Tai-Horng Young, I-Jong Wang, Fung-Rong Hu, Tsung-Jen Wang. Fabrication of a bioengineered corneal endothelial cell sheet using chitosan/polycaprolactone blend membranes. Colloids Surf B Biointerfaces. 2014;116:403-10.

23. Lawrence BD, Marchant JK, Pindrus MA, Omenetto FG, Kaplan DL. Silk film biomaterials for cornea tissue engineering. Biomaterials. 2009;30(7):1299-308.

24. Crabb RA, Chau EP, Evans MC, Barocas VH, Hubel A. Biomechanical and microstructural characteristics of a collagen film-based corneal stroma equivalent. Tissue Eng. 2006;12(6):1565-75.

25. Ozcelik B, Brown KD, Blencowe A, Ladewig K, Stevens GW, Scheerlinck JP, et al. Biodegradable and biocompatible poly(ethylene glycol)-based hydrogel films for the regeneration of corneal endothelium. Adv Healthc Mater. 2014; 3(9):1496-507.

26. Bernards DA, Bhisitkul RB, Wynn P, Steedman MR, Lee OT, et al. Ocular biocompatibility and structural integrity of micro- and nanostructured poly(caprolactone) films. J Ocul Pharmacol Ther. 2013;29(2):249-57.

27. Huang SF, Chen JL, Yeh MK, Chiang CH. Physicochemical properties and in vivo assessment of timolol-loaded poly(D,L-lactide-co-glycolide) films for long-term intraocular pressure lowering effects. J Ocul Pharmacol Ther. 2005;21(6):445-53.

28. Okuda T, Higashide T, Fukuhira Y, Sumi Y, Shimomura M, Sugiyama K. A thin honeycomb-patterned film as an adhesion barrier in an animal model of glaucoma filtration surgery. J Glaucoma. 2009;18(3): 220-6.

29. Okuda T, Higashide T, Fukuhira Y, Kaneko H, Shimomura M, Sugiyama K. Suppression of avascular bleb formation by a thin biodegradable film in a rabbit filtration surgery with mitomycin C. Graefes Arch Clin Exp Ophthalmol. 2012; 250(10):1441-51.

30. Liu H, Wu L, Fu S, Hou Y, Liu P, Cui H, et al. Polylactide-glycoli acid and rapamycin coating intraocular lens prevent posterior capsular opacification in rabbit eyes. Graefes Arch Clin Exp Ophthalmol. 2009; 247(6):801-7.

31. Liu H, Zhang Y, Ma H, Zhang C, Fu S. Comparison of posterior capsule opacification in rabbit eyes receiving different administrations of rapamycin. Graefes Arch Clin Exp Ophthalmol. 2014;252(7):1111-8.

32. Yoshiyuki Kubo, Ken-ichi Hosoya. Inner Blood-Retinal Barrier Transporters: Relevance to Diabetic Retinopathy. Diabetic Retinopathy, Dr. Mohammad Shamsul Ola (Ed.), ISBN: 978-953-51-0044-7, InTech; 2012.

33. Kim JH, Kim JH, Park JA, Lee SW, Kim WJ, Yu YS, et al. Bloodneural barrier: intercellular communication at glio-vascular interface. Journal of Biochemstry and Molecular Biology. 2006;39:339-345.

34. Wolburg H, Noell S, Mack A, Wolburg-Buchholz K, Fallier-Becker P. Brain endothelial cells and the glio-vascular complex. Cell and Tissue Research. 2009; 335:75-96.

35. Klein R, Klein BE, Jensen SC, Meuer SM. The five-year incidence and progression of age-related maculopathy: the Beaver Dam Eye Study. Ophthalmology. 1997;104:7-21.

36. Ferris FL, Fine SL, Hyman L. Age-related macular degeneration and blindness due to neovascular maculopathy. Arch Ophthalmol. 1984;102:1640-2.

37. Turowski P, Adamson P, Santhia J, Moss SE, Aylward GW, Hayes MJ, et al. Basement membrane-dependent modification of phenotype and gene expression in human retinal pigment epithelial ARPE-19 cells. Invest Ophthalmol Vis Sci. 2004;45:2786-94

38. Thomson RC, Giordano GG, Collier JH, Ishaug SL, Mikos AG, Lahir-Munir D, et al. Manufacture and characterization of poly(α-hydroxy ester) thin films as temporary substrates for retinal pigment epithelium cells. Biomaterials. 1996;17(3): 321-7

39. Golgolewski S, Jovanoric M, Perren SM, Dillon JG, Hughes MK. Tissue response an in vivo degradation of selected polyhydroxyacids: polylactides (PLA), poly(3-hydroxybuterate) (PHB), and poly(3-hydroxybuterate-co-3-hydroxyvalerate (PHB/VA). J Biomed Mater Res. 1993;27: 1135-1148.

40. Gilding DK. Biodegradable polymers. In: Williams DF, ed. Biocompatibility of clinical implant materials (vol 2). Boca Raton, FL: CRC Press. 1981;209-232.

41. Vert M, Christel P, Chabot F, Leray J. Bioresorbable plastic materials for bone surgery. In: Hastings GW, Ducheyne P, eds. Macromolecular Biomaterials. Boca Raton, FL: CRC Press. 1984;119-142.

42. Lu L, Nyalakonda K, Kam L, Bizios R, Gopferich A, Mikos A. Retinal pigment epithelial cell adhesion on novel micropatterned surfaces fabricated from synthetic biodegradable polymers. Biomaterials. 2001;22:291-7.

43. Lu L, Carcia CA, Mikos AG. Retinal pigment epithelium cell culture on thin biodegradable poly(DL-lactic-co-glycolic acid) films. J Biomater Sci Polym Edn. 1998;9:1187-205.

44. Tezcaner A, Bugra K, Hasirci V. Retinal epithelium cell culture on surface modified poly(hydroxybutyrate-co-hydroxyvalerate) thin films. Biomaterials. 2003;24:4573-83.

45. Lu J, Lee CJ, Bent SF, Fishman HA, Sabelman EE. Thin collagen film scaffolds for retinal epithelial cell culture. Biomaterials. 2007;28:1486-94.

46. Da Silva GR, Da SC Junior A. Saliba JB, Berdugo M, Goldenberg BT, Naud MC, Ayres E, et al. Polyurethanes as supports for human retinal pigment epithelium cell growth. Int J Artif Organs. 2011;34:198-209.

47. Ayres E, Orefice RL, Yoshida MI. Phase morphology of hydrolysable polyurethanes derived from aqueous dispersions. Eur Polym J. 2007;43:3510-21

48. Da Silva GR, Silva-Cunha AJ, Ayres E, Orefice RL. Effect of the macromolecular architecture of biodegradable polyurethanes on the controlled delivered of ocular drugs. J Mater Sci Mater Med. 2009;20:481-7.

25

Post-stroke Visual Impairment: A Systematic Literature Review of Types and Recovery of Visual Conditions

Lauren R. Hepworth[1], Fiona J. Rowe[1*], Marion F. Walker[2], Janet Rockliffe[3], Carmel Noonan[4], Claire Howard[5] and Jim Currie[6]

[1]Department of Health Services Research, University of Liverpool, Liverpool L69 3GB, United Kingdom.
[2]Department of Rehabilitation and Ageing, University of Nottingham, Nottingham NG7 2UH, United Kingdom.
[3]Speakability (North West Development Group), 1 Royal Street, London SE1 7LL, United Kingdom.
[4]Department of Ophthalmology, Aintree University Hospital NHS Foundation Trust, L9 7AL, United Kingdom.
[5]Department of Orthoptics, Salford Royal NHS Foundation Trust, Manchester M6 8HD, United Kingdom.
[6]Different Strokes (London South East), 9 Canon Harnett Court, Wolverton Mill, MK12 5NF, United Kingdom.

Authors' contributions

This work was carried out in collaboration between all authors. Author LRH ran searches, identified relevant studies, acted as first review author, extracted data, entered data, provided content expertise and co-wrote the final drafts. Author FJR lead this review, provided methodological expertise, acted as a second review author, carried out analyses, and co-wrote the final drafts. Authors MFW, JR, CN, CH and JC provided additional content expertise, read and commented on final drafts and acted as additional reviewers where there was uncertainty or disagreement. All authors read and approved the 'final manuscript.

<u>Editor(s):</u>
(1) Yüksel Totan, Department of Ophthalmology, Turgut Özal University, Turkey.
<u>Reviewers:</u>
(1) Arturo Solís Herrera, Human Photosynthesis Study Center, Mexico.
(2) Italo Giuffre, Catholic University of Roma, Italy.

Corresponding author: E-mail: rowef@liverpool.ac.uk

ABSTRACT

Aim: The aim of this literature review was to determine the reported incidence and prevalence of visual impairment due to stroke for all visual conditions including central vision loss, visual field loss, eye movement problems and visual perception problems. A further aim was to document the reported rate and extent of recovery of visual conditions post stroke.

Methods: A systematic review of the literature was conducted including all languages and translations obtained. The review covered adult participants (aged 18 years or over) diagnosed with a visual impairment as a direct cause of a stroke. Studies which included mixed populations were included if over 50% of the participants had a diagnosis of stroke. We searched scholarly online resources and hand searched journals and registers of published, unpublished and ongoing trials. Search terms included a variety of MESH terms and alternatives in relation to stroke and visual conditions. The quality of the evidence was assessed using key reporting guidelines, e.g. STROBE, CONSORT.

Results: Sixty-one studies (n=25,672) were included in the review. Overall prevalence of visual impairment early after stroke was estimated at 65%, ranging from 19% to 92%. Visual field loss reports ranged from 5.5% to 57%, ocular motility problems from 22% to 54%, visual inattention from 14% to 82% and reduced central vision reported in up to 70%. Recovery of visual field loss varied between 0% and 72%, with ocular motility between 7% and 92% and visual inattention between 29% and 78%.

Conclusion: The current literature provides a range of estimates for prevalence of visual impairment after stroke. Visual impairment post stroke is a common problem and has significant relevance to the assessment and care these patients receive. Prospective figures regarding incidence remain unknown.

Keywords: Incidence; prevalence; visual impairment; stroke; recovery; review.

1. INTRODUCTION

Types of visual impairment following stroke can be complex including ocular as well as cortical damage [1-6]. Visual impairment can have a wide ranging impact on activities of daily living, independence and quality of life. Links with depression have also been found [7-11]. Many studies provide information on prevalence of various visual conditions from their sample based on cross section and case note observation studies [12-17]. Accurate estimates of prevalence or incidence of visual impairment for stroke survivors remains unknown. Determination of prevalence of visual impairment in a stroke unit is important in order to enable appropriate planning of efficacious referrals to an eye specialist for assessment, treatment and targeted advice [6,18,19].

The aim of this systematic literature review was to provide a comprehensive synthesis and exploration of reported evidence relating to visual problems after stroke with specific attention to incidence and prevalence.

1.1 Visual Impairment Definitions

Visual impairment is a deficit of visual function and includes abnormalities of peripheral vision, central vision, eye movements and a variety of perception problems [1,3,4,20].

Visual field loss is loss of a section of the field of vision and can either be central or peripheral. Following stroke visual field loss is frequently homonymous, with a loss in the same half of the visual field of both eyes. The types of visual field loss can include, hemianopia, quadrantanopia, constriction and scotomas [20,21]. It is also possible to have a loss of the central area of vision.

There are a wide range of ocular motility problems which can occur as a result of stroke including strabismus, cranial nerve palsies, gaze palsies, vergence abnormalities and nystagmus [22]. Strabismus is the misalignment of the eyes, which can be longstanding from childhood or occur as a result of an insult to the extra-ocular muscles or the cranial nerves supplying them. Eye movement palsies or pareses following stroke can include cranial nerve palsy, horizontal gaze palsy and/or vertical gaze palsy. Nystagmus is a continuous oscillatory movement of the eyes and is frequently associated in which both eyes move symmetrically. It may occur in every position of gaze or only be present in certain gaze positions. A further consideration is that patients commonly have multiple defects concurrently [23].

There are a number of different perceptual problems which can occur after stroke. The most recognised is visual inattention/neglect, in which the individual does not respond or attend to visual stimuli on the affected side. Other perceptual problems are also reported such as agnosia, visual hallucinations and image movement problems [24].

2. METHODS

We conducted an integrative review, aiming to bring together all evidence relating to incidence, prevalence and recovery from stroke-related visual problems. The review observed and is reported according to the PRISMA guidelines (Appendix 1). This review was not registered with PROSPERO [25].

2.1 Inclusion Criteria for Considering Studies for This Review

2.1.1 Types of studies

The following types of studies were included: randomised controlled trials, controlled trials, prospective and retrospective cohort studies and observational studies. Case reports and case-controlled studies were excluded, as they specifically look at selected cases and are therefore unable to report incidence or prevalence. All languages were included and translations obtained when necessary.

2.1.2 Types of participants

We included studies of adult participants (aged 18 years or over) diagnosed with a visual impairment as a direct result of a stroke. Studies which included mixed populations were included if over 50% of the participants had a diagnosis of stroke and data were available for this subgroup.

2.1.3 Types of outcome and data

We defined incidence as the number of new cases of any visual condition occurring during a certain period in a stroke survivor population. We defined prevalence as the number of cases of any visual condition present in a stroke survivor population at a certain time. We defined a measure of recovery as being present if prevalence figures were available at more than one time point post stroke. The visual impairments included are defined below.

2.2 Visual Impairment Definitions

Visual impairment is a deficit of visual function and includes abnormalities of peripheral vision, central vision, eye movements and a variety of perception problems [1,3,4,20].

Visual field loss is loss of a section of the field of vision and can either be central or peripheral. Following stroke visual field loss is frequently homonymous, with a loss in the same half of the visual field of both eyes. The types of visual field loss can include, hemianopia, quadrantanopia, constriction and scotomas [20,21]. It is also possible to have a loss of the central area of vision.

There are a wide range of ocular motility problems which can occur as a result of stroke including strabismus, cranial nerve palsies, gaze palsies, vergence abnormalities and nystagmus [22]. Strabismus is the misalignment of the eyes, which can be longstanding from childhood or occur as a result of an insult to the extra-ocular muscles or the cranial nerves supplying them. Eye movement palsies or paresis following stroke can include cranial nerve palsy, horizontal gaze palsy and/or vertical gaze palsy. Nystagmus is a continuous oscillatory movement of the eyes and is frequently associated in which both eyes move symmetrically. It may occur in every position of gaze or only be present in certain gaze positions. A further consideration is that patients commonly have multiple defects concurrently [23].

There are a number of different perceptual problems which can occur after stroke. The most recognised is visual inattention/neglect, in which the individual does not respond or attend to visual stimuli on the affected side. Other perceptual problems are also reported such as agnosia, visual hallucinations and image movement problems [24].

2.3 Search Methods for Identification of Studies

We used systematic strategies to search key electronic databases and contacted known individuals conducting research in stroke and visual impairment. We searched Cochrane registers and electronic bibliographic databases (Appendix 2). In an effort to identify further published, unpublished and ongoing trials, we searched registers of ongoing trials, hand-searched journals and conference transactions, performed citation tracking using Web of Science Cited Reference Search for all included studies, searched the reference lists of included trials and review articles about vision after acquired brain injury and contacted experts in the field (including authors of included trials, and excluded studies identified as possible preliminary or pilot work). Search terms included a comprehensive range of MeSH terms and alternatives in relation to stroke and visual conditions (Appendix 2).

2.4 Selection of Studies

The titles and abstracts identified from the search were independently screened by two authors (FR, LH) using the pre-stated inclusion criteria. The full papers of any studies considered potentially relevant were then considered and the selection criteria applied independently by two reviewers (FR, LH). In the case of disagreement for inclusion of studies, an option was available to obtain a third author opinion (CN).

2.5 Data Extraction

A pre-designed data extraction form was used which gathered information on sample size, study design, assessments undertaken, visual conditions reported, timing of assessment and population type. Data was extracted and documented by one researcher (LH) and verified by another (FR).

2.6 Data Analysis

Due to the heterogeneous nature of the studies, a narrative analysis was undertaken. The exception to this was a calculation to estimate the prevalence of overall visual impairment following stroke. Strict criteria of only studies using consecutive recruitment from a stroke population and reporting an overall prevalence for visual impairment were used for the mean prevalence calculation.

2.7 Quality Assessment

To assess the quality of the studies included in this review, two checklists were considered relevant to the study designs in our inclusion criteria: the STROBE (Strengthening the Reporting of Observational Studies in Epidemiology) checklist [26,27]. The checklist was adapted as the original was designed to assess the quality of reporting rather than the potential for bias within a study. There is currently no 'gold standard' quality assessment tool for observational studies [28]. The STROBE Statement covers 22 items covering the whole of the articles from introduction, method, results and discussion, which are important to consider when assessing the quality of observation studies (including cohort, case-control and cross-sectional studies). The adapted version used in this review included 18 items; only the information which is pertinent to quality appraisal of the studies was included. Using Boyle's recommendations for the evaluation of prevalence studies, the items exclude which were not considered relevant information, such as the title, abstract, background, setting and funding [29].

3. RESULTS OF THE SEARCH

The search results are outlined in Appendix 3. Sixty-four articles (26,321 participants) were included. Of the 64 included studies, none of which were RCTs, 52 were prospective observational studies and 12 were retrospective analyses. Consequently quality of study was assessed using the STROBE checklist. Although none of the studies were RCTs, one study was a retrospective analysis of data from an RCT archive [30]. Studies excluded from this review are outlined in a Appendix 4. Quality appraisal using the adapted STROBE checklist is outlined in a Appendix 5.

Seven of the studies (14,573 participants) reported on overall visual impairment. Nineteen of the studies (17,924 participants) reported on visual field defects; 22 of the studies (4330 participants) reported on ocular alignment and motility defects; nine of the studies (2097 participants) reported on central vision problems; and 13 of the studies (2885 participants) reported on types of perceptual visual deficits following stroke (including visual neglect/inattention, visual hallucinations, agnosia and reduced stereopsis). Several studies reported on two or more of these categories.

None of the studies included had a specific primary aim to calculate either prevalence or incidence of visual impairment following stroke. Fifty five studies were studies specifically investigated visual impairment following stroke, this included studies looking at specific visual problems such as visual inattention. The remaining 16 studies investigated symptoms and signs of stroke, which included reported visual impairment.

4. QUALITY OF THE EVIDENCE

Three paper reported 100% of the items requested by the adapted STROBE checklist [31]. Sixteen papers reported 90% or more of the requested items, 51 papers reported 75% or more. Sixty-one reported 50% or more and three papers failed to reach 50%, achieving 17%, 33% and 39% [32-34]. Only 36% of papers reported limitations of their studies. Results from all papers were reported and the individual results for each paper are outlined in a Appendix 5.

5. PREVALENCE AND INCIDENCE

5.1 Visual Impairment

Our search of the literature did not reveal any studies that specifically aimed to assess the incidence of visual impairment following stroke. We identified a number of studies that report an overall figure of prevalence for visual impairment. All these studies, however, were judged to have limitations relating to the methods of recruitment or assessment. Thus a calculation of incidence was not possible and estimates are calculated for prevalence.

Three prospective studies of stroke populations (n=709) report an average prevalence of visual impairment post stroke of 65% ranging from 62-71% (Table 1) [32,33,35]. These studies evaluated a general stroke population including medical and orthoptic assessments undertaken during the acute stroke phase within one week of onset to three months post stroke onset. Further to these three studies of general stroke populations, one prospective study (n=915) recruited a sub population of stroke survivors with suspected visual impairment who received full orthoptic assessment, typically within three weeks of stroke onset [6]. They reported a prevalence of 92% visual impairment. It is unknown what was missed from the general stroke population as not all individuals can report visual symptoms and referrals were evaluated to be more accurate when visual symptoms were taken into consideration in addition to ocular signs in comparison to ocular signs alone [36]. Ali et al., analysed results from a database for stroke survivors recruited to a variety of stroke-related clinical trials and reported a baseline prevalence of 60% visual impairment [30]. This cohort would typically include those who are able and willing to participate in a clinical trial and are therefore, not representative of the whole population, for example individuals with cognitive impairment and aphasia are less likely to be recruited [37].

Three studies (n=13,541) used a stroke assessment tool (NIHSS ± status questionnaire) which only partly assesses visual function [30,31,38]. The National Institute of Health Stroke Scale (NIHSS) is an assessment tool that only assesses for the presence of visual field loss and horizontal gaze problems [39]. Thus it is not a full assessment of the possible visual problems which can manifest as a result of stroke. It can therefore be argued that the numbers presented by these studies are not a true measure of overall incidence of visual impairment following stroke. In addition to the NIHSS, the Questionnaire for Verifying Stroke-free Status (QVSFS) was used. However this questionnaire only asks the patient about painless complete or partial vision loss [40]. The range of overall incidence of visual problems was 19-25.9% from these studies which was considerably less than studies with more comprehensive vision assessment methods.

5.2 Visual Field Loss

The reported prevalence of visual field loss after stroke varies considerably in the literature from 5.5% to 57% (Table 2) and most probably due to its dependence on the type and affected area of a stroke, inclusion criteria and the timing of assessments and the method of testing used [41-44].

Seven studies (n=1210) recruited stroke patients consecutively either as they were admitted to hospital acute stroke units or rehabilitation wards. Assessment of visual fields by confrontation and/or perimetry on admission after stroke onset detected visual field loss in up to 57% [32,33,41,45-48]. The mean prevalence of visual field loss after stroke was calculated as 31% [32,33,41,45-48]. These studies typically assessed patients in the acute phase with homonymous hemianopia or quadrantanopia defects most frequently detected.

In addition to the above studies, seven prospective studies (n=15,388) of stroke sub-populations report prevalence of visual field loss [21,30,43,49-51]. These sub-populations typically include only stroke survivors with hemianopic or quadrantanopic field loss or with suspected visual impairment of any type, or do not recruit consecutively. Thus reported prevalence is not representative of the full stroke population.

Prevalence of visual field loss has been described based on symptom reporting by patients in four studies (n=1362) ranging from 14.6 to 22.7% [42,52-54]. These reports are considerably lower and likely reflecting the poor reliability of detection by patient reported symptoms. In addition to those formally diagnosed with visual field loss following stroke, it is important to consider how many patients are unaware of their visual loss. Celesia et al. conducted a prospective observation study (n=32) to investigate the presence of hemianopic anosognosia [54]. From a sample of thirty two patients with homonymous visual field loss, 62% were unaware of their visual deficit. In a recent paper it was reported that only 45% of participants with visual field loss reported symptoms of the visual field loss [36]. It is important to note that not all patients had isolated visual field loss. Multiple visual impairments caused by stroke were reported such as visual acuity loss, eye movement abnormalities and perceptual difficulties. This discrepancy between those who do not complain of symptoms and have a diagnosis of visual field loss may highlight an under estimation in the incidence in this and other studies.

For studies whose population samples have solely included patients with visual field loss post stroke, it is not possible to establish prevalence. However, several of these studies have shown almost equal numbers suffering right or left defects [34,44,55,56].

5.3 Ocular Motility/Strabismus

Three prospective studies (n=1262) reported an average prevalence of all ocular motility problems as 33% (Table 3) with a range from 22% to 54%, [18,35,57]. Assessments were usually within the acute period and two studies used detailed orthoptic evaluation of eye movements and binocular vision [18,35]. Methods of ocular motility assessment are important to the accuracy of identification of eye movement abnormalities to ensure full detection of deficits in various gaze positions.

5.3.1 Eye alignment

Strabismus may occur as an isolated finding or in association with ocular motility problems and is reported in 16.5% to 52% of stroke survivors recruited to three prospective observation studies (n=626), with an average prevalence of 38% [32,35,58]. These studies used validated

orthoptic assessments to detect presence of strabismus, increasing their accuracy of detection. In a sub-population prospective multi-centre observational study, 19% of the sample were identified with strabismus [23]. Pre-existing strabismus was acknowledged in 2.5%, thus 16.5% were considered to be a direct result of stroke. The cause of the strabismus in 70% of cases was an ocular motility defect. Only 36% were symptomatic with diplopia, which highlights an issue in relying purely on symptoms alone. This study has a risk of under-estimating the prevalence, as the sample is not representative of the whole stroke population.

Diplopia is reported as a symptom in many papers which is a result of a misalignment of the eyes and a disruption of binocular vision. Other studies have highlighted the discrepancy between patients who do or do not report diplopia in the presence of strabismus or ocular motility defects. There is a risk that a proportion is not captured, if the symptom of diplopia is relied upon to identify ocular motility defects. The majority of studies reporting the incidence of diplopia limit recruitment to include strokes affecting specific areas of the brain [43,59,60], are retrospective [42,53] or required informed consent [61]. These studies cannot be generalised to the whole stroke population and also carry a risk of under estimating the true prevalence of strabismus.

5.3.2 Eye movement palsy

Seven studies (n=2783) report figures for gaze palsies including horizontal and/or vertical gaze positions and have a mean prevalence following stroke of 26% (range 18-44%) [22,32,35,43, 57,62,63]. These defects may occur in isolation or in conjunction with other visual problems, and are the most common of all ocular motility abnormalities [22,57]. Horizontal gaze palsies are more prevalent than vertical and complete palsies more prevalence than partial [22,32,35,63].

Cranial nerve palsies affecting the ocular motor muscles include third, fourth and sixth nerves with a mean post-stroke prevalence of 16% (range 3 to 39%) from three studies (n=2329) [18,32,43,57]. Third nerve and sixth nerve palsies are reported as being more prevalent than fourth nerve palsies in these stroke populations [18,32,64]. Where ocular movement assessment only tests horizontal gaze (such as with the NIHSS screening tool) the identification of all ocular cranial nerve palsies is limited. It is likely that more subtle nerve palsies and those involving the vertical muscles may be missed.

5.3.3 Nystagmus

Following stroke, nystagmus is reported in an average of 11% (range 4 to 48%) in three studies (n=438) [35,62,65]. In most prospective and retrospective studies reporting nystagmus, the specific types of nystagmus are not reported. This, in addition to lack of information regarding the method of assessment, makes it difficult to assess if the more subtle types, or nystagmus not present in primary position, have been missed. These factors increase the risk of an underestimation of prevalence. When reported, common types of acquired nystagmus are gaze evoked, multi-vector and upbeat [66]. The studies described to date, frequently report when the stroke has affected the posterior circulation, including the cerebellum [42,60,67,68]. No studies have reported the prevalence of nystagmus in anterior circulation strokes in isolation. It is, therefore not possible to estimate the proportion of cases which are potentially missed by restricting populations to posterior circulation strokes only.

5.3.4 Vergence

Clisby (n=140) reported 55% of patients to have reduced convergence and/or stereopsis [32]. Rowe et al. (n=243) reported reduced convergence from the initial ten month data set of the Vision in Stroke (VIS) study [69]. Using the gold standard 'normal' attainment for convergence of 6cm, 54% were judged to have reduced convergence. However, they also reported that 26% had convergence reduced less than 10cm, which could be judged to be a more appropriate standard for an older group of patients. Siong et al. reported 21% of the recruited population to have convergence reduced less than 15 cm [61].

5.4 Visual Acuity and Central Vision Deficit

Clinical assessment of visual acuity has been used to identify those with reduced vision and up to 70% of stroke survivors (Table 4) have been noted to have poor central vision [32,36,64,70]. The mean prevalence of reduced visual acuity post-stroke was calculated from three studies

(n=270) as 53% [32,64,70]. Methods include visual acuity assessment at near, a 3 or 6 metre distance. Further retrospective studies (n=447) provide information on the prevalence of patients reporting symptoms associated with a reduction of visual acuity [42,53]. A key issue identified by three studies (n=1045) related to patient glasses [36,64,70]. These were frequently reported as missing, or the glasses present were dirty, broken or the wrong prescription.

An important component of central visual function is contrast sensitivity, the reduction of which can deform image perception. Contrast sensitivity function has been reported to be abnormal in 62% of stroke patients (n=16) [71]. Different areas of the spectrum are impaired depending on the lesion site. For example, participants with parietal and temporal lesions have been reported to have reduced detection of low spatial frequencies whereas those with occipital and occipito-temporal lesions had difficulty with medium to high spatial frequencies [71]. Furthermore, reduced contrast sensitivity in stroke survivors, particularly those with severe functional difficulties, has been found to be associated with reduced activities of daily living [72].

Central vision is key to activities such as reading. However, reading difficulties may be caused by a wide range of visual impairments in addition to reduced visual acuity. Rowe et al. (n=915) reported difficulties with reading occurred in 19.3% of the sample [19]. The three largest associations with reading difficulties were visual field loss (61.6%, the majority of which were complete homonymous hemianopia), reduced convergence of less than 6 cm (45.8%) and saccadic abnormalities (45.0%). Other visual impairments associated with reading difficulties included reduced visual acuity (22.5%), perceptual deficits (22%), including 16.5% with visual inattention, nystagmus (12.4%) and diplopia (8.5%).

5.5 Visual Perception Abnormalities

The commonest form of visual perception disorder following stroke is visual neglect or inattention. The literature reporting the prevalence of visual neglect/inattention can be difficult to interpret. Often the different types of inattention (e.g. auditory, visual, and spatial) are not separated, so it is not always possible to isolate visual inattention.

Table 1. Overall visual impairment prevalence

Study	Design	Population	Time of vision assessment	Sample size (n=)	Prevalence of visual issue (%)	Co-existent ocular condition	Method of visual assessment
1974; Isaeff et al. [33]	Prospective observation	General stroke	Median within 3 months of onset	322	62	Yes	Medical
1987; Freeman & Rudge [35]	Prospective observation	General stroke	Median within 1 week of onset	247	63	Yes	Medical Orthoptic
1995; Clisby [32]	Prospective observation	General stroke	Acute period on stroke unit	140	71	Yes	Orthoptic
2007; Barrett et al. [38]	Prospective observation	General stroke	Unknown	505	19	Unknown	NIHSS and Questionnaire for verifying stroke-free status
2009; Rowe et al. [6]	Prospective observation	Stroke survivors with suspected visual issues	Median within 3 weeks of onset	323	92	Yes	Orthoptic
2013; Ali et al. [30]	Trial data	Acute stroke	Median within 1 week of stroke onset	11900	60	Unknown	NIHSS
2010; Gall et al. [31]	Retrospective	General stroke	Unknown	1136	25.9 23—male 29—female	Unknown	NIHSS

Table 2. Visual field loss prevalence

Study	Design	Population	Time of vision assessment	Sample size (n=)	Prevalence of visual issue (%)	Co-existent ocular condition	Method of visual field assessment
1973; Haerer et al. [47]	Prospective observation	General stroke	Unknown	265	25 – homonymous hemianopia/quadrantanopia	Unknown	Confrontation
1974; Isaeff et al. [33]	Prospective observation	General stroke	Median within 3 months of onset	322	17 – visual field loss	Ocular pathology	Confrontation
1989; Gray	Prospective observation	General stroke	Followed every 24 hours for 4 days	174	56.9 – homonymous hemianopia	Ocular pathology	Confrontation

Study	Design	Population	Time of vision assessment	Sample size (n=)	Prevalence of visual issue (%)	Co-existent ocular condition	Method of visual field assessment
et al. [41]			and max to 28 days		46.6 – hemianopia 10.3 – quadrantanopia		
1993; Benedetti et al. [48]	Prospective observation	General stroke	Median within 48 hours of admission	94	19.1 – homonymous hemianopia	Unknown	Unknown
1995; Clisby [32]	Prospective observation	General stroke	Acute period on stroke unit	140	47 – visual field loss	Ocular pathology	Confrontation Campimetry
1997; Agrell et al. [45]	Prospective observation	General stroke	Median within 3 months of onset	67	30 – homonymous hemianopia	Visual inattention	Confrontation
1997; Celesia et al. [54]	Prospective observation	Stroke survivors with hemianopia	Median within 24 hours of onset	32	100 – homonymous hemianopia 62 – asymptomatic	Unknown	Kinetic perimetry
2000; Lotery et al. [64]	Prospective observation	General stroke	Median within 3 months of onset	77	19.5 – visual field loss ¾ hemianopia	Ocular pathology	Unknown
2001; Cassidy et al. [46]	Prospective observation	General stroke	Median within 3 months of onset	148	50.6 - visual field loss	Ocular pathology	Confrontation Perimetry
2007; Townsend et al. [51]	Prospective observation	General stroke excluding receptive aphasia and cognitive impairment	Within 9 months of onset	61	16 – homonymous hemianopia	Unknown	Static perimetry
2009; Rowe et al. [6]	Prospective observation	Stroke survivors with suspected visual issues	Median within 3 weeks of onset	915	49.5 – visual field loss ⅔ hemianopia ½ asymptomatic	Ocular pathology Visual inattention	Confrontation Kinetic perimetry Static perimetry
2012; Tao et al. [43]	Prospective observation	General stroke: anterior vs posterior circulation	Median within 3 months of onset	1174	6.9 – visual field loss Hemianopia: 4.3 – posterior circulation 1.3 – anterior circulation Quadrantanopia:1.3 – posterior circulation	Unknown	NIHSS Confrontation

Study	Design	Population	Time of vision assessment	Sample size (n=)	Prevalence of visual issue (%)	Co-existent ocular condition	Method of visual field assessment
2013; Ali et al. [30]	Prospective trial data	General stroke	Median within 1 week of stroke onset	11900	51 – visual field loss: majority hemianopia	Unknown	NIHSS Confrontation
2013; Rowe et al. [21]	Prospective	Stroke survivors with suspected visual impairment	Variable over 2 weeks to 6 months	915	52.3 – visual field loss 54 – complete homonymous hemianopia 19.5 – partial homonymous hemianopia 15.2-homonymous quadrantanopia 0.2 – temporal crescent 9.2– constricted fields 5.1 – scotomas 1.7 – bilateral hemianopia	Yes	Confrontation Static perimetry Kinetic perimetry
2014; Siong et al. [61]	Prospective observation	General stroke	10 days to 26 years post stroke onset	113	26.5 – monocular defects 11.5 – binocular defect	Ocular pathology	Confrontation
2001; Lawrence et al. [49]	Retrospective	Stroke register	Median within 3 months of onset	1136	26.1 – visual field loss	Unknown	Unknown
2002; Rathore et al. [52]	Retrospective	Database stroke cohort	Unknown	474	14.6 – homonymous hemianopia	Unknown	Unknown
2005; Ng et al. [50]	Retrospective	Posterior circulation strokes	Unknown	89	53 – visual field loss	Unknown	Unknown
2011; Jerath et al. [53]	Retrospective	General stroke Male vs female	Unknown	449	22.7 – visual field loss (female) 20.9 – visual field loss (male)	Unknown	Neurology Accident & Emergency assessment Non-standardised
2012; Searls et al. [42]	Retrospective	Posterior circulation stroke	Unknown	407	22 – visual field loss	Unknown	Neurology assessment of signs and symptoms

Table 3. Eye movement disorder prevalence

Study	Design	Population	Time of vision assessment	Sample size (n=)	Prevalence of visual issue (%)	Co-existent ocular condition	Method of assessment
1975; Yap et al. [57]	Prospective observation	General stroke	Median within 2 days of onset	100	44 – ocular motility disorders 28 – gaze palsy 11 – impaired VOR 6 – cranial nerve palsy	Unknown	Unknown
1982; De Renzi et al. [62]	Prospective observation	General stroke	Follow-up every 3-4 days for 2 weeks post onset	91	28 – horizontal gaze palsy 7 - nystagmus	Unknown	NIHSS
1987; Freeman & Rudge [35]	Prospective observation	General stroke	Median within 1 week of onset	247	22 – ocular motility disorders 35 – strabismus (additional 6% pre-existent) 18 – palsies (skew deviation:3 1 ½ syndrome 6 Horizontal gaze palsy 57% Vertical gaze palsy 20%] 23 - nystagmus	Yes	Medical Orthoptic
1995; Clisby [32]	Prospective observation	General stroke	Acute period on stroke unit	140	52 – strabismus 44 – gaze palsy: 90 – horizontal with right hemisphere stroke 73 – horizontal with left hemisphere stroke 39 – cranial nerve palsy (mainly III) 55- reduced vergence and stereoacuity	Ocular pathology	Orthoptic
1996; Fowler et al. [58]	Prospective observation	Mixed neurological on	Median within 2 months of	239 (54% stroke)	26 – stroke-related strabismus	Unknown	Orthoptic

Study	Design	Population	Time of vision assessment	Sample size (n=)	Prevalence of visual issue (%)	Co-existent ocular condition	Method of assessment
2000; Lotery et al. [64]	Prospective observation	rehabilitation unit	admission	77	2.6 – third nerve palsy	Yes	Ophthalmology and optometric
2006; Singer et al. [63]	Prospective	Sub population excluding haemorrhagic stroke and posterior circulation ischaemia	Within 6 hours of onset	116	26.7 – complete gaze palsy 0.6 – partial gaze palsy	Unknown	NIHSS
2007; Rowe et al. [70]	Prospective observation	Stroke survivors with suspected visual impairment	Median within 3 weeks of onset	243	54 – reduced convergence <6cms. 26 – reduced convergence <10cms.	Yes	Orthoptic
2008; Rowe et al. [66]	Prospective observation	Stroke survivors with suspected visual impairment	Median within 3 weeks of onset	323	12 – nystagmus N=2 – pre-existent N=18 – oscillopsia/vertigo symptoms	Yes	Orthoptic
2009; Siddique et al. [65]	Prospective	General stroke	Acute period	100	4 - nystagmus	Unknown	Unspecified protocol
2009; Akhtar et al. [68]	Prospective	Posterior circulation stroke only	Acute period	116	48 – nystagmus	Unknown	Unknown
2009; Rowe et al. [24]	Prospective observation	Stroke survivors with suspected visual impairment	Median within 3 weeks of onset	323	54 – reduced convergence <6cms 26 – reduced convergence <10cms	Yes	Orthoptic
2010; Rowe et al. [23]	Prospective observation	Stroke survivors with suspected visual impairment	Median within 3 weeks of onset	512	19 – strabismus 16.5 – new onset 2.5 – pre-existent	Yes	Orthoptic
2011; Rowe et al.	Prospective observation	Stroke survivors with suspected	Median within 3 weeks of onset	915	54 – ocular motility disorders	Yes	Orthoptic

Study	Design	Population	Time of vision assessment	Sample size (n=)	Prevalence of visual issue (%)	Co-existent ocular condition	Method of assessment
[18, 19]		visual impairment			2/3 – diplopia 19 – strabismus (2.5% pre-existent) 10 – cranial nerve palsy (VI>III>IV) 58 - VI 26 - III		
2011; Baier & Dieterich [67]	Prospective	Cerebellar stroke	Mean within 6 days	21	33 – nystagmus	Unknown	Eye movement recording
2012; Maeshima et al. [59]	Prospective observation	Pontine stroke	Unknown	68	15.9 – diplopia	Unknown	Unknown
2012; Tao et al. [43]	Prospective observation	General stroke: Anterior vs posterior circulation stroke	Acute period	1174	8 – diplopia: 7.3 posterior circulation 0.7 anterior circulation 13.5 – gaze palsy: 11 – anterior circulation 2.6 – posterior circulation 4 – cranial nerve palsy: posterior circulation	Unknown	NIHSS
2013; Su & Young [60]	Prospective observation	Posterior fossa stroke: vertigo clinic	Unknown	70	31 – ocular motility disorders 45 – diplopia N=22 – nystagmus [45.5% multidirectional 54.5 unidirectional 86 - reduced OKN]	Unknown	Nystagmus – eye movement recordings
2013; Rowe et al. [22]	Prospective observation	Stroke survivors with suspected visual impairment	Median within 3 weeks of onset	915	23 – gaze defect: 15.9 – horizontal and vertical gaze palsy 69.7 – complete 13.5 – saccadic palsy 22.2 – smooth pursuit	Yes	Orthoptic

Study	Design	Population	Time of vision assessment	Sample size (n=)	Prevalence of visual issue (%)	Co-existent ocular condition	Method of assessment
					palsy 22.2 – impaired gaze holding 3.9 – Parinaud's syndrome 9.7 – INO 1.4 – one and a half syndrome		
2014; Siong et al. [61]	Prospective observation	General stroke	10 days to 26 years post stroke onset	113	53.1 – jerky eye movements 11.5 – restricted ocular motility 20 – reduced convergence (<15cm)	Yes	Optometrist
2011; Jerath et al [53]	Retrospective	General stroke Male vs female	Unknown	449	7.8 – diplopia (7.1% male, 0.7% female) 17.5 – nystagmus (4.6 male, 12.9 female)	Unknown	Neurology Accident & Emergency assessment Non-standardised
2012; Searls et al. [42]	Retrospective	Posterior circulation stroke	Unknown	407	20 – ocular motility disorders 15 – diplopia 25 – nystagmus	Unknown	Neurology assessment of signs and symptoms

Table 4. Central visual deficit prevalence

Study	Design	Population	Time of vision assessment	Sample size (n=)	Prevalence of visual issue (%)	Co-existent ocular condition	Method of assessment
1989; Bulens et al. [71]	Prospective observation	General stroke	Days to years post onset	16	62 – reduced contrast sensitivity	No	Ophthalmology
1995; Clisby [32]	Prospective observation	General stroke	Acute period on stroke unit	140	58 – reduced visual acuity	Excluded ocular pathology	Orthoptic with adapted visual acuity assessment for dysphasia
2000; Lotery et al. [64]	Prospective observation	General stroke	Median within 2 weeks of onset	77	30 – visual acuity ≤6/12 27 – no glasses available, dirty or damaged lenses	Yes	Ophthalmology and optometric
2006; Edwards et al. [70]	Prospective observation	General stroke with exclusions if unable to hold a pencil or severe motor or language deficits	Median within 15 days of onset	53	70 – reduced visual acuity 30 – 6/7.5-6/15 4 – 6/21-6/30 36 – 6/60-6/120 54 – no glasses available	Unknown	Near visual acuity
2011; Rowe et al. [19]	Prospective observation	Stroke survivors with suspected visual impairment	Median within 3 weeks of onset	915	19.3 – reading impairment: 61.6 – field loss 45.8 – reduced convergence 45 – saccadic defects 22.5 – reduced visual acuity 22 – perceptual defect	Yes	Orthoptic
2013a; Rowe et al. [36]	Prospective observation	Stroke survivors with suspected visual impairment	Median within 3 weeks of onset	915	31 – reduced visual acuity	Yes	Orthoptic

Study	Design	Population	Time of vision assessment	Sample size (n=)	Prevalence of visual issue (%)	Co-existent ocular condition	Method of assessment
2011; Jerath et al. [53]	Retrospective	General stroke Male vs female	Unknown	449	27 – loss of vision reported: 15.8 - male 10.3 - female 19 – visual disturbance reported: blurred vision, focus difficulty, photophobia, visual hallucinations	Unknown	Neurology Accident & Emergency assessment Non-standardised
2012; Searls et al. [42]	Retrospective	Posterior circulation stroke	Unknown	407	20 – blurred vision	Unknown	Neurology assessment of signs and symptoms
2012; dos Santos & Andrade [72]	Retrospective	General stroke with haemorrhagic stroke excluded		40	100 – reduced contrast in comparison to controls	Excluded ocular pathology	Ophthalmology
2014; Siong et al. [61]	Prospective observation	General stroke	10 days to 26 years post stroke onset	113	29.8 – vision worse than 0.3 LogMAR 11.5 – mild reduced vision (worse than 0.5 LogMAR) 1.8 – moderate reduced vision (worse than 1.0 LogMAR)	Yes	Optometrist

Visual inattention has been reported on average in 32% (range 14% to 82%) (Table 5) of stroke survivors from five studies (n=1800) [56,73-76]. These studies have recruited participants consecutively and have used a range of tests or tools for visual inattention including cancellation tests and the Behavioural Inattention Test. Studies (n=1335) using cancellation tests alone reported prevalence of 15% to 26% [73,75,77]. Those using a variety of assessments (n=991) for visual inattention reported a prevalence of 14% to 82% [56,74,78-81]. Discrepancies in the wide range of prevalence figures typically related to the timing of assessment plus inclusion/exclusion criteria of left versus right sided stroke lesions and severe cognitive and/or communication deficits. As expected, there was a greater prevalence of left versus right sided inattention.

In addition to visual neglect/inattention, the prevalence of other perceptual deficits are reported in the literature. Perceptual deficits, such as object agnosia, colour detection difficulties have been reported in the literature in very small numbers [19,23,24,81]. Our literature search found four studies reporting an estimated prevalence for different visual perceptual deficits following stroke [24]. Beaudoin et al. (n=189) reported an overall prevalence of visual perception deficits as 49.2% [82]. Rowe et al. (n=323) estimated the prevalence as 20%, of which the prevalence of visual hallucinations after stroke was 4% and visual agnosia was 2.5% [24]. It was reported that patients with visual hallucinations and other perceptual deficits frequently do not disclose these symptoms. This, in addition to the method of recruitment could result in an under-estimation of the true prevalence. Yang et al. (n=82) reported 50% of participants had pathologic (>3°) subjective visual vertical tilt following brainstem stroke [83]. Chechlacz et al. (n=454) reported 28% of participants with right hemisphere stroke showed left visual extinction versus 6.8% of participants with left hemisphere stroke showed right visual extinction [84].

Freeman and Rudge reported 79% of participants to have defective stereopsis [35]. Stereopsis was only tested in the pilot study (n=26), therefore the number of participants tested was limited to 19. It was also purposely not tested on participants with manifest strabismus even those which were a direct result of the stroke. The majority of those with strabismus would not demonstrate any

stereopsis. This would result in an underestimation of those suffering reduced or absent stereopsis as a direct result of stroke.

6. RECOVERY OF VISUAL FUNCTION

Our literature search identified just one study that appears to report the recovery of overall visual problems following stroke (Table 6). The majority that report recovery do so for visual field loss (Table 7). Ali et al. had the largest sample for tracking recovery of multiple visual problems following stroke [30]. However, not all visual problems were included due to the use of the NIHSS which limits assessment to visual field loss and horizontal gaze paresis. There was a variable sample size at the three time points used (baseline, 30 days and 90 days post stroke). The authors reported a reduction of visual problems to 28.2% at 30 days and a further reduction to 20.5% at 90 days, compared to the initial 60.5% at baseline. The sample size considerably decreased between baseline (n=11,900) to 30 days post stroke (n=4,965).

6.1 Visual Field Loss

Recovery of visual field loss is reported by a number of studies but across variable time periods (Table 7). The percentage of patients recovering from visual field loss ranges from 0% to 44% for complete recovery and up to 72.2% for partial recovery (n=6656) [30,35,41,46,55, 85-87]. Variability in recovery rates appears to be dependent on time of baseline assessment and length of follow-up, accuracy of visual field assessment methods and their sensitivity to detection of change, prospective versus retrospective studies and exclusions of severe neurological and communication defects.

Gray et al. (n=174) documented recovery in 47.8% of their sample, with a slightly higher proportion of 56.5% who had suffered a right hemianopia [41]. The macula was involved in 56.3% of the sample; 72.2% seeing an improvement in this and surrounding areas. They noted four different patterns of recovery, the most common (34.4%) of which was recovery of the lower quadrant. This was followed by complete recovery (25%), recovery of the upper quadrant (21.9%) and finally improvement in both quadrants with some residual defect (18.7%). They found that most improvement occurred between 6 and 25 days post stroke. Cassidy et al. (n=19) reported that of those patients who demonstrated some recovery, only 15.8%

achieved complete recovery at four weeks [46]. The majority of 42.1% had some central recovery and the remainder had quadrantic recovery. For a patient with complete homonymous hemianopia the recovery of the macula area can appear to be only a small recovery. However, this can have a considerable functional impact such as with reading ability. They were also able to demonstrate the reduced sensitivity of the confrontation method at detecting areas of recovery. Variances in reports related to whether the baseline visual field loss was complete or partial and/or congruous versus incongruous loss along with stroke-specific or mixed populations.

6.2 Ocular Motility Abnormalities and Strabismus

Less has been reported on the recovery of ocular alignment and motility problems following a stroke (Table 8). The percentage of patients which were reported to recover ranged from 7% to 28.5% for full recovery and up to 92% for partial recovery (n=6047) [18,22,30,35,62,66]. The greatest recovery was for reduced stereoacuity at 92% [35]. Sixth nerve palsies were reported to have the highest incidence of complete recovery of cranial nerve palsies at 28.5% [18]. At least one third showed no recovery across ocular motility conditions of gaze palsy, nystagmus, cranial nerve palsy and strabismus [18,19,35,66].

6.3 Visual Acuity and Central Vision Deficit

Little is reported on the recovery of vision following stroke (Table 9). We found one study (n=247) that outlined the recovery of reduced vision following stroke [35]. The majority (71%) showed some recovery. It is not clear from this paper what extent of recovery was made and whether this had been achieved at the one or six month follow-up.

Rowe et al. (n=915) reported the recovery rates for a group of participants suffering reading difficulties [19]. The data from follow-up visits was available for 42.9% of the participants. Of these, 10.5% had complete resolution of their symptoms, and 43.4% showed some improvement. A similar proportion of 44.7% saw no change in their symptoms and only 1.3% experienced deterioration in their condition.

6.4 Visual Perception abnormalities

6.4.1 Visual inattention

Four studies (n=5286) have reported recovery of visual neglect/inattention [30,35,79,88]. The percentage of recovery reported in the literature ranges from 29% to 78% (Table 10). In contrast to other visual impairments, patients suffering with visual neglect were more likely to require a longer stay in hospital and have a poorer prognosis for recovering function [73]. Recovery is mostly seen within 3 months post onset [30,35,79] with approximately 10% full recovery within the first 2 weeks [90].

6.4.2 Other perceptual deficits

One study (n=140) was found to report the recovery of visual hallucinations [89]. The authors reported that visual hallucinations (Charles Bonnet syndrome) persisted for several days or weeks after the onset of stroke before gradually subsiding. The median duration of visual hallucinations was 28 days and they stated that the first 90 days is when spontaneous recovery is most likely to occur.

7. LIMITATIONS AND RECOMMENDATIONS FOR FUTURE INCIDENCE, PREVALENCE AND RECOVERY STUDIES

None of the studies provided information about stroke survivors who were not admitted to a stroke unit/ward/rehabilitation unit. It is acknowledged that a proportion of stroke survivors have visual impairment only (usually occipital infarcts) but the numbers of these remain unknown.

The time of visual examination post stroke has a direct effect on the estimate of prevalence of visual problems that occur due to stroke. As recovery of visual conditions can occur rapidly in some cases during the first weeks post stroke, studies that assess visual function later than this early two week period are likely to detect those with persistent visual impairment. The extent of visual impairment for those with persistent visual conditions may also be misrepresented as these individuals may have had substantial improvement with only partial deficits remaining. Thus there is considerable potential for an underestimation of stroke related visual impairment.

Table 5. Visual perceptual impairment prevalence

Study	Design	Population	Time of vision assessment	Sample size (n=)	Prevalence of visual issue (%)	Co-existent ocular condition	Method of assessment
1987; Freeman & Rudge [35]	Prospective observation	General stroke	Median within 1 week of onset	247	79 – reduced stereoacuity	Yes	Orthoptic
1993; Stone et al. [56]	Prospective	General stroke	Median within 3 days of onset	171	82 – visual neglect [right hemisphere] 65 – visual neglect [left hemisphere] 28 – anosognosia [right hemisphere] 5 – anosognosia [left hemisphere]	Unknown	Modified behavioural inattention test
1997; Pedersen et al. [73]	Prospective	General stroke	At admission	1014	23 – visual neglect [42 – right hemisphere, 8 – left hemisphere]	Unknown	Cancellation tasks
1998; Cassidy et al. [79]	Prospective	General stroke with left hemisphere lesions excluded	Within 7 days and monthly follow-up	66	40.9 – visual neglect 74 – visual field loss	Unknown	Behavioural inattention test
1999; Cassidy et al. [80]	Prospective	General stroke with left hemisphere lesions excluded	Within 7 days and monthly follow-up	44	61.4 – visual neglect	Unknown	Behavioural inattention test
2002; Appleros et al. [74]	Prospective retrospective cases	General stroke	Unknown	279	23 – visual neglect [62 – right hemisphere] 74 – anosognosia	Unknown	Test battery
2006; Linden et al. [75]	Prospective	General stroke	At 20 months of onset	243	15 – visual neglect	Unknown	Star cancellation
2007; Becker & Karnath [76]	Prospective	General stroke	Median within 3 days of onset	93	26.2 – visual neglect [right hemisphere] 24.3 – visual extinction	Unknown	Cancellation tasks

Study	Design	Population	Time of vision assessment	Sample size (n=)	Prevalence of visual issue (%)	Co-existent ocular condition	Method of assessment
2009; Lee et al. [78]	Prospective	General stroke Left hemisphere excluded	Median within 2 months of onset	138	2.4 – visual neglect [left hemisphere] 4.9 – visual extinction 58 – visual neglect 22.5 – neglect dyslexia	Unknown	Test battery
2009; van Nes et al. [77]	Prospective	General stroke Excluded aphasia, gaze palsy, cognitive issues	Median within 2 weeks of onset	78	21.8 – visual neglect 88 – right hemisphere	Gaze paresis excluded	Cancellation tasks
2009; Rowe et al. [6,24]	Prospective	Stroke survivors with suspected visual defect	Median within 3 weeks of onset	323	14 – visual neglect 4 – visual hallucinations 2.5 – visual agnosia	Yes	Test battery
2013; Beaudoin et al. [82]	Prospective longitudinal	General stroke	At discharge to home	189	49.2 – visual perceptual defect	Unknown	Motor-free visual perceptual test- vertical version
2014; Chechlacz et al. [84]	Prospective observational	Sub-acute stroke	2.5 – 27.3 days	454	9.1 – left visual extinction 4.6 right visual extinction	Unknown	Confrontation extinction
2014; Siong et al. [61]	Prospective observational	General stroke	10 days to 26 years post stroke onset	113	5.3 visual neglect	Yes	Line bisection
2014; Yang et al. [83]	Prospective observational	Brainstem infarction	Less than 10 days post symptom onset	82	50 – pathologic subjective visual vertical tilt (>3°) 76 – ipsiversive 24 – contraversive 54.7 – abnormal torsion	Unknown	Computerised assessment

Table 6. Recovery of visual impairment

Study	Design	Population	Time of vision assessment	Sample size (n=)	Prevalence of visual issue (%)	Assessment
2013; Ali et al. [30]	Prospective	Stroke trial database	Baseline, 30 days and 90 days	11900 at baseline 4965 at follow-up	28.2 – visual impairment at 30 days 20.5 – visual impairment at 90 days Versus 60.6 at baseline	NIHSS

Table 7. Recovery of visual field loss

Study	Design	Population	Time of vision assessment	Sample size (n=)	Prevalence of visual issue (%)	Assessment
1987; Freeman & Rudge [35]	Prospective	General stroke	Mean 73 day follow-up 1 week to 6 months	247	33 – improvement (22 full, 11 partial) 25 – stable field	Confrontation
1989; Gray et al. [41]	Prospective	General stroke	Followed every 24 hours for 4 days and max to 28 days	174	Complete hemianopia: 17 – full resolution within 2-10 days 27 – partial improvement 39 – stable field Partial hemianopia: 44 – full resolution within 48 hours 28 – full resolution within 14 days 17 – stable field	Confrontation
1991; Tiel & Kolmel [85]	Prospective	Posterior circulation stroke Excluded communication difficulty and severe neurological deficits	Daily follow-up within 3 weeks of onset	125	47.8 – improvement within 6-25 days 56.5 for right hemianopia 56.3 – macula involved with 72.2 improvement of this 34.4 – recovery of lower quadrant 25 – full recovery 21.9 – recovery of upper quadrant 18.7 – partial recovery	Confrontation
2001; Cassidy et	Prospective	General stroke	4 week intervals up to 12 weeks	19	15.8 – full recovery at 4 weeks 42.1 – central recovery	Perimetry

Study	Design	Population	Time of vision assessment	Sample size (n=)	Prevalence of visual issue (%)	Assessment
al. [46]					11.1 - stable	
2013; Ali et al. [30]	Prospective	Stroke trial database	Baseline, 30 days and 90 days	11900 at baseline 4965 at follow-up	Complete hemianopia: 13 at 30 days 10 at 90 days Versus 35% at baseline Partial hemianopia: 11 at 90 days Versus 14.5% at baseline	NIHSS Confrontation
2006 Zhang et al. [87]	Retrospective	Mixed population	Median 3 months of onset Change at 3 and 6 months	254	3 – full recovery 34 – partial 63 – stable field	Perimetry Central 30 or 24 degrees
2007; Schmielau & Wong [86]	Prospective	Mixed population	Change at 1 through to 105 months post onset	20	61.5 – improvement	Kinetic perimetry
2007; Kedar et al. [55]	Retrospective	Mixed population	Median 3 days post onset	852	Congruous hemianopia: 38.1 – improvement 58.5 – stable field 3.4 – deteriorated Incongruous hemianopia: 39.6 – improvement 41.5 – stable field 18.9 – deteriorated	Perimetry Central 30 or 24 degrees
2013c; Rowe et al. [21]	Prospective	Stroke survivors with suspected visual impairment	Variable over 2 weeks to 6 months	915	7.5 – full recovery 39.2 – partial recovery 1 – deterioration 52.3 – static	Confrontation Static perimetry Kinetic perimetry

Table 8. Recovery of eye movement deficits

Study	Design	Population	Time of vision assessment	Sample size (n=)	Prevalence of visual issue (%)	Assessment
1982; De Renzi et al. [62]	Prospective	General stroke	Follow-up every 3-4 days for 2 weeks post onset	91	8.6 days - mean duration to improvement with left stroke 14.9 – mean duration to improvement with right stroke	NIHSS
1987; Freeman & Rudge [35]	Prospective	General stroke	Up to 12 months post onset	76	7 – full improvement 50 – partial improvement 43 – stable 92 – improvement in stereoacuity within 1 month	Orthoptic
2011; Rowe et al. [18]	Prospective	Stroke survivors with suspected visual impairment	Variable over 2 weeks to 6 months	915	Cranial nerve palsy: 22.5 – full improvement 43 – partial improvement 3.5 – deterioration Nystagmus: 42 – partial improvement 24 – stable Gaze palsy: 4 – full improvement 66 – partial improvement 30 - stable	Orthoptic
2013; Ali et al. [30]	Prospective	Stroke trial database	Baseline, 30 days and 90 days	11900 at baseline 4965 at follow-up	Complete gaze palsy: - at 30 days Versus 14.5% at baseline Partial gaze palsy: 9 – at 30 days Versus 31% at baseline	NIHSS Confrontation

Table 9. Recovery of central vision deficit

Study	Design	Population	Time of vision assessment	Sample size (n=)	Prevalence of visual issue (%)	Assessment
1987; Freeman & Rudge [35]	Prospective observation	General stroke	Median within 1 week of onset	247	71 – improvement	Medical Orthoptic
2011; Rowe et al. [19]	Prospective	Stroke survivors with suspected visual impairment	Variable over 2 weeks to 6 months	915	10.5 – full improvement 43.4 – partial improvement 44.7 – stable 1.3 - deteriorated	Orthoptic

Table 10. Recovery of visual perceptual impairment

Study	Design	Population	Time of vision assessment	Sample size (n=)	Prevalence of visual issue (%)	Assessment
1987; Freeman & Rudge [35]	Prospective	General stroke	Up to 4 months post onset	247	Visual neglect: 29 – complete recovery 57 - stable	Medical Orthoptic
1998; Cassidy et al. [79]	Prospective	General stroke with left hemisphere lesions excluded	Monthly follow-up	66	9.1 – visual neglect at 3 months Versus 40.9% at baseline	Behavioural inattention test
2004; Farne et al. [88]	Prospective	R hemisphere only	Follow-up at 2 weeks and 3 months post onset	33 at baseline 8 at 3 months	43 – improvement at 2 weeks [9 – full] 63 – improvement at 3 months	Behavioural inattention test
2007; Poggel et al. [89]	Prospective	Post-geniculate lesions	Mean 36 months (7-189 months), up to 6 months follow-up.	19	Visual hallucinations persisted for several days/weeks and then gradually subsided	Interview
2007; Poggel et al. [89]	Retrospective questionnaire	Mixed population	Up to 6 months follow-up	121	Mean duration of 28 days	Questionnaire
2013; Ali et al. [30]	Prospective	Stroke trial database	Baseline, 30 days and 90 days	11900 at baseline 4965 at follow-up	0.6 – visual neglect at 90 days Versus 27.7% at baseline	NIHSS Confrontation

Accuracy of non-specialist vision assessments and accuracy of screening tools and scores is likely to impact on reported prevalence figures. Where basic screening is undertaken, it is possible to miss subtle visual problems whose ocular signs are not included in the screening assessment. Thus there is the potential for underdiagnoses when the assessment is performed by the stroke team rather than an eye team specialist or where screening tools are used which only measure specific features of vision, e.g. detection of hemianopia or horizontal gaze defects only as with the NIHSS, or reliance on basic confrontation assessment rather than detailed confrontation or perimetry assessment.

Studies that report sub populations of stroke survivors are also prone to reporting bias for visual problems. Despite large sample sizes in studies that have included sub populations of stroke survivors, such as the VIS study of those already suspected of having visual impairment or studies of clinical trial databases, these studies are unlikely to be representative of the general stroke population [6, 30]. These estimates are potential under- or over-representations of the true prevalence of visual problems across all stroke survivors.

The time of the baseline assessment is crucial for studies tracking the recovery of visual impairment. If the baseline assessment is delayed, complete or partial recovery may have already taken place. Furthermore, it has not yet been accurately established at what time point recovery of each visual problem following stroke can be expected. If a study only has short period of follow-up, recovery could continue after the participant has completed the study. Both factors result in under-estimation of recovery of stroke-related visual impairment.

Future studies are required to establish the incidence for post-stroke visual impairment in the early acute period within the first week of onset. Such studies should involve a full stroke cohort with no exclusions so that visual impairment rates are comprehensively evaluated. These patients require follow-up at regular time intervals to plot change in visual impairment over the first week, first month and longer term after stroke onset to provide information on trajectory of improvement, if any, and rates for full, partial or no recovery. At baseline and follow-up visits, full specialist assessment is required such that subtle visual deficits that can cause visual impairment are not missed.

8. CONCLUSIONS

The literature currently available for review does not include any studies whose primary aim was to determine incidence or prevalence of visual impairment post stroke. Thus, this review can only provide estimates of prevalence for individual stroke related visual problems. The estimation of the overall prevalence of visual impairment was approximately 65% at baseline assessment. A reduction to approximately 20% is seen by three month post stroke, due to factors such as recovery, adaptation and death. The figures reported cover a wide range of prevalence for each visual problem. A variety of factors may be the cause of this wide range of figures including; the different study aims, research methods used, baseline assessments being conducted at different time points and different methods assessment. The prevalence is reported as being highest for eye movement defects, visual field loss and visual inattention. The existing literature regarding the recovery of visual problems following stroke is scarce for both individual deficits and overall visual recovery. Further prospective studies are required to establish the incidence of post-stroke visual impairment, the prevalence at various time periods post stroke and trajectory of improvement.

ETHICAL APPROVAL

It is not applicable.

ACKNOWLEDGEMENTS

This review was supported by funding from the Stroke Association and Thomas Pocklington Trust. We acknowledge the advice received from Professor Rumona Dickson, University of Liverpool, and Dr Alex Pollock, Glasgow Caledonian University.

COMPETING INTERESTS

Authors have declared that no competing interests exist.

REFERENCES

1.   Pollock A, et al. Interventions for disorders of eye movement in patients with stroke. Cochrane Database of Systematic Reviews. 2011;10.

2.   Pollock A, et al. Interventions for visual field defects in patients with stroke. Cochrane Database of Systematic Reviews. 2011;10.

3.   Pollock A, et al. Interventions for age-related visual problems in patients with stroke. Cochrane Database of Systematic Reviews. 2012;3.

4.   Bowen A et al. Cognitive rehabilitation for spatial neglect following stroke. Cochrane Database of Systematic Reviews. 2013;7.

5.   Jones SA, Shinton RA. Improving outcome in stroke patients with visual problems. Age & Ageing. 2006;35(6):560-565.

6.   Rowe F et al. Visual impairment following stroke: do stroke patients require vision assessment? Age & Ageing. 2009;38(2): 188-193.

7.   Granger CV et al. Functional assessment scales: A study of persons after stroke. Archives of Physical Medicine & Rehabilitation. 1993;74(2):133-138.

8.   Nelles G, et al. Compensatory visual field training for patients with hemianopia after stroke. Neuroscience Letters. 2001;306(3): 189-192.

9.   Ramrattan RS, et al. Prevalence and causes of visual field loss in the elderly and associations with impairment in daily functioning: The rotterdam study. Archives of Ophthalmology. 2001;119(12): 1788-1794.

10. West CG, et al. Is vision function related to physical functional ability in older adults? Journal of the American Geriatrics Society. 2002;50(1):136-145.

11. Tsai SY, et al. Association between visual impairment and depression in the elderly. Journal of the Formosan Medical Association. 2003;102(2):86-90.

12. Maberley DAL, et al. The prevalence of low vision and blindness in Canada. Eye. 2006;20(3):341-346.

13. Hyman L, et al. Prevalence and causes of visual impairment in the Barbados eye study1. Ophthalmology. 2001;108(10): 1751-1756.

14. Hsu WM, et al. Prevalence and causes of visual impairment in an elderly Chinese population in Taiwan1: The shihpai eye study. Ophthalmology. 2004;111(1):62-69.

15. Rodriguez J, et al. Causes of blindness and visual impairment in a population-based sample of U.S. Hispanics. Ophthalmology. 2002;109(4):737-743.

16. Klein R, Klein BEK, Lee KE. Changes in visual acuity in a population. Ophthalmology. 1996;103(8):1169-1178.

17. Marmamula S, et al. A cross-sectional study of visual impairment in elderly population in residential care in the South Indian state of Andhra Pradesh: A cross-sectional study. BMJ Open. 2013;3(3).

18. Rowe F. Prevalence of ocular motor cranial nerve palsy and associations following stroke. Eye. 2011;25(7):881-887.

19. Rowe F, et al. Reading difficulty after stroke: Ocular and non ocular causes. International Journal of Stroke. 2011;6(5): 404-411.

20. Pollock A, et al. Interventions for visual field defects in patients with stroke. Stroke. 2012;43(4):e37-e38.

21. Rowe F et al. A prospective profile of visual field loss following stroke: Prevalence, type, rehabilitation and outcome. Bio Med Research International; 2013.

22. Rowe F, et al. Profile of gaze dysfunction following cerebro vascular accident. ISRN Ophthalmology; 2013.

23. Rowe F, et al. The profile of strabismus in stroke survivors. Eye. 2010;24(4):682-685.

24. Rowe F. Visual perceptual consequences of stroke. Strabismus. 2009;17(1):24-28.

25. University of York centre for reviews and dissemination. PROSPERO: International prospective register of systematic reviews. 2013;27:2015. Available:http://www.crd.york.ac.uk/PROSPERO/

26. Von Elm E, et al. Strengthening the reporting of observational studies in epidemiology (STROBE): Guidelines for reporting observational studies. Plos Medicine. 2007;4(10):1623-1627.

27. Vandenbroucke JP, et al. Strengthening the reporting of observational studies in epidemiology (STROBE): Explanation and elaboration. Plos Medicine. 2007;4(10): 1628-1654.

28. Sanderson S, Tatt ID, Higgins JP. Tools for assessing quality and susceptibility to bias in observational studies in epidemiology: A systematic review and annotated bibliography. International Journal of Epidemiology. 2007;36(3):666-676.

29. Boyle MH, Guidelines for evaluating prevalence studies. Evidence-Based Mental Health. 1998;1(2):37-39.

30. Ali M, et al. Recovery from poststroke visual impairment: Evidence from a clinical

trials resource. Neurorehabilitation & Neural Repair. 2013;27(2):133-141.

31. Gall SL, et al. Sex differences in presentation, severity, and management of stroke in a population-based study. Neurology. 2010;74(12):975-981.

32. Clisby C. Visual assessment of patients with cerebrovascular accident on the elderly care wards. British Orthoptic Journal. 1995;52:38-41.

33. Isaeff WB, Wallar PH, Duncan G. Ophthalmic findings in 322 patients with a cerebral vascular accident. Annals of Ophthalmology. 1974;6(10):1059-1064.

34. Trobe JD, Lorber ML, Schlezinger NS. Isolated homonymous hemianopia. A review of 104 cases. Archives of Ophthalmology. 1973;89(5):377-381.

35. Freeman CF, Rudge NB. The orthoptist's role in the management of stroke patients. in 6th International Orthoptic Congress. Harrogate, UK; 1987.

36. Rowe F, et al. Symptoms of stroke-related visual impairment. Strabismus. 2013;21(2):150-154.

37. Rothwell PM, External validity of randomised controlled trials: "To whom do the results of this trial apply?" The Lancet. 2005;365(9453):82-93.

38. Barrett KM, et al. Sex differences in stroke severity, symptoms, and deficits after first-ever ischemic stroke. Journal of Stroke & Cerebrovascular Diseases. 2007;16(1):34-39.

39. Lyden P, et al. Underlying structure of the national institutes of health stroke scale: Results of a factor analysis. Stroke. 1999;30(11):2347-2354.

40. Jones WJ, Williams LS, Meschia JF, Validating the questionnaire for verifying stroke-Free status (Qvsfs) by neurological history and examination. Stroke. 2001;32(10):2232-2236.

41. Gray CS, et al. Recovery of visual fields in acute stroke: Homonymous hemianopia associated with adverse prognosis. Age and Ageing. 1989;18(6):419-421.

42. Searls DE, et al. Symptoms and signs of posterior circulation ischemia in the new England medical center posterior circulation registry. Archives of Neurology. 2012;69(3):346-351.

43. Tao WD, et al. Posterior versus anterior circulation infarction: How different are the neurological deficits? Stroke. 2012;43(8):2060-2065.

44. Zhang X, et al. Homonymous hemianopias: Clinical-anatomic correlations in 904 cases. Neurology. 2006;66(6):906-910.

45. Agrell BM, Dehlin OI, Dahlgren CJ. Neglect in elderly stroke patients: A comparison of five tests. Psychiatry and Clinical Neurosciences. 1997;51(5):295-300.

46. Cassidy TP, Bruce DW, Gray CS, Visual field loss after stroke: Confrontation and perimetry in the assessment of recovery. Journal of Stroke and Cerebrovascular Diseases. 2001;10(3):113-117.

47. Haerer AF. Visual field defects and the prognosis of stroke patients. Stroke. 1973;4(2):163-168.

48. Benedetti MD, et al. Short term prognosis of stroke in a clinical series of 94 patients. The Italian Journal of Neurological Sciences. 1993;14(2):121-127.

49. Lawrence ES, et al. Estimates of the prevalence of acute stroke impairments and disability in a multiethnic population. Stroke. 2001;32(6):1279-1284.

50. Ng YS, et al. Clinical characteristics and rehabilitation outcomes of patients with posterior cerebral artery stroke. Archives of Physical Medicine and Rehabilitation. 2005;86(11):2138-2143.

51. Townend BS, et al. Perimetric homonymous visual field loss post-stroke. Journal of Clinical Neuroscience.2007;14(8):754-756.

52. Rathore SS, et al. Characterization of incident stroke signs and symptoms: Findings from the atherosclerosis risk in communities study. Stroke. 2002;33(11):2718-2721.

53. Jerath NU, et al. Gender differences in presenting signs and symptoms of acute ischemic stroke: A population-based study. Gender Medicine. 2011;8(5):312-319.

54. Celesia GG, Brigell MG, Vaphiades MS, Hemianopic anosognosia. Neurology. 1997;49(1):88-97.

55. Kedar S, et al. Congruency in homonymous hemianopia. American Journal of Ophthalmology. 2007;143(5):772-780.

56. Stone SP, Halligan PW, Greenwood RJ, The incidence of neglect phenomena and related disorders in patients with an acute right or left hemisphere stroke. Age & Ageing. 1993;22(1):46-52.

57. Yap MHL, Loong SC, Nei IP. Eye signs in strokes. Annals of the Academy of Medicine Singapore. 1975;4(2):133-137.

58. Fowler MS, et al. Squints and diplopia seen after brain damage. Journal of Neurology. 1996;243(1):86-90.

59. Maeshima S, et al. Functional outcome in patients with pontine infarction after acute rehabilitation. Neurological Sciences. 2012;33(4):759-764.

60. Su CH, Young YH, Clinical significance of pathological eye movements in diagnosing posterior fossa stroke. Acta Oto-Laryngologica. 2013;133(9):916-923.

61. Siong KH, et al. Prevalence of visual problems among stroke survivors in Hong Kong Chinese. Clinical and Experimental Optometry. 2014;97:433-441.

62. De Renzi E, et al. Conjugate gaze paresis in stroke patients with unilateral damage. An unexpected instance of hemispheric asymmetry. Archives of Neurology. 1982; 39(8):482-486.

63. Singer OC, et al. Conjugate eye deviation in acute stroke: Incidence, hemispheric asymmetry, and lesion pattern. Stroke. 2006;37(11):2726-2732.

64. Lotery AJ, et al. Correctable visual impairment in stroke rehabilitation patients. Age and Ageing. 2000;29(3):221-222.

65. Siddique MAN, et al. Clinical presentation and epidemiology of stroke - A study of 100 cases. Journal of Medicine. 2009; 10(2):86-89.

66. Rowe F, et al. The spectrum of nystagmus following cerebro-vascular accident. British and Irish Orthoptic Journal. 2008;5:22-25.

67. Baier B, Dieterich M. Incidence and anatomy of gaze-evoked nystagmus in patients with cerebellar lesions. Neurology. 2011;76(4):361-365.

68. Akhtar N, et al. Ischaemic posterior circulation stroke in State of Qatar. European Journal of Neurology. 2009; 16(9):1004-1009.

69. Rowe F, et al. Visual impairment in stroke survivors: A prospective multi-centre trial. in 31st European Strabismological Association. Mykonos, Greece; 2007.

70. Edwards DF, et al. Screening patients with stroke for rehabilitation needs: Validation of the post-stroke rehabilitation guidelines. Neurorehabilitation and Neural Repair. 2006;20(1):42-48.

71. Bulens C, et al. Spatial contrast sensitivity in unilateral cerebral ischaemic lesions involving the posterior visual pathway. Brain. 1989;112(Pt 2):507-520.

72. Dos Santos NA, Andrade SM. Visual contrast sensitivity in patients with impairment of functional independence after stroke. BMC Neurology. 2012;12:90.

73. Pedersen PM, et al. Hemi neglect in acute stroke--incidence and prognostic implications. The Copenhagen Stroke Study. American Journal of Physical Medicine & Rehabilitation. 1997;76(2):122-127.

74. Appelros P, et al. Neglect and anosognosia after first-ever stroke: Incidence and relationship to disability. Journal of Rehabilitation Medicine. 2002; 34(5):215-220.

75. Linden T, et al. Visual neglect and cognitive impairment in elderly patients late after stroke. Acta Neurologica Scandinavica. 2005;111(3):163-168.

76. Becker E, Karnath HO. Incidence of visual extinction after left versus right hemisphere stroke. Stroke. 2007;38(12):3172-3174.

77. Van Nes IJ, et al. Is visuospatial hemineglect really a determinant of postural control following stroke? An acute-phase study. Neurorehabilitation & Neural Repair. 2009;23(6):609-614.

78. Lee BH, et al. Neglect dyslexia: Frequency, association with other hemispatial neglects, and lesion localization. Neuropsychologia. 2009;47(3):704-710.

79. Cassidy TP, Lewis S, Gray CS. Recovery from visuospatial neglect in stroke patients. Journal of Neurology, Neurosurgery & Psychiatry. 1998;64(4): 555-557.

80. Cassidy TP, et al. The association of visual field deficits and visuo-spatial neglect in acute right-hemisphere stroke patients. Age & Ageing. 1999;28(3):257-260.

81. Shrestha GS, et al. Ocular-visual defect and visual neglect in stroke patients - A report from Kathmandu, Nepal. Journal of Optometry. 2012;5(1):43-49.

82. Beaudoin AJ, et al. Visuoperceptual deficits and participation in older adults after stroke. Australian Occupational Therapy Journal. 2013;60(4):260-266.

83. Yang TH, et al. Topology of brainstem lesions associated with subjective visual vertical tilt. Neurology. 2014;82:1968-1975.

84. Chechlacz M, et al. The frequency and severity of extinction after stroke affecting different vascular territories. Neuropsychologia. 2014;54:11-17.

85. Tiel K, Kolmel HW. Patterns of recovery from homonymous hemianopia subsequent to infarction in the distribution of the posterior cerebral artery. Neuro-Ophthalmology. 1991;11(1):33-39.

86. Schmielau FEK, Wong Jr. Recovery of visual fields in brain-lesioned patients by reaction perimetry treatment. Journal of Neuro Engineering and Rehabilitation. 2007;4.

87. Zhang X, et al. Natural history of homonymous hemianopia. Neurology. 2006;66: 901-905.

88. Farne A, et al. Patterns of spontaneous recovery of neglect and associated disorders in acute right brain-damaged patients. Journal of Neurology, Neurosurgery & Psychiatry. 2004;75(10):1401-1410.

89. Poggel DA, et al. Visual hallucinations during spontaneous and training-induced visual field recovery. Neuropsychologia. 2007;45(11):2598-2607.

APPENDIX

Appendix 1 – PRISMA 2009 Checklist

Title

Title	1	Identify the report as a systematic review, meta-analysis, or both.	1

Abstract

Structured summary	2	Provide a structured summary including, as applicable: background; objectives; data sources; study eligibility criteria, participants, and interventions; study appraisal and synthesis methods; results; limitations; conclusions and implications of key findings; systematic review registration number.	1

Introduction

Rationale	3	Describe the rationale for the review in the context of what is already known.	2
Objectives	4	Provide an explicit statement of questions being addressed with reference to participants, interventions, comparisons, outcomes, and study design (PICOS).	2

Methods

Protocol and registration	5	Indicate if a review protocol exists, if and where it can be accessed (e.g., Web address), and, if available, provide registration information including registration number.	N/A
Eligibility criteria	6	Specify study characteristics (e.g., PICOS, length of follow-up) and report characteristics (e.g., years considered, language, publication status) used as criteria for eligibility, giving rationale.	2-3
Information sources	7	Describe all information sources (e.g., databases with dates of coverage, contact with study authors to identify additional studies) in the search and date last searched.	Appendix 2
Search	8	Present full electronic search strategy for at least one database, including any limits used, such that it could be repeated.	Appendix 2
Study selection	9	State the process for selecting studies (i.e., screening, eligibility, included in systematic review, and, if applicable, included in the meta-analysis).	2-3
Data collection process	10	Describe method of data extraction from reports (e.g., piloted forms, independently, in duplicate) and any processes for obtaining and confirming data from investigators.	4
Data items	11	List and define all variables for which data were sought (e.g., PICOS, funding sources) and any assumptions and simplifications made.	3-4
Risk of bias in individual studies	12	Describe methods used for assessing risk of bias of individual studies (including specification of whether this was done at the study or outcome level), and how this information is to be used in any data synthesis.	4 Appendix 5
Summary measures	13	State the principal summary measures (e.g., risk ratio, difference in means).	N/A
Synthesis of results	14	Describe the methods of handling data and combining results of studies, if done, including measures of consistency	N/A

		(e.g., I^2) for each meta-analysis.	
Risk of bias across studies	15	Specify any assessment of risk of bias that may affect the cumulative evidence (e.g., publication bias, selective reporting within studies).	4
Additional analyses	16	Describe methods of additional analyses (e.g., sensitivity or subgroup analyses, meta-regression), if done, indicating which were pre-specified.	N/A
Results			
Study selection	17	Give numbers of studies screened, assessed for eligibility, and included in the review, with reasons for exclusions at each stage, ideally with a flow diagram.	4, Appendix 3
Study characteristics	18	For each study, present characteristics for which data were extracted (e.g., study size, PICOS, follow-up period) and provide the citations.	Tables 1 to 10
Risk of bias within studies	19	Present data on risk of bias of each study and, if available, any outcome level assessment (see item 12).	4 Appendix 5
Results of individual studies	20	For all outcomes considered (benefits or harms), present, for each study: (a) simple summary data for each intervention group (b) effect estimates and confidence intervals, ideally with a forest plot.	Tables 1 to 10
Synthesis of results	21	Present results of each meta-analysis done, including confidence intervals and measures of consistency.	N/A
Risk of bias across studies	22	Present results of any assessment of risk of bias across studies (see Item 15).	4
Additional analysis	23	Give results of additional analyses, if done (e.g., sensitivity or subgroup analyses, meta-regression [see Item 16]).	N/A
Discussion			
Summary of evidence	24	Summarize the main findings including the strength of evidence for each main outcome; consider their relevance to key groups (e.g., healthcare providers, users, and policy makers).	5-24
Limitations	25	Discuss limitations at study and outcome level (e.g., risk of bias), and at review-level (e.g., incomplete retrieval of identified research, reporting bias).	24-25
Conclusions	26	Provide a general interpretation of the results in the context of other evidence, and implications for future research.	25
Funding			
Funding	27	Describe sources of funding for the systematic review and other support (e.g., supply of data); role of funders for the systematic review.	25

From: Moher D, Liberati A, Tetzlaff J, Altman DG, The PRISMA Group (2009). Preferred Reporting Items for Systematic Reviews and Meta-Analyses: The PRISMA Statement. PLoS Med 6(6): e1000097. DOI: 10.1371/journal.pmed1000097. Available: www.prisma-statement.org

Appendix 2. Search Options and Search Terms

Databases:

- Cochrane Stroke Group Trials Register
- The Cochrane Eyes and Vision Group Trials Register
- The Cochrane Central Register of Controlled Trials (CENTRAL) (*The Cochrane Library*, latest issue);
- MEDLINE (1950 to April 2015);
- EMBASE (1980 to April 2015);
- CINAHL (1982 to April 2015);
- AMED (1985 to April 2015);
- PsycINFO (1967 April 2015);
- Dissertations & Theses (PQDT) database (1861 to April 2015);
- British Nursing Index (1985 to April 2015);
- PsycBITE (Psychological Database for Brain Impairment Treatment Efficacy, www.psycbite.com).

Registers:

- ClinicalTrials.gov (http://clinicaltrials.gov/);
- Current Controlled Trials (www.controlledtrials. com);
- Trials Central (www.trialscentral.org);
- Health Service Research Projects in Progress (wwwcf.nlm.nih.gov/hsr_project/home_proj.cfm);
- National Eye Institute Clinical Studies Database (http://clinicalstudies.info.nih.gov/cgi/protinstitute.cgi?NEI.0.html)
- British and Irish Orthoptic Journal, Australian Orthoptic Journal, and proceedings of the European Strabismological Association (ESA), International Strabismological Association (ISA), International Orthoptic Association (IOA) (http://pcwww.liv.ac.uk/~rowef/index_files/Page646.htm)
- Proceedings of Association for Research in Vision and Ophthalmology (www.arvo.org);

Terms:

Cerebrovascular disorders/	Eye Movements/
Brain ischaemia/	Eye/
Intracranial Arterial Disease	Eye Disease/
Intracranial Arteriovenous Malformations/	Visually Impaired Persons/
"Intracranial Embolism and Thrombosis*/	Vision Disorders/
Stroke/	Blindness/
	Diplopia/
	Vision, Binocular/
	Vision, Monocular/
	Visual Acuity/
	Visual Fields/
	Vision, Low/

	Ocular Motility Disorders/
	Blindness, Cortical/
	Hemianopsia/
	Abducens Nerve Diseases/
	Abducens Nerve/
	Oculomotor Nerve/
	Trochlear Nerve/
	Visual Perception/
	Nystagmus
	strabismus
	smooth pursuits
	saccades depth perception
	stereopsis gaze disorder
	internuclear opthalmoplegia
	Parinaud's syndrome
	Weber's syndrome
	skew deviation
	conjugate deviation oscillopsia
	visual tracking agnosia hallucinations
OR	OR
AND	

Appendix 3. Flowchart of Pathway for Inclusion of Articles

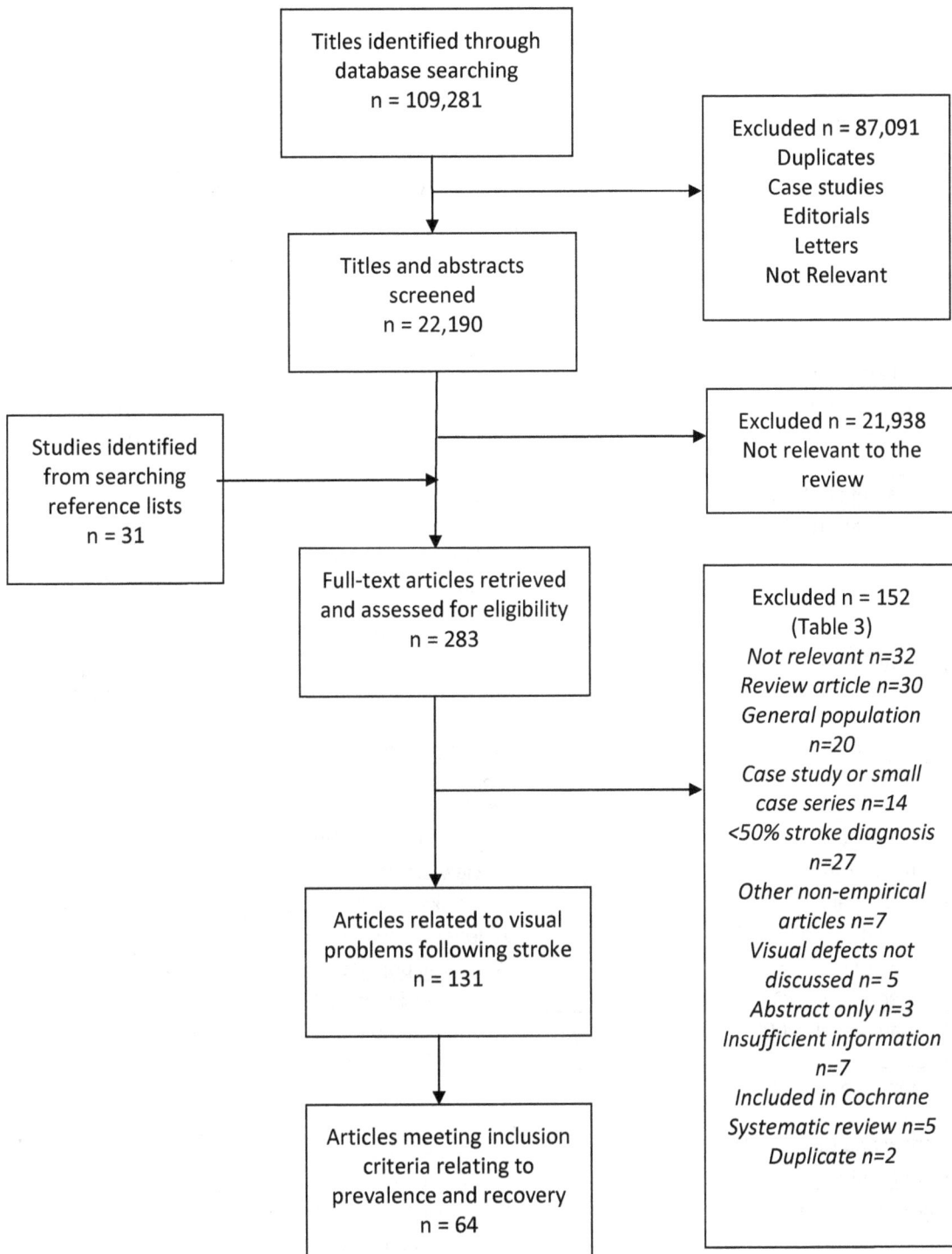

Titles identified through
database searching
n = 109,281

Excluded n = 87,091
Duplicates
Case studies
Editorials
Letters
Not Relevant

Titles and abstracts
screened
n = 22,190

Excluded n = 21,938
Not relevant to the
review

Studies identified
from searching
reference lists
n = 31

Full-text articles retrieved
and assessed for eligibility
n = 283

Excluded n = 152
(Table 3)
Not relevant n=32
Review article n=30
*General population
n=20*
*Case study or small
case series n=14*
*<50% stroke diagnosis
n=27*
*Other non-empirical
articles n=7*
*Visual defects not
discussed n= 5*
Abstract only n=3
*Insufficient information
n=7*
*Included in Cochrane
Systematic review n=5*
Duplicate n=2

Articles related to visual
problems following stroke
n = 131

Articles meeting inclusion
criteria relating to
prevalence and recovery
n = 64

Appendix 4. Excluded Articles

Study	Reason for exclusion
Ajina and Kennard, 2012	Review article
Al-Khayat et al., 2005	No stroke patients included
Anderson and Rizzo, 1994	Case report
Anderson and Rizzo, 1995	Review article
Baier at al., 2010	Not relevant to the review – preselected cases
Barker et al., 2012	Not relevant to the review – assessment of neuropsychology
Barnes et al., 2006	Unable to distinguish number of stroke patients
Barrett, 2009	Review article
Bartolomei et al., 1998	No stroke patients included
Beran and Murphy-Lavoie, 2009	Not related to stroke
Beck and Harris, 1994	Not related to stroke – general population
Behrmann et al., 2004	Not relevant to the review – addresses different types of search patterns in neglect
Biousse et al., 1998	Only reported on three patients
Blythe et al., 1987	Not relevant to the review – preselected cases assessed for blindsight
Bodis-Wollner and Diamond, 1973	Unable to establish the proportion of participants were post-stroke, participants reported to have cerebral lesions.
Bodis-Wollner and Diamond, 1976	Unable to establish the proportion of participants were post-stroke, participants reported to have cerebral lesions.
Bombois et al., 2007	Stroke patients excluded
Bronstein et al., 1990	Unable to establish the proportion of participants were post-stroke
Brown Jr et al., 1998	A general population sampled
Brunette, 1967	Review article
Bulsara et al., 2007	No stroke patients included
Bunce and Wormald, 2008	A general population sampled
Bunce et al., 2010	A general population sampled
Büttner and Grundei, 1995	Sample included 50% or fewer stroke patients
Buxbaum et al., 2008	Not relevant to the review – performance on wheelchair navigation
Caneman et al., 1992	Not relevant to the review – performance on maze test
Carlow and Bicknell, 1981	Review article
Carman-Merrifield, 2005	Review article
Cheek et al., 1965	Sample included 50% or fewer stroke patients
Cheung et al., 2008	Not relevant to the review - discussed retinal pathology
Chia et al., 2004	A general population sampled
Ciuffreda et al., 2006	Sample included 50% or fewer stroke patients
Ciuffreda et al., 2007	Sample included 50% or fewer stroke patients

Clenet, 2011	Case study
Cockburn, 1983	A general population sampled
Colombo et al., 1981	Not relevant to the review – preselected cases from a larger cohort
Cooper, 1971	Not relevant to stroke
Cooper et al., 2012	Only reported on two patients
Crews et al., 2006	Sample included 50% or fewer stroke patients
Danta et al., 1978	Sample included 50% or fewer stroke patients
Das et al., 2007	Review article
Dennis et al., 1990	Not relevant to the review – transient ischaemic attacks
Di Legge et al., 2004	Correspondence to the editor
Dulli et al., 1998	No reference to visual problems
François, 1975	Review article
Fraser et al., 2011	Review article
Galanth et al., 2014	Visual problems of stroke patients not discussed
Gállego et al., 2008	Review article
Gamio and Melek, 2003	Case report
George et al., 2011	Protocol article
Georgiadis et al., 1999	No reference to visual problems
Gilhotra et al., 2002	A general population sampled
Gilhotra et al., 2002	A general population sampled
Giroud et al., 1994	Not relevant to review - focused on seizures after stroke
Globe et al., 2005	A general population sampled
Goldstein and Simel, 2005	Review article
Good et al., 2001	Not relevant to review - paediatric population
Gottlieb and Miesner, 2004	Review article
Grunda et al., 2013	Review article
Guenther et al., 2009	Not relevant to the review – evaluating prediction model
Habekost and Starrfelt, 2006	Case report
Hankey, 1997	A general population sampled
Hofman et al., 2007	A general population sampled and study protocol update
Hofman et al., 2011	A general population sampled and study protocol update
Horton, 2005	Editorial
Howard et al., 2006	Unable to establish the proportion of participants were post-stroke
Jagger et al., 1989	No stroke patients included
Jarvis et al., 2012	Not relevant to the review – information provided to the stroke team
Jensen et al., 2009	Case study
Jin et al., 2010	No stroke patients included
Jobke et al., 2009	Already included in a Cochrane Systematic Review

Jones and Shinton, 2006	Review article
Jungehülsing et al., 2008	A general population sampled
Kasten et al., 2007	Sample included 50% or fewer stroke patients
Kasten et al., 2006	Sample included 50% or fewer stroke patients
Kerkhoff and Stögerer, 1994	No stroke patients included
Kim and Kim, 2005	Not relevant to the review – restricted to midbrain stroke only
Kissel et al., 1983	No stroke patients included
Klavora and Warren, 1998	Not relevant to the review - overview of equipment, no participant data presented
Książkiewicz and Sobczak-Kamińska, 1998	Not relevant to the review - eye assessment related to level of consciousness
Kumar, 2006	News article
Kuppersmith et al., 1996	No stroke patients included
Lamoreux et al., 2008	A general population sampled
Langelaan et al., 2007	A general population sampled
Leff et al., 2000	Sample included 50% or fewer stroke patients
Leff and Behrmann, 2008	Review article
Leśniak and Seniów, 2007	Review article
Lessell, 1975	Review article
Levine, 2006	Letter to editor
Lisabeth et al., 2009	Unable to distinguish with numbers of stroke and TIA patients
Macfarlane and Jolly, 1995	Not relevant to the review – role of the orthoptist
Markowitz, 2009	Review article
Marshall et al., 2008	Not relevant to the review - fMRI study
Marx et al., 1992	A general population sampled
McKean et al., 2014	Not relevant to the review – predicting factors on imaging of stroke
Mead et al., 2002	Visual problems of stroke patients not discussed
Merten, 2001	Review article
Mitchell et al., 1996	A general population sampled
Nazerian et al., 2014	Sample included 50% or fewer stroke patients
Nazzarko, 2007	Review article
Neikter, 1999	Only conference abstract available
Nelles et al., 2009	Not relevant to the review – training effects on neural plasticity
Niu et al., 2005	Not relevant to the review – examines location of lesion for neglect
Olbert, 1985	Case study
O'Neill et al., 2011	Sample included 50% or fewer stroke patients
Pambakian et al., 2005	Review article
Patel et al., 2004	Sample included 50% or fewer stroke patients
Patino et al., 2010	A general population sampled
Pelak et al., 2007	Review article
Peli, 2000	Sample included 50% or fewer stroke patients

Petzold et al., 2013	Not related to stroke patients
Piechocki, 2004	News article
Poggel et al., 2004	Already included in a Cochrane Systematic Review
Proto et al., 2009	Review article
Purvin, 1996	Review article
Purvin, 2004	Review article
Racette and Casson, 2005	Not relevant to the review – impact on driving
Rafałowska et al., 1972	Only reported on three patients
Ramrattan et al., 2001	A general population sampled
Riise, 1969	No stroke patients included
Ritchie at al., 2012	Only reported on two patients
Ross, 1983	Not relevant to the review – selected sample
Rossi et al., 1990	Already included in a Cochrane Systematic Review
Rowe, 2009	Duplicate – subset sample
Rowe, 2010	Not relevant to the review
Rutner et al., 2006	Sample included 50% or fewer stroke patients
Sabel and Kasten, 2000	Review article
Sabel and Mueller, 2005	Only abstract available
Sabel and Trauzettal-Klosinksi, 2005	Expert debate
Sahraie et al., 2010	Case study
Sand et al., 2013	Review article
Schofield and Leff, 2009	Review article
Schwartz et al., 2012	Not relevant to the review –assessment of eye position using CT scan
Shiraishi et al., 2004	Stroke patients not identified separately
Simon et al., 2003	Not relevant to the review –assessment of eye position using CT scan
Spitzyna et al., 2007	Already included in a Cochrane Systematic Review
Suchoff et al., 2008	Sample included 50% or fewer stroke patients
Tsai et al., 2003	Sample included 50% or fewer stroke patients
Unwin et al., 1999	Only conference abstract available
Vahlberg and Hellström, 2008	Review article
van der Graaff et al., 2000	Case study
Viken et al., 2014	Not relevant to the review – predicting functional outcomes
Weinberg et al., 1977	Already included in a Cochrane Systematic Review
Williams et al., 2003	Visual problems not discussed
Wolter and Preder, 2006	Review article
Woo and Mandelman, 1983	Case report
Zhang et al., 2006	Duplicate report of study already included in the review
Zhou et al., 2013	A general population sampled
Zihl, 1980	Only reported on three patients
Zihl et al., 1988	Not relevant to the review
Zihl and Hebel, 1997	Sample included 50% or fewer stroke patients
Zihl et al., 2009	Not relevant to the review – selected sample

Appendix 5. Quality Appraisal of Papers Using the STROBE Checklist

	Introduction	Methods							Results						Discussion			
	3	4	6	7	8	9	10	11	12	13	14	15	16	17	18	19	20	21
Agrell et al., 1997 [45]	+	+	+	+	+	+	+	+	?	-	+	+	+	+	+	-	+	-
Akhtar et al., 2009 [68]	+	+	+	+	+	-	+	+	+	-	+	+	+	n/a	+	-	-	+
Ali et al., 2013 [30]	+	+	+	+	+	-	+	-	-	?	?	+	+	+	+	+	+	+
Appelros et al., 2002 [74]	+	+	+	+	+	+	+	+	+	+	+	+	+	+	+	+	+	+
Baier and Dieterich, 2011 [67]	-	+	+	+	+	-	-	-	-	+	+	+	+	n/a	+	-	+	+
Barrett et al., 2007 [38]	+	+	+	+	-	+	-	+	+	+	+	+	+	+	+	+	+	-
Beaudoin et al., 2013 [82]	+	+	+	+	+	+	-	-	-	+	+	+	+	n/a	+	+	+	+
Becker and Karnath, 2007 [76]	+	+	+	+	+	-	+	+	-	+	+	+	+	n/a	+	-	-	-
Benedetti et al. 1993 [48]	+	+	+	+	+	-	+	+	-	+	+	+	+	+	+	+	+	+
Bulens et al 1989 [71]	-	+	+	+	-	-	-	+	-	-	+	+	+	+	+	-	-	-
Cassidy et al., 1998 [79]	+	+	+	+	+	-	+	+	-	+	+	+	+	n/a	+	+	+	+
Cassidy et al. 1999 [80]	+	+	+	+	+	-	-	+	-	+	-	+	+	n/a	+	-	+	-
Cassidy et al., 2001 [46]	+	+	+	+	+	+	+	+	-	+	-	+	+	+	+	+	+	-

	3	4	6	7	8	9	10	11	12	13	14	15	16	17	18	19	20	21
Celesia et al., 1997 [54]	+	+	+	+	+	-	+	+	-	+	+	+	+	+	+	-	+	-
Chechlacz et al., 2014 [84]	-	+	-	+	+	+	+	+	+	+	+	+	+	+	+	+	+	+
Clisby, 1995 [32]	+	-	-	-	+	-	+	-	-	+	-	+	-	-	-	-	-	-
De Renzi et al., 1982 [62]	-	+	+	+	+	+	+	+	-	+	+	+	+	n/a	+	+	+	-
Dos Santos et al., 2012 [72]	+	-	+	+	+	+	-	+	+	+	+	+	+	n/a	+	+	+	+
Edwards et al., 2006 [70]	+	+	+	+	+	+	-	+	+	+	+	+	+	+	+	-	+	+
Farné et al., 2004 [89]	+	+	-	+	+	-	+	+	+	+	+	+	+	+	+	-	-	-
Fowler et al., 1996 [58]	+	+	+	+	+	-	+	+	-	+	+	+	+	n/a	+	+	+	-
Freeman and Rudge, 1987 [35]	+	+	+	+	+	-	+	+	-	+	+	+	+	n/a	+	-	-	-
Gall et al., 2010 [31]	+	+	+	+	+	+	+	+	+	+	+	+	+	n/a	+	+	+	+
Gray et al., 1989 [41]	+	+	+	+	+	+	+	+	-	+	+	+	+	n/a	+	-	-	+
Haerer, 1973 [47]	+	+	+	+	-	-	+	-	-	+	+	+	+	n/a	+	+	+	-
Isaeff et al., 1974 [33]	-	+	?	-	-	-	-	+	-	+	+	+	+	n/a	-	-	-	-
Jerath et al., 2011 [53]	+	+	+	+	+	+	+	+	+	+	+	+	+	n/a	+	+	+	+
Kedar et al., 2007 [55]	+	+	+	+	+	+	+	+	+	+	+	+	+	+	+	+	+	-
Lawrence et al., 2001 [49]	+	+	+	+	-	-	+	+	+	+	+	+	+	+	+	-	+	-

	3	4	6	7	8	9	10	11	12	13	14	15	16	17	18	19	20	21
Lee et al., 2009 [78]	-	+	+	+	+	-	+	+	-	+	+	+	+	+	+	-	+	-
Linden et al., 2006 [75]	+	+	+	+	+	-	+	+	+	+	+	+	+	n/a	+	-	+	-
Lotery et al., 2000 [64]	+	+	+	+	-	-	-	+	-	+	+	+	+	n/a	+	-	-	-
Maeshima et al., 2012 [59]	-	+	+	+	+	-	+	+	+	+	+	+	+	n/a	+	-	-	-
Ng et al., 2005 [50]	+	+	+	+	+	-	+	+	+	+	+	+	+	+	+	+	+	+
Pedersen et al., 1997 [73]	+	+	+	+	+	-	+	+	+	+	+	+	+	+	+	-	-	-
Poggel et al., 2007 [89]	-	+	+	+	+	-	+	+	+	+	+	+	+	+	+	-	-	-
Rathore et al., 2002 [52]	-	-	+	+	-	-	+	+	+	+	+	+	+	+	+	+	+	-
Rowe, 2007 [69]	+	+	+	+	-	-	+	+	-	+	+	+	+	+	+	-	+	+
Rowe et al., 2008 [66]	+	+	+	+	-	-	+	+	-	+	+	+	+	+	+	-	+	+
Rowe et al., 2009 [24]	+	+	+	+	+	-	+	+	-	+	+	+	+	+	+	-	+	+
Rowe et al., 2009 [6]	+	+	+	+	-	-	+	+	-	+	+	+	+	+	+	+	+	+
Rowe et al., 2010 [23]	+	+	+	+	+	-	+	+	+	+	+	+	+	+	+	-	+	-
Rowe et al., 2011 [18]	+	+	+	+	+	-	+	+	+	+	+	+	+	+	+	+	+	+
Rowe et al., 2011 [19]	+	+	+	+	+	-	+	+	+	+	+	+	+	+	+	+	+	-
Rowe et al., 2013 [36]	+	+	+	+	+	-	+	+	+	+	+	+	+	+	+	-	+	-

	3	4	6	7	8	9	10	11	12	13	14	15	16	17	18	19	20	21
Rowe et al., 2013 [22]	+	+	+	+	-	-	+	+	+	+	+	+	+	+	+	+	+	-
Rowe et al., 2013 [21]	+	+	+	+	+	-	+	+	+	+	+	+	+	+	+	+	+	+
Schmielau and Wong Jr, 2007 [86]	+	-	+	+	+	-	-	+	-	+	+	+	+	+	+	-	-	-
Searls et al., 2012 [42]	+	+	+	+	-	-	+	+	+	+	+	+	+	+	+	-	-	-
Shrestha et al., 2012 [81]	+	+	+	+	+	-	+	+	+	+	+	+	+	+	+	-	-	-
Siddique et al., 2009 [65]	-	+	+	-	-	-	+	+	-	+	+	+	+	+	+	-	+	+
Singer et al., 2006 [63]	-	+	+	+	+	-	+	+	+	+	+	+	+	+	+	+	+	+
Siong et al., 2014 [61]	+	+	+	+	+	+	+	+	+	+	+	+	+	+	+	+	+	+
Stone et al., 1993 [56]	+	+	+	+	+	-	+	+	+	+	+	+	+	+	+	-	-	-
Su and Young, 2013 [60]	-	+	+	+	+	-	+	+	-	+	+	+	-	-	+	+	+	-
Tao et al., 2012 [43]	+	+	+	+	-	-	+	+	+	+	+	+	+	+	+	+	+	-
Tiel and Kölmel, 1991 [85]	-	+	+	+	-	-	+	+	-	+	+	+	-	n/a	+	-	-	-
Townsend et al., 2007 [51]	+	+	+	+	+	+	+	+	+	+	+	+	+	n/a	+	-	-	+
Trobe et al., 1973 [34]	+	+	+	-	-	-	+	-	-	+	+	+	-	-	+	-	-	-
van Nes et al., 2009 [77]	+	+	+	+	+	+	+	+	+	+	+	+	+	+	+	-	-	-
Yang et al., 2014 [83]	+	+	+	+	+	+	+	+	+	+	+	+	+	+	+	-	-	-

	3	4	6	7	8	9	10	11	12	13	14	15	16	17	18	19	20	21
Yap et al., 1975 [57]	+	+	+	+	-	-	+	+	-	+	+	+	-	n/a	+	-	-	-
Zhang et al., 2006a [44]	+	+	+	+	+	+	+	+	-	+	+	+	+	+	+	-	+	+
Zhang et al., 2006b [87]	+	+	+	+	+	+	+	+	-	+	+	+	-	n/a	+	+	+	+

- = Not reported; ? = Unclear; + = Reported

26

A Comparative Study of Pterygium Excision Using Autologous Blood versus Sutures; a Study from Remote Eastern Bihar, India

P. Peeush[1*] **and S. Sarkar**[1]

[1]*Department of Ophthalmology, M.G.M Medical college Kishanganj, Bihar, India.*

Authors' contributions

This work was carried out in collaboration between both authors. Author SS designed the study. Author PP wrote the protocol, and wrote the first draft of the manuscript. Both authors read and approved the final manuscript.

Editor(s):
(1) Ahmad M. Mansour, Department of Ophthalmology, American University of Beirut, Lebanon.
Reviewers:
(1) Anonymous, Mansoura University, Egypt.
(2) Anonymous, Gaziantep University, Gaziantep, Turkey

ABSTRACT

Aims: The study was undertaken to assess the surgical modalities for treatment of Pterygium in rural population.
Study Design: Prospective study.
Place and Duration of Study: Study was conducted in the Department of Ophthalmology for a period of July to December 2013.
Methodology: All the grade 1 and 2 patients between age group 25-50years without any history of diabetes and /or oral anticoagulant agent intake were included in this study while others were excluded. The patients were randomly divided into two groups for pterygium excision with autograft using either autologous blood or sutures. Post operatively, these patients were then observed for presence of pain, irritation and graft failure on day 1, day 7 and 1month.
Results: The surgical rate of success was better for sutures compared with autologous blood in rural eastern population.
Conclusion: Autologous conjunctival graft with sutures was found to have better outcome in terms of surgical success when compared with a new approach of autologous blood especially in the areas with patients of poor compliance.

*Corresponding author: E-mail: parimalpeeush@gmail.com

Keywords: Pterygium; autologous blood; sutures.

1. INTRODUCTION

A pterygium is a degenerative condition of the sub-conjunctival tissue which proliferates as vascularized granulation tissue to invade the cornea destroying the superficial layers of stroma and Bowman's membrane, the whole being covered by conjunctival membrane. It varies from small, atrophic quiescent asymptomatic lesions to large, aggressive, rapidly growing fibro-vascular lesions that cause impairment of vision by covering the pupillary area of the cornea and also by altering the curvature of the cornea due to fibrosis, causing astigmatism. It may also invade the cornea leading to corneal opacity. [1,2] For treatment of this condition various treatment modalities are available but surgery still remains gold standard. During the past decade, debate over the best approach to pterygium surgery was centered on sutures and fibrin glue to affix the conjunctival graft but recent introduction of patient's own blood (autologous blood) for fixation of conjunctival flap has proven to be better over the previous two approaches. Although, none of the approaches have been tested in the rural settings.

In this study, we are comparing two patient groups who had pterygium excision with autograft using either sutures or autologous blood in rural eastern India where majority of the population are outdoor workers like farmers, labourers etc and have a predilection for developing pterygium.

2. MATERIALS AND METHODS

The present study was conducted at the Department of Ophthalmology. A total number of 50 cases with pterygium classified as grade 1 or 2 were selected from out-patient department (OPD) for surgical intervention during the period of 6 months from July to December 2013. The following points were tabulated as under name, age, sex, address, occupation, history, general examination, local examination. Informed consent was taken from the patient before performing the surgery. The patients were randomly divided into two groups for pterygium excision with autograft using either autologous blood or sutures. Post operatively, the eye was patched overnight, and it was treated subsequently with topical antibiotics and anti-inflammatory drops and/or ointments. These patients were then observed for presence of pain, irritation and graft failure on day 1, day 7 and 1month. Surgical success was taken as presence of graft in place, no recurrence of pterygium and no signs of inflammation at the end of 1 month. Statistical analysis of the data was performed using chi-square test.

2.1 Inclusion Criteria

All the grade 1 and 2 patients between age group 25-50 years without any history of diabetes and /or oral anticoagulant agent intake were included in this study. [The grading of pterygium is given in Table 1]

2.2 Exclusion Criteria

All patients more than 50 or less than 25 years or with grade 3 pterygium between age group 25-50 years, any history of diabetes and /or oral anticoagulant agent intake were excluded from this study.

3. RESULTS AND DISCUSSION

3.1 Results

Males (88%) and females (12%) were randomly distributed in the study for pterygium excision via autologous blood and sutures (Table 2).

All the patients belonged to lower socio-economic group and were outdoor workers. Majority of the pterygium examined were nasal in both the study groups. Grade 1 was observed in 19(38%) whereas grade 2 was seen in 31(62%) (Table 3).

All these patients were post-operatively observed for day 1, 7 and at 1 month (Table 4).

Post operative examination of the two groups showed that twenty-three patients had successful grafting in which sutures were used compared to fourteen patients who were treated with autologous blood. The rate of surgical success was 68% in autologous blood compared to 100% when sutures were used (Table 5).

But post-operative pain, foreign body sensation was seen in patients with sutures. Surgical failures were seen on post-operative day 1 in patients were autologous blood was used. Statistical analysis by Chi-square test shows that the p-value is less than 0.001, hence using sutures for the patient compared to autologous blood is better.

3.2 Discussion

Pterygia are characterized by elastotic degeneration of collagen and fibrovascular proliferation, with an overlying covering of epithelium. Histopathology of the abnormal collagen in the area of elastotic degeneration shows basophilia with hematoxylin and eosin stain. Pterygium is commonly seen in patients above 20 years with highest prevalence in more than 40 years of age. The incidence of pterygium was 4% in the age group of less than 30 years and reaches maximum of 32% in the age of 30-39 years and then it gradually declines. Male gender and high sun exposure are strong and independent factors related to development of pterygium. Majority of patients were in our study were outdoor workers like farmers, labourers etc. The incidence was found to be maximum among farmers (40%) followed by labourers (20%). Globally, prevalence rates vary depending on the latitudes. [3,4] Nasal presentation being more common is seen due to transmission of UV light from temporal side of cornea through the stroma on to the nasal aspect of eye, perhaps explaining why these lesions are more common nasally. Various treatment modalities are available but conjunctival autografts using sutures remains the gold standard. These grafts are stable with acceptable cosmetic results. Studies were done using fibrin, including lamellar corneal grafting and the closure of corneal perforations as it is a faster and simpler with less postoperative pain and

Table 1. Shows grading of pterygium

Grade	Description
1	Extends less thasn 2 mm onto the cornea.
2	Involves upto 4 mm of the cornea and may be primary or recurrent following surgery
3	Encroaches onto more than 4 mm of the cornea and involves the visual axis.

Table 2. Showing the distribution of males and females into two groups

| | Group 1 (sutures) total -25 | | Group 2 (autologous blood) total-25 | |
	Males	Females	Males	Females
Number	21	4	23	2
Percentage	84 %	16 %	86%	8%

Table 3. Showing distribution of stage of pterygium in the two study groups

| | Group 1(sutures) total-25 | | Group 2 (autologous blood) total-25 | |
	Stage 1	Stage 2	Stage 1	Stage 2
Number	10	15	9	16
percentage	40%	60%	36%	64%

Table 4. Showing post operative follow-up of the two study groups for pain and foreign body sensation

	Autologous blood	Sutures
Total no. of patients	25	25
Pain and irritation at day 1	15 (60%)	25 (100%)
Pain and irritation at day 7	8 (32%)	10 (40%)
Post-operative 1 month	8 (32%)	-

Table 5. Showing surgical success in two study groups

Patient group	With sutures	With autologous blood
Surgical success	25 (100%)	17 (68%)
Failure	-	8 (32%)

discomfort [5]. The newest approach is autoblood graft fixation, a technique also known as suture- and glue-free autologous graft. Autologous blood is natural, has no extra cost or associated risks, and can overcome the postoperative irritations to a great extent. [6] However in the present study, 100% surgical success was seen in conjunctival graft with sutures whereas only 68% surgical success was seen those patients with autologous blood. This is different from the findings of a cross-sectional study performed in the United Kingdom, 15 eyes received grafts affixed with autologous blood. No transplant dislocations or failures occurred. [7] Patients who regularly take aspirin or other blood thinners—or who suffer from a coagulation factor deficiency would not be good candidates for autologous blood graft fixation. In the present study, patients on asprin and other anti-coagulants were excluded so there was no evident reason for graft failure in autologous blood grafts. The reason hypothesized was that they were not compliant with the post operative precautions that were ought to be followed. Similar observation was found in other studies where graft retraction was seen in more patients in fibrin glue group than suture group. The surgeon concluded that this can be due to movement of the graft due to lid movement causing displacement of the graft [8-10].

The main disadvantage of the autologous blood is the risk of graft loss in the immediate postoperative period. Graft loss is usually seen in first 24 to 48 hours. One of the important advantages seen with autologous blood was that this procedure was cosmetically better, pain and foreign body sensation was less prominent in early post operative period as compared to autograft with sutures. Limitation of the study is that only one month follow-up was performed and true recurrence could only be assessed after a follow up of 1 year. In the current clinical settings of rural India, patients are difficult to follow-up for a long period of time due to various financial and logistical limitations which makes it difficult to assess true recurrence. In India, majority of the population resides in the rural area; hence more study needs to be done in the area.

4. CONCLUSION

Autologous conjunctival graft with sutures was found to have better outcome in terms of surgical success when compared with a new approach of autologous blood especially in the areas with patients of poor compliance.

CONSENT

All authors declare that 'written informed consent was obtained from the patient for publication.

ETHICAL APPROVAL

Not applicable.

COMPETING INTERESTS

Authors have declared that no competing interests exist.

REFERENCES

1. Coroneo MT, Di Girolamo N, Wakefield D. The pathogenesis of pterygia. Curr Opin Ophthalmol. 1999;10:282-8.

2. Elliot R. The aetiology of pterygium. Trans Ophthalmol Soc NZ. 1961;13:22.

3. Saw SM, Tan D. Pterygium: prevalence, demography and risk factors. Ophthalmic Epidemiol. 1999;6:219-28.

4. Threlfall TJ, English DR. Sun exposure and pterygium of the eye: a dose-response curve. Am J Ophthalmol. 1999;128:280-7.

5. Sarnicola V, Vannozzi L, Motolese PA. Recurrence rate using fibrin glue-assisted ipsilateral conjunctival autograft in pterygium surgery: 2-year follow-up. Cornea. 2010;29(11):1211e1214.

6. Singh PK, Singh S, Vyas C, Singh M. Conjunctival autografting without fibrin glue or sutures for pterygium surgery. Cornea. 2013;32:104-7.

7. De Wit D, Athanasiadis I, Sharma A, Moore J. Sutureless and glue-free conjunctival autograft in pterygium surgery: a case series. 2010;24:1474-1477

8. Cohen RA, McDonald MB. Fixation of conjunctival autografts with an organic tissue adhesive [letter]. Arch Ophthalmol. 1993;111:1167e1168.

9. Harvey SU, Reyes JM, Flore JD, Lim-Bon-Siong R. Comparison of fibrin glue and sutures for attaching conjunctival autografts after pterygium excision. Ophthalmology. 2005;112:667e671.

10. Korangy G, Seregard S, Kopp ED. The cut and paste method for primary surgery: long- term follow- up. Acta Opthalmol Scand. 2005;83:298e301.

27

Comparison of Ocular and Developmental Outcomes in Laser-and Bevacizumab-treated Infants with Retinopathy of Prematurity

Lingkun Kong[1][*], Kimberly L. Dinh[2], Sid A. Schechet[1], David K. Coats[1], Robert G. Voigt[3], Ann B. Demny[3] and Paul G. Steinkuller[1]

[1]*Department of Ophthalmology, Baylor College of Medicine, Houston, Texas, USA.*
[2]*Department of Pharmacy, Baylor College of Medicine, Houston, Texas, USA.*
[3]*Department of Pediatrics, Baylor College of Medicine, Houston, Texas, USA.*

Authors' contributions

This work was carried out in collaboration between all authors. Authors LK, PGS, KLD, RGV, ABD and DKC designed the study, wrote the protocol, and wrote the first draft of the manuscript. Author SAS managed the literature searches and data collection. All authors read and approved the final manuscript.

<u>Editor(s):</u>
(1) Rachid Tahiri Joutei Hassani, Ophthalmology Department III, XV – XX National Ophthalmologic Hospital, France.
<u>Reviewers:</u>
(1) Anonymous, Dicle University, Turkey.
(2) Francisco J. Sepúlveda-Cañamar, Ophtalmology and Nephrology Services, Unidad Médica de Atención Ambulatoria, Instituto Mexicano del Seguro Social, San Pedro Garza García, México.
(3) Anonymous, Dr. A.Y. Ankara Oncology Training and Research Hospital, Turkey.
(4) A. S. Alhomida, Biochemistry, King Saud University, Riyadh, Saudi Arabia.

ABSTRACT

Purpose: To compare vision and developmental outcomes in infants who were treated with intravitreal bevacizumab injection (IVB) versus laser for retinopathy of prematurity (ROP).
Methods: Forty-two infants were enrolled in this study and treated with either IVB at 0.625 mg per eye, per dose (22 patients, 43 eyes), or laser (20 patients, 37 eyes) for type I ROP. Systemic complications were compared between these two groups. Structural examinations and cycloplegic refractions were performed at age 1 year. Body weight gains were collected from birth to 36 weeks of postnatal age. Neurodevelopmental assessment was done at 1 year chronological age.
Results: At 1 year of age, four eyes (10.8%) in the laser-treated group and none (0.0%) in the IVB-treated group had unfavorable structural outcome; ten (30%) eyes in the IVB-treated group and 17

*Corresponding author: E-mail: lkong@bcm.edu

(53%) eyes in the laser-treated group were myopic, $p =0.03$; the mean spherical equivalent was -0.03 diopter (D) in the IVB-treated group and -2.94 D in the laser-treated group, $p=0.02$. The mean visual acuity in LogMar was 0.54 (SD, 0.34) and 0.58 (SD, 0.52) in the IVB- and laser-treated groups, respectively (p=0.31). The average weekly weight gain continued at normal rates in both groups after treatment. Seven of ten patients (70%) in the IVB-treated group and six of nine patients (67%) in the laser-treated group were categorized as severely developmentally delayed.
Conclusions: Bevacizumab intravitreal injection had similar short-term efficacy compared to laser treatment with regard to treatment of type I ROP but was associated with a lower prevalence of high myopia.

Keywords: Retinopathy of prematurity; laser; intravitreal injection; neurodevelopment.

1. INTRODUCTION

Retinopathy of prematurity (ROP) is a leading cause of childhood blindness in the United States and worldwide [1]. Laser photocoagulation of the peripheral avascular retina is currently the standard treatment when type I ROP is diagnosed. Potential acute and long-term complications of laser treatment include pain, cataract, high myopia, and progression of the disease despite timely treatment. A treatment failure rate of approximately 9.1% has been reported with laser treatment, and additional treatment or surgery is sometimes required [2]. Recent reports have suggested that bevacizumab has a beneficial effect on advanced ROP, and the agent is being used as monotherapy in several centers around the world [3-8]. Data published from a multicenter clinical trial study showed that intravitreal bevacizumab (IVB) monotherapy, as compared with conventional laser treatment, in infants with stage 3+ ROP showed a significant benefit for zone I but not for zone II disease [7]. Immunohistology and pathology studies have demonstrated no obvious short-term toxicity to the retina, optic nerve, or other ocular tissues [4].

The expression of vascular endothelial growth factor (VEGF) appeared not to be uniformly blocked in the developing tissues, allowing maturation of the mid-peripheral retina while restricting abnormal neovascularization [4]. However, questions have arisen about bevacizumab regarding short- and long-term safety to ocular tissues, other organs, and, especially, neurological development [6,9-11].

The purpose of this study was to compare ocular and developmental outcomes and systemic complications in infants who were treated with either IVB injection or laser for Type I ROP.

2. METHODS

2.1 Study Subjects

This is a cohort study to evaluate the efficacy and safety of IVB vs. laser for the treatment of severe ROP. The study was approved by the Institutional Review Board of Baylor College of Medicine/Texas Children's Hospital.

All infants with type I or severe zone 3 ROP who were treated with 0.625 mg IVB injection or laser from September 2010 to December 2012 were enrolled in this study. At the time of diagnosis of type I ROP, a full discussion of both treatment options was conducted with the parents in a manner intended to be completely unbiased. The advantages and disadvantages of each form of treatment were explained carefully, especially issues of the unknown possible late ocular and systemic side effects of IVB injection. The parents were provided with a written version of the issues discussed. The parents made the final decision regarding treatment. The following data were collected: gestational age (GA), birth weight (BW), primary diagnosis, duration of stay in the hospital, post-procedure pain management, systemic complications, vision outcomes, and development outcomes.

Diagnosis and treatment of type I ROP followed ET ROP guidelines [12]. Laser treatment was performed in the operating room under general anesthesia, and IVB injection was administered at the bedside under sterile conditions, using topical anesthesia and IV sedation with fentanyl if needed. Bevacizumab (Avastin®, Genentech Inc.) was injected into the vitreous of the affected eye (s) at 0.625 mg (in 0.025 mL solution) per eye, per dose. The injection procedure followed the protocol established by Mintz-Hittner (personal communication before the 2011 publication of the BEAT-ROP study results) [7].

2.2 Ocular Outcomes

Infants were followed closely after treatment to monitor resolution of the disease and to watch for the recurrence of vision-threatening ROP, until ROP was fully regressed and no abnormal vascular tissue was present that was capable of reactivation and progression [13]. The definitions for treatment failure were: 1) recurrence of type I ROP or 2) stage 4A or higher retinal detachment. In both groups, if ROP recurred and met the treatment failure criteria, laser was used for type I or stage 4A ROP and intraocular surgery was used for stage 4B or higher retinal detachment.

Structural outcomes of all eyes were documented with dilated fundus examinations at 1 year chronological age. The definition of favorable vs. unfavorable structural outcome from the ET-ROP study was applied [2]. The best corrected visual acuity (VA) of each eye was measured at 2 years chronological age with Teller Acuity Cards. Unfavorable vision outcome was defined as best corrected VA of 20/200 or worse. Full cycloplegic refractive error was measured at 1 and 2 years chronological age. We used the standard definition of myopia and high myopia as in the ET-ROP study [14].

2.3 Systemic and Developmental Outcomes

Systemic complications were documented and compared between the treatment groups. Short-term systemic events such as gastrointestinal bleeding, necrotizing entercolitis, and hypertension (requiring treatment with anti-hypertensive medications) were documented. Body weight was documented weekly from birth to 36 weeks of postnatal age. Neurodevelopmental assessments were done between 6 to 12 months chronological age. Neurodevelopmental assessments were performed by board-certified, developmental-behavioral pediatric and neurodevelopmental disability pediatricians. Each neurodevelopmental assessment included a developmental history, direct behavioral observations, and direct developmental testing using the Revised Gesell Developmental Schedules; the Motor Quotient [14] was used to assess gross motor development; and the Capute Scales [15], consisting of the Cognitive Adaptive Test and the Clinical Linguistic and Auditory Milestone Scale, was used to assess non-verbal, visual-motor problem-solving development and speech and language

development. Developmental age equivalents derived from the developmental measures were converted to developmental quotient scores ([developmental age ÷ chronologic age] x 100) for gross motor development, visual motor problem-solving development, language development, and overall cognitive development. A developmental quotient score of 85 or more is considered normal; 71-84 is considered mild-to-moderate delay; and less than 70 is considered severe delay [28,16].

2.4 Statistical Analysis

Statistical analyses were performed using the IBM SPSS software version 20 (New York, USA). A p-value less than 0.05 was considered statistically significant. Demographic and clinical variables were summarized with descriptive statistics. Duration of stay was analyzed for inborn patients only. Two-tailedt-test was used for comparing group means. Chi-square and Fisher's exact test were used for proportions. Linear regression analysis was used to fit the growth model of body weight. The neurodevelopmental data were analyzed with student t-test matched paired and Wilcoxon signed-rank test with SPSS software.

3. RESULTS

3.1 Patient Characteristics

A total of 42 infants were included in our analysis: 22 patients (43 eyes) in the IVB-treated group and 20 patients (37 eyes) in the laser group. The clinical characteristics of the patients are listed in (Table 1). Both groups were similar in baseline demographics in terms of APGAR (Appearance, Pulse, Grimace, Activity, and Respiration) scores, incidence of co-morbidities, the mean gestational age and body weight at birth, and the mean postmenstrual age (PMA) and body weight at the time of treatment for type I ROP. Post-operative pain and sedation management was required for 3of 22(14%) patients in the IVB-treated group and 13of 20(65%) patients in laser-treated group (p=0.009). There was no significant difference in the length of hospital stay (p=0.78; Table 1).

3.2 Ocular Outcomes

The severity of ROP in the affected eyes at the time of treatment was similar in these two groups (Table 2). There were no intraocular infections in either group. Laser treatment (and lid speculum time) for ROP took 20-30 minutes per eye, and IVB injection required use of a lid speculum for 1-2 minutes. We did not routinely check intraocular pressure (IOP) with equipment unless there was reason to suspect an increase in IOP by tactile palpation or cloudy cornea. By assessment of tactile tension and corneal clarity, none of the patients in this study developed increased IOP after undergoing the procedure.

3.2.1 IVB-treated eyes

In the IVB-treated group, there were seven eyes (3 right eyes; 4 left eyes) with zone I disease and 36 eyes (19 right eyes; 17 left eyes) with zone II disease (Table 2). All zone I ROP regressed fully after one injection. Of the 36 eyes with zone II disease, three eyes (8.3%) underwent laser treatment for recurrence of type I ROP. One patient was born at 24 weeks GA and treated with IVB initially for zone II/stage 2+ ROP in both eyes. The plus disease disappeared within 3 days after the injection and ROP regressed two weeks after the injection. However, type I ROP recurred bilaterally 84 days after the initial injection and was rescued with laser treatment. Another patient was born at 22 weeks GA and was initially treated with IVB for zone II/stage 3+ ROP in both eyes. The plus disease got better 2 days after injection and ROP started regressing in both eyes initially. However, the regression stopped in the right eye 13 days later and type I ROP recurred 18 days after the injection. This eye was rescued by laser. All ROP in the IVB-treated group eventually regressed fully. No patient in the IVB-treated group developed a retinal fold involving the macula.

3.2.2 Laser-treated eyes

In the laser-treated group, there were four eyes (1 right eye; 3 left eyes) with zone I disease, 31 eyes (16 right eyes; 15 left eyes) with zone II and 2 eyes (right eye) with zone III disease (Table 2). Two of the four eyes (from one patient, 50%) with zone I disease required surgery for development of stage 5 ROP, 53 daysafter the initial laser treatment. Two of the 31 eyes (6.5%) with zone II (zone II) disease required surgery for stage 5 ROP 44 days after receiving the initial laser treatment. Of these re-treated patients, one was born at 23 weeks GA (inborn, zone I/stage 2+) and the other one was born at 24 weeks GA (transferred from the other hospitals for the treatment of ROP, posterior zone II/stage 3+).

At 1 year of age, no eyes in the IVB-treated group and four eyes (zone I=2; zone II=2; 10.8% total) in the laser-treated group had unfavorable structural outcomes according to the ET-ROP definition (Table 3).

3.2.3 Primary outcomes

At age 1 year, in IVB-treated group, two patients died and three patients lost follow-ups. One IVB patient died from an acute cardiopulmonary arrest and suspected myocardial infarction 142 days after the injection. The other IVB patient died from multi-system complications 151 days after the injection. In laser-treated group, two patients died and two patients lost follow-ups. One laser patient died 92 days after laser treatment from multi-system failure with concomitant patchy pulmonary interstitial glycogenesis. The other laser treated patient died 180 days after laser as a result of an acute decompensation with bradycardia and desaturations. Thirty-three eyes in IVB-treated group and 31 eyes in laser-treated group had cycloplegic retinoscopy examination at 1and 2 years chronological age; the refractive error (RE) results are shown in (Table 4). In laser-treated group, one patient developed unilateral secondary cataract and had cataract surgery. This aphakic eye (RE +16.00) was eliminated from the statistical analysis. At age 1 year, the eyes treated with laser were significantly more myopic than were those treated with IVB (p=0.03) (Table 4). The proportion of patients who had high myopia was significantly higher in laser-treated group. At the age of 2 years, both groups showed progression of myopia, but the laser-treated group experienced more progression of myopia than did the IVB group. The distributions of the spherical equivalent (SE) at 1 and 2 years are shown in (Table 4).

Vision testing with Teller acuity cards was performed on 28 eyes in the IVB-treated group and 25 eyes in the laser-treated group at age 2 years. Two eyes (7%) in the IVB-treated group and four eyes (16%) in the laser-treated group had the best corrected VA below 20/200, p=0.21. In the IVB-treated group, one child (2 eyes) had an unfavorable visual outcome: light perception vision due to severe periventricular leukomalacia (PVL) and optic pathway hypoplasia. For this child, the ROP was fully regressed and no retinal structural abnormality was seen at age 2 years. The mean VA in LogMar was 0.54 (SD, 0.34) and 0.58 (SD, 0.52) in the IVB- and laser-treated groups, respectively (p=0.31).

Table 1. Comparison of risk factors and other characteristics of patients with type I retinopathy of prematurity in bevacizumab and laser treated groups

	IVB (n=22)	Laser (n=20)	P value
Birth weight, grams	645±135	669±145	0.59
Gestational age, weeks	24.3±1.3	24.8±1.8	0.46
Gender, male (%)	13 (59)	6 (30)	0.19
APGAR at 1 minute, median (range)	4 (1-8)	4 (2-8)	0.82
APGAR at 5 minutes, median (range)	7 (3-9)	7 (5-9)	0.80
Respiratory distress syndrome, n (%)	21 (95)	19 (95)	0.14
Bronchopulmonary dysplasia, n (%)	20(91)	16 (80)	0.47
Patent ductusarteriosus, n (%)	21 (95)	18 (90)	0.72
Culture-proven sepsis, n (%)	8 (36)	3 (15)	0.68
Intraventricular hemorrhage Grade 1 to 4, n (%)	16 (73)	13(65)	0.94
PMA at treatment, weeks	35.7±2.2	37.4±3.9	0.09
Body weight at treatment, grams	2046±485	2347±940	0.19
Post-operative pain and sedation management, n (%)	3 (14)	13 (65)	0.009
Duration of hospitalization, days	153±52	158±58	0.78

IVB = Intravitreal Bevacizumab; APGAR=an acronym for Appearance, Pulse, Grimace, Activity, and Respiration; PMA = postmenstrual age (gestational age + weeks since birth)

Table 2. Comparison of status of type I retinopathy of prematurity at the time of treatment

	IVB (n=22)	Laser (n=20)	P value
Right eye only, n(%)	1 (5)	2 (10)	0.53
Left eye only, n of patients(%)	0(0)	1(5)	0.29
Both eyes, n of patients (%)	21(95)	17 (85)	0.28
Right eye, n of patients (%)			
Zone 1	3 (14)	1 (5)	0.33
Zone 2	19 (86)	16 (84)	0.86
Zone 3	0(0)	2 (11)	0.12
Plus disease	21 (95)	19 (100)	0.34
Stage 2	6 (27)	4 (21)	0.65
Stage 3	16 (73)	15 (79)	0.43
Left eye, n of patients (%)			
Zone 1	4 (19)	3 (17)	0.49
Zone 2	17 (81)	15 (83)	0.87
Zone 3	0 (0)	0 (0)	
Plus disease	21 (100)	18 (100)	0.34
Stage 2	10 (48)	10 (56)	0.61
Stage 3	11 (52)	8 (44)	0.64

IVB = Intravitreal Bevacizumab

3.3 Growth Curve

Body weight was measured weekly, from birth to 36 weeks postnatal age. The growth curve for each group was plotted with mean body weight of the same postnatal age. The growth curves were obtained for pre- and post-treatment. The body weight showed linear increase with age in all groups. The correlation coefficient (r^2) between the average body weight and postnatal age was 0.97 (p=0.005, pre-treatment) and 0.98 (p=0.001, post-treatment) in the IVB-treated group, and was 0.93 (p=0.05, pre-treatment) and 0.92 (p=0.007, post-treatment) in the laser-treated group. The two groups had similar growth curves for both before and after treatment. The average weight gain before ROP treatment was 126.9g/week (SE,7.7) in the IVB-treated group and 128.1 g/week (SE, 6.1) in the laser-treated group, p=0.16. After receiving treatment for ROP, the average weight gain was 137.4g/week (SE, 3.0) in the IVB-treated group and 143.1g/week (SE, 4.6) in the laser-treated group, p=0.10. Faster weight gain occurred after treatment in both groups compared to pre-treatment, $p=0.007$ in the IVB-treated group and $p=0.003$ in the laser-treated group.

3.4 Neurodevelopmental Assessments

Ten patients from the IVB-treated group and nine patients from the laser-treated group underwent neurodevelopmental assessments at 6 to 12 months chronological age. (Table 5) shows the history of seizures, GA and mean developmental quotient scores in the IVB- and laser-treated groups. The ranges of developmental quotient scores in all tested subgroups were broad, ranging from 17 to 84 in the IVB-treated group and from 20 to 80 in the laser-treated group. Seven of ten patients (70%) in the IVB-treated group and six of nine patients (67%) in the laser-treated group were categorized as severely developmentally delayed (developmental quotient score less than 70) according to the gross motor developmental quotient scores.

Table 3. Structural outcomes at ages 1 and 2 Years for bevacizumab- and laser-treated infants with type I retinopathy of prematurity

ROP	Retreated eyes N (%)			Unfavorable structural outcomes at age 1 year[a] N (%)		
	IVB (n=43 eyes)	Laser (n=37 eyes)	P value	IVB (n=43 eyes)	Laser (n=37 eyes)	P value
Zone 1 ROP	0(0)	2(50)	0.0001	0 (0)	2(50)	0.0001
Zone 2 ROP	3(8.3)	2(6.5)	0.83	0(0)	2(6.5)	0.04
Zone 3 ROP	-	0(0)	N/A	-	0(0)	N/A
Total	3(7.0)	4(10.8)	0.33	0(0)	4 (10.8)	0.02

IVB = Intravitreal Bevacizumab; [a] the unfavorable structural outcomes at age 2 years remained same as age 1

Table 4. Percentage of eyes with myopia and high myopia in the bevacizumab and laser treated groups at age 1 and 2 years

Refractive status	IVB	Laser	P value
Eyes with any myopia ≥0.25 D,n//N (%)			
1 year	10/33 (30)	17/31 (55)	0.03
2 years	16/28 (57)	20/25 (80)	0.002
Eyes with high myopia ≥5 D, n/N (%)			
1 year	3/33 (9)	10/31 (32)	0.006
2 years	3/28 (11)	14/25 (56)	0.0005
Refractive errors, SE Mean±SD (range)			
1 year	-0.03±2.91 (-7.00 to+4.00)	-2.94±4.42 (-12.0 to +5.00)	0.02
2 years	-1.22±2.95 (-7.50 to 4.00)	-5.61±4.50 (-16 to 1.0)	0.03

IVB: intravitreal Bevacizumab; SE: spherical equivalent; D = diopter; SD =standard deviation; n= number of eyes with myopia; N=total number of eyes examined

Table 5. Developmental assessment for infants treated with bevacizumab and laser for type I retinopathy of prematurity

	IVB N=10	Laser N=9	P
Gestational age	24.6 ±1.2	24.0±0.0	0.67
IVH grade 3-4, n (%)	5 (50%)	4 (44%)	0.79
Hydrocephalus with VP shunt, n (%)	4 (40%)	2 (22%)	0.41
History of seizure, n (%)	1 (10%)	1 (11%)	0.94
Developmental quotient scores			
Gross motor	55.7±25.9	53.2±21.2	0.78
Visual motor	49.4±20.5	51.4±23.3	0.84
Language	47.8±19.8	50.4±20.8	0.84
Cognitive	48.6±19.6	50.9±21.7	0.83

IVB= intravitreal Bevacizumab; IVH = Intraventricular hemorrhage; VP = Ventriculoperitoneal

4. DISCUSSION

Several multicenter clinical trials have analyzed the efficacy of different interventions proposed to minimize the negative visual outcomes associated with ROP [7,17,18,19,20]. VEGF is an important component of the pathogenesis of ROP. Anti-VEGF therapy by IVB emerged as a potential therapy in 2007 [3,7]. However, studies showed that bevacizumab leaks into the blood stream and reduces the serum level of VEGF [21], which could potentially cause systemic complications with a negative impact on neurodevelopment. In this study, we found no post-treatment hypertension or exacerbation of NEC in either group. In both groups, the mortality rates were lower than the national rates reported for premature infants with BWs less than 1500g in the 2007 linked file: 17.8% for GA <32 weeks and 24.5% for BW <1500 grams [22].

In this study, we used body weight gain as one of the development parameters to assess the effect of systemically absorbed bevacizumab on general growth. The typical pattern of weight changes in infants is a variable degree of initial weight loss, followed by limited weight gain (70–150g) between 10 and 20 days. Growth velocity, the change in growth over time, is a more sensitive index of growth than is a single measurement. Normal full-term infants lose 10% of body weight in the first 2 weeks after birth; they then gain an average of 30 grams (1% of body weight) per day until they reach 3 months of age, and then 20 grams per day until they are 6 month of age [23-25]. In low-birth-weight preterm infants, an absolute growth rate is a reliable indicator of the weight growth pattern during the first year of life, and there is no significant difference in gender [26]. Studies have shown that preterm infants who were born at less than 30 weeks postmenstrual age with BW less than 1250 grams have an average weight gain of 16 grams per day [26]. In our study, the absolute weight gains in both groups before treatment were similar and consistent with the published data [26]. After treatment, significantly faster weight gain occurred in both groups, compared to pre-treatment, $p=0.007$ in the IVB-treated group and $p=0.003$ in the laser-treated group. There was no significant difference of the rate of body weight gain between the two groups, $p=0.1$. Our hypothesis is that the faster weight gain experienced after receiving the IVB injection and laser treatment was possibly due to up-regulation of insulin like growth factor (IGF-1).

This study didn't detect differences in developmental quotient scores. The Gessell Developmental Schedule is used by pediatricians to identify infants at risk for neurological impairment and mental development delay. An uncorrected developmental quotient score is suggested to be a more sensitive index for identifying abnormalities in preterm infants [27,28]. A low developmental quotient score is often related to intraventricular hemorrhage with or without ventricular dilation [28,29]. Although early developmental tests have limited ability to predict future Intelligence Quotient (IQ), their predictive power is better for children with significant developmental delays. Tests of early child development, such as the Capute Scales and Bayley Scales, were designed to separate normal from abnormal, not to separate subtle degrees of normality. However, infants and children without disabilities have greater variability and less stability of developmental scores over time than do children with cognitive disabilities. In this study, half of the infants had developmental assessment at between 6 to 12 months of chronological age. We are not able to draw any meaningful conclusion due to the small sample size and the broad range of developmental quotient in each group. However, these data could provide important information for the planning and justification of a randomized controlled multicenter trial in the future.

Laser surgery has been confirmed as a safe and effective treatment for ROP [12,30]. The postoperative inflammation and the need for post-operative analgesics is significantly less compared to cryotherapy [31]. The results from this study showed that the need for post-treatment pain management in the IVB-treated group was significantly less than in the laser-treated group. Previous reports indicate that although VEGF inhibition for treatment of ROP is promising and can allow further retinal vascularization, late recurrences of ROP are possible [32,33]. In this study, 3 of 43 eyes (6.9%) in the IVB-treated group needed laser rescue after one IVB injection. In one patient, type I ROP recurred 84 days after the initial injection, suggesting that long-term postoperative follow-ups should be considered in certain IVB-treated patients.

For the majority of the patients, and all with zone I disease, type I ROP resolved fully after one IVB injection. Although 3 (7.0%) patients in the IVB-treated group required laser rescue, ROP resolved eventually without unfavorable structural changes. The unfavorable structural outcome in our laser-treated group is 10.8%; in the ET-ROP study, 14% of patients with type I ROP showed unfavorable structural outcome at age 9 month.

Our study applied the same injection dose as in the BEAT-ROP study. Reducing the bevacizumab dose could decrease the potential risk for systemic complications. Future studies are necessary to address these questions: 1) Is the commonly used dose (0.625mg per eye per injection) the proper one? And2) How can we optimally select the ideal dose for the individual patient? Serum VEGF levels or serum levels of other growth factors may provide useful information, potentially leading to individualized treatment.

5. CONCLUSION

Our pilot study showed that IVB is comparable to laser therapy for treatment of type I ROP, especially for zone I disease. IVB had a more favorable side effect profile than did laser therapy, and that the prevalence rates of high myopia were lower in the IVB-treated group, compared with the laser-treated group. The potential for delayed complications from anti-VEGF therapy remains a major concern. A large, randomized, controlled trial is necessary to answer these concerns.

CONSENT

All subjects signed the consent forms for treatment and study.

ETHICAL APPROVAL

The study protocol was approved by institutional review board.

ACKNOWLEDGEMENTS

We thank Petros Carvounis, M.D and Michele Parker for their invaluable assistance with the study patients in the neonatal intensive care unit, Texas Children's Hospital, Baylor College of Medicine. We thank O'Brian E. Smith, Ph.D, Baylor College of Medicine for his statistics consultation, and B. Lee Ligon, Ph.D., Baylor College of Medicine, for editorial assistance.

COMPETING INTERESTS

Authors have declared that no competing interests exist.

REFERENCES

1. Kong L, Fry M, Al-Samarraie M, Gilbert C, Steinkuller PG. An update on progress and the changing epidemiology of causes of childhood blindness worldwide. J AAPOS. 2012;16:501-7.

2. Good WV. Final results of the early treatment for retinopathy of prematurity (ETROP) randomized trial. Trans Am Ophthalmol Soc. 2004;102:233-50.

3. Chung EJ, Kim JH, Ahn HS, Koh HJ. Combination of laser photocoagulation and intravitreal bevacizumab (Avastin) for aggressive zone I retinopathy of prematurity. Graefes Arch Clin Exp Ophthalmol. 2007;245:1727-30. Epub 2007 Aug 10.

4. Kong L, Mintz-Hittner HA, Penland RL, Kretzer FL, Chevez-Barrios P. Intravitreous bevacizumab as anti-vascular endothelial growth factor therapy for retinopathy of prematurity: a morphologic study. Arch Ophthalmol. 2008;Aug126:1161-3.

5. Kusaka S, Shima C, Wada K, Arahori H, Shimojyo H, Sato T, et al. Efficacy of intravitreal injection of bevacizumab for severe retinopathy of prematurity: a pilot study. Br J Ophthalmol. 2008;92:1450-5. Epub 2008 Jul 11.

6. Lim LS, Mitchell P, Wong TY, Gole GA, Camuglia JE, Ells AL. Bevacizumab for retinopathy of prematurity. N Engl J Med. 2011;364:2360. Author reply 1-2.

7. Mintz-Hittner HA, Kennedy KA, Chuang AZ. Efficacy of intravitreal bevacizumab for stage 3+ retinopathy of prematurity. N Engl J Med. 2011;364:603-15.

8. Wutthiworawong B, Thitiratsanont U, Saovaprut C, Subhangkasen I, Geyuraphun B, Ampornprut A, et al. Combine intravitreal bevacizumab injection with laser treatment for aggressive posterior retinopathy of prematurity (AP-ROP). J Med Assoc Thai. 2011;Aug 94:15-21.

9.   Gilbert CE, Zin A, Darlow B, Lim LS, Mitchell P, Wong TY, et al. Bevacizumab for retinopathy of prematurity. N Engl J Med. 2011;364:2359-60. Author reply 61-2.

10. Gole GA, Camuglia JE, Ells AL. Bevacizumab for retinopathy of prematurity. N Engl J Med. 2011;364:2360-1. Author reply 2.

11. Good WV, Palmer EA, Gilbert CE, Zin A, Darlow B, Lim LS, et al. Bevacizumab for retinopathy of prematurity. N Engl J Med. 2011;364:2359. Author reply 61-2.

12. Good WV. Final results of the early treatment for retinopathy of prematurity (ETROP) randomized trial. Trans Am Ophthalmol Soc. 2004;102:233-48. Discussion 48-50.

13. Pediatrics SoOAAo, Ophthalmology AAo, Strabismus AAfPOa, Article J, Guideline P, States U, et al. Screening examination of premature infants for retinopathy of prematurity. Pediatrics. 2006;117:572-6.

14. Knobloch H. Manual of developmental diagnosis: The administration and interpretation of the revised gesell and amatruda developmental and neurological examination. Maryland: Harper & Row, Publisher Inc. 1980;56-78.

15. Knobloch H, Pasamanick B. Gesell and amatruda's developmental diagnosis. New York: Harper & Row; 1974.

16. Mao C, Guo J, Chituwo BM. Intraventricular haemorrhage and its prognosis, prevention and treatment in term infants. J Trop Pediatr. 1999;45:237-40.

17. Multicenter trial of cryotherapy for retinopathy of prematurity. Preliminary results. Cryotherapy for Retinopathy of Prematurity Cooperative Group. Arch Ophthalmol. 1988;106:471-9.

18. Repka MX, Tung B, Good WV, Capone A, Jr., Shapiro MJ. Outcome of eyes developing retinal detachment during the Early Treatment for Retinopathy of Prematurity study. Arch Ophthalmol. 2011;129:1175-9.

19. Supplemental Therapeutic Oxygen for Prethreshold Retinopathy Of Prematurity (STOP-ROP), a randomized, controlled trial. I: primary outcomes. Pediatrics. 2000;105:295-310.

20. Sears JE, Pietz J, Sonnie C, Dolcini D, Hoppe G. A change in oxygen supplementation can decrease the incidence of retinopathy of prematurity. Ophthalmology. 2009;116:513-8. DOI: 10.1016/j.ophtha.2008.09.051. Epub 9 Jan 20.

21. Sato T, Wada K, Arahori H, Kuno N, Imoto K, Iwahashi-Shima C, et al. Serum concentrations of bevacizumab (Avastin) and vascular endothelial growth factor in infants with retinopathy of prematurity. Am J Ophthalmol. 2011;17:17.

22. Mathews TJ, MacDorman MF. Infant mortality statistics from the 2007 period linked birth/infant death data set. Natl Vital Stat Rep. 2011;59:1-30.

23. Crossland DS, Richmond S, Hudson M, Smith K, Abu-Harb M. Weight change in the term baby in the first 2 weeks of life. Acta Paediatr. 2008;97:425-9.

24. Macdonald PD, Ross SR, Grant L, Young D. Neonatal weight loss in breast and formula fed infants. Arch Dis Child Fetal Neonatal Ed. 2003;88:472-6.

25. Boom JA. Normal growth patterns in infants and prepubertal children. Jun 19, 2012 ed: UpToDate; 2012.

26. Casey PH, Kraemer HC, Bernbaum J, Tyson JE, Sells JC, Yogman MW, et al. Growth patterns of low birth weight preterm infants: A longitudinal analysis of a large, varied sample. J Pediatr. 1990;117:298-307.

27. Miller G, Dubowitz L, Palmer P. Follow-up of pre-term infants: Is correction of the developmental quotient for prematurity helpful? Early Hum Dev. 1984;9:137-44.

28. Palmer P, Dubowitz LMS, Levene MI, Dubowitz V. Developmental and neurological progress of preterm infants with intraventricular haemorrhage and ventricular dilatation. Archives of Disease in Childhood. 1982;57:748-53.

29. Thorburn RJ, Lipscomb AP, Stewart AL, Reynolds EO, Hope PL, Pape KE. Prediction of death and major handicap in very preterm infants by brain ultrasound. Lancet. 1981;1:1119-21.

30. Axer-Siegel R, Snir M, Cotlear D, Maayan A, Frilling R, Rosenbaltt I, et al. Diode laser treatment of posterior retinopathy of prematurity. Br J Ophthalmol. 2000;84:1383-6.

31. Allegaert K, Van de Velde M. Blunted inflammatory and faster clinical recovery following laser treatment compared to cryotherapy. Arch Dis Child. 2007;92:655.

32. Patel RD, Blair MP, Shapiro MJ, Lichtenstein SJ. Significant treatment failure with intravitreous bevacizumab for retinopathy of prematurity. Arch Ophthalmol. 2012;130:801-2.

33. Hu J, Blair MP, Shapiro MJ, Lichtenstein SJ, Galasso JM, Kapur R. Reactivation of retinopathy of prematurity after bevacizumab injection. Arch Ophthalmol. 2012;130:1000-6.

28

Ocular Involvement in Patients with Rheumatoid Arthritis

Artur Zoto[1][*] and Brikena Selimi[2]

[1]Department of Rheumatology, University Hospital Center "Mother Teresa", Tirana, Albania.
[2]Department of Ophthalmology, University Hospital Center "Mother Teresa", Tirana, Albania.

Authors' contributions

This work was carried out in collaboration between both authors. Author AZ designed the study, wrote the protocol, and wrote the first draft of the manuscript. Author BS managed the literature searches. Both authors read and approved the final manuscript.

<u>Editor(s):</u>
(1) Jimmy S. M. Lai, Department of Ophthalmology, The University of Hong Kong, Hong Kong and Honorary Consultant Ophthalmologist, Queen Mary Hospital, Hong Kong, China.
(2) Li Wang, Department of Ophthalmology, Cullen Eye Institute, Baylor College of Medicine, USA.
<u>Reviewers:</u>
(1) Anonymous, Şevket Yılmaz Training and Research Hospital, Turkey.
(2) A. P. Vignesh, Jawaharlal Institute of Postgraduate Medical Education and Research, India.
(3) Anonymous, Dicle University, Turkey.
(4) Enzo Maria Vingolo, Ophthalmology University, Italy.
(5) Carolina P. B. Gracitelli, Federal University of Sao Paulo, Brazil.
(6) Anonymous, Pamukkale University, Turkey.

ABSTRACT

Aim: The aim of this study was to find out the prevalence of various ocular involvements in patients with rheumatoid arthritis and to asssess the relation to immunological alterations.
Methods: This is a cross-sectional study involving 70 patients with rheumatoid arthritis. All patients fulfill the criteria of American College of Rheumatology and the European League against Rheumatism for the diagnosis of rheumatoid arthritis. Serum samples for rheumatoid factor and anti-cyclic citrullinated peptide antibody were obtained. The lacrimal secretion was measured in all patients by Schirmer's test. The patients were referred to the Ophthalmologist for examination of the eyes and interpretation of the related findings.
Results: Ocular manifestations were identified in 13 (19%) of patients with rheumatoid arthritis. Keratoconjunctivitis sicca was identified in 9 (13%) patients, episcleritis in 2 (3%) patients and scleritis in 2 (3%) patients. Patients with positive rheumatiod factor and anti-cyclic citrullinated peptide antibody, were 42 (100.0%) of whom 10 (23.8%) represent ocular lesions, while in the

*Corresponding author: E-mail: turi3@mail.com

other group of 28 (100.0%) patients seronegative only 3 (10.7%) patients have ocular lesions. **Conclusion:** Ocular involvement are common in rheumatoid arthrits. Keratoconjunctivitis sicca, episcleritis and scleritis are ocular manifestations that occur in rheumatoid arthritis. The most common ocular manifestation was keratoconjunctivitis sicca. Immunological alterations are important factors in ocular manifestations.

Keywords: Ocular; keratoconjunctivitis sicca; episcleritis; scleritis.

1. INTRODUCTION

Rheumatoid arthritis is a systemic autoimmune and inflammatory disease that affects not only the articulations but may involve a multiplicity of organs and are of diverse severity [1]. Ocular involvement is one of the extra-articular manifestation of rheumatoid arthritis and can cause morbidity in these patients. Ocular manifestations in rheumatoid arthritis are diverse and include dry eye, episcleritis, scleritis and peripheral ulcerative keratitis [2]. Ocular involvement, severe dry eye or keratoconjunctivitis sicca in particular, may exist independently from severe rheumatoid arthritis presentations and the eyes should be evaluated in all patents with rheumatoid arthritis, regardless of whether ocular manifestations are present [3]. Dry eye diagnosis is based on the clinical features and some diagnostic tests. Schirmer test is one of the diagnostic tools in evaluating ocular surface status. Episcleritis and scleritis are describe as inflammation of the eye and frequently occur as ocular complications of rheumatoid arthritis. Extra-articular manifestations of rheumatoid arthritis are generally more often seen in patients with rheumatoid factor positive and anti-cyclic citrullinated peptide antibody positive [4,5]. In clinical practice the most common diagnostic test for rheumatoid arthritis is rheumatoid factor and anti-cyclic citrullinated peptide and is generally accepted by the majority of rheumatologists and recommended by the European League of Arthritis and Rheumatism [6].

The aim of this study was to find out the prevalence of various ocular manifestations in patients with rheumatoid arthritis and to assess the relation to immunological alterations.

2. MATERIALS AND METHODS

This is a cross-sectional study involving 70 patients with rheumatoid arthritis. All patients fulfill the criteria of American College of Rheumatology and the European League against Rheumatism for the diagnosis of rheumatoid arthritis [7]. These patients were hospitalized in the clinic of Rheumatology or followed as outpatients. All patients were treated with Methotrexate 10-15 mg weekly for at least 3 months and received weekly folic acid 10 mg, low doses of glucocorticoid ≤7.5 mg per day and non steroidal anti inflammatory drugs in function of disease activity as is usual in clinical practice. Patients with rheumatoid arthritis who suffering from other diseases such as infectious (e.g. viral infection, bacterial, fungal or parasitic infection) or miscellaneous disease (e.g. atopic syndrome, rosacea, secondary to foreign bodies, chemical lesions or drugs such as alendronate, risedronate, zoledronic acid, ibandronate) which may influence the ocular lesions were excluded from the study [8]. We excluded also patients with prior eye surgery, contact lenses users, those taking medications such as anticholinergics, antihistamine, antidepressants, diuretics, etc.

Patients were examined by laboratory tests such as rheumatoid factor and anti-cyclic citrullinated peptide antibody.

A number of diagnostic tests have been performed to establish the diagnosis of keratoconjuctivitis sicca such as Schirmer's test, tear film break up time test and rose Bengal staining. We chose the Schirmer test even though the Schirmer test is used as one of the six major criteria for Sjögren's syndrome diagnosis based on the American-European Consensus Criteria for Sjögren's syndrome [9]. The patients were referred to the Ophthalmologist for examination of the eyes and interpretation of the related findings.

The lacrimal secretion was measured in all patients by Schirmer's test. It is performed by first drying the tear film, then inserting a Schirmer strip which was 5 mm x 35 mm into the lower conjunctival cul-de-sac toward the temporal aspect of the lower lid. Both eyes were tested simultaneously. The patient were asked to keep eyes closed. After 5 minutes we removed the strip and wrote down the millimeters moistened in the part of the strip that wasn't inside the eye. The wet portion of the strip was measured in millimeters with the scale. If the strip measures less than 10 mm of wetting the lacrimal glands are not functioning correctly. Episcleritis and scleritis are distinguished on the basis of appearance, symptoms and slit lamp microscopic examination. The diagnosis of episcleritis and scleritis is mainly clinical. Symptoms of episcleritis and scleritis can include redness, pain, tearing or photophobia, tenderness.

To determine if alterations of immunological examinations are associated with ocular manifestations, patients were classified into two groups. The first group included patients with rheumatoid factor and anti-cyclic citrullinated peptide antibody positive, the second group included patients seronegative.

2.1 Statistical Analysis

Continuous variables were expressed as mean values and their respective standard deviations. Categorical variables were presented in absolute values and their respective percentages. Differences between the categorical variables were assessed with Chi square test.

The P value ≤ 0,05 was considered a statistically significant. Data were analyzed using the Statistical Package for the Social Sciences software, version 19.0

3. RESULTS

The mean age of the patients was 46.17 (±8.75) years. The mean duration of disease was 9.21 (±3.54) years. Female patients are 52 (74.3%) and male patients are 18 (25.7%). Ocular manifestations were identified in 13 (19%) patients with rheumatoid arthritis. Keratoconjunctivitis sicca, was identified in 9 (13%) patients, episcleritis in 2 (3%) patients and scleritis in 2 (3%) patients (Table 1). Patients with positive rheumatiod factor and anti-cyclic citrullinated peptide, were 42 (100.0%) of whom 10 (23.8%) represent ocular manifestations (group 1), while in the other group (group 2) of 28 (100.0 %) patients seronegative only 3 (10.7%)

patients have ocular manifestations (Table 2). Ocular involvement were more frequent in patients with positive immunological tests. In patients with positive immunological tests, keratoconjunctivitis sicca is found in 8 patients, episcleritis in 1 patients and scleritis in 1 patient. Ocular manifestations in patients with positive immunological tests are significant versus patients with negative immunological tests $P = 0.02$.

4. DISCUSSION

In our study ocular manifestations were found in 19 % of patients and in our opinion these ocular lesions are frequent in this group of patients with rheumatoid arthritis. This indicates that ocular lesions are important extra-articular manifestations in rheumatoid arthritis. The extra-articular complications of rheumatoid arthritis include ophthalmological manifestations, which can in some cases be the first signs of the disease [10]. Approximately 25% of patients with rheumatoid arthritis have ocular symptoms [11]. The most common manifestation of ocular involvement in our study was keratoconjunctivitis sicca in 13% of patients. The incidence of keratoconjunctivitis sicca is between 15% to 25%, in literature and in patients with positive immunological tests at least 10% of their [12-14]. Keratoconjunctivitis sicca is the most frequent complication in rheumatic diseases and is particularly common in rheumatoid arthritis and Sjögren syndrome [12]. Episcleritis and scleritis are described in patients with rheumatoid arthritis. Studies have shown that patients with rheumatoid arthritis associated scleritis have more widespread systemic disease and a higher mortality rate than those without scleritis [15,16].

Table 1. Ocular involvement in rheumatoid arthritis

Condition	Number of patients	Percentage (%)
Keratoconjunktivitis sicca	9	13
Episcleritis	2	3
Scleritis	2	3

Table 2. Ocular involvement by immunological alterations

Patients group	Total	Normal	Oculare involvement	P-value
Group 1	42 (100.0)	32 (76.2)	10 (23.8)	0.02
Group 2	28 (100.0)	25 (89.3)	3 (10.7)	

Absolute numbers and row percentage (in parentheses)

In the present study 3% of patients had episcleritis and 3% of patients had scleritis. In others study scleritis and episcleritis in patients with rheumatoid arthritis is found at a prevalence rate of 4% to 10% [17]. The prevalence of scleritis on rheumatoid arthritis is reported to be 0.67% to 6.3% [18]. Another finding of this study is that ocular involvement in rheumatoid arthritis occurs more frequently in patients with alterations of the immune system. According to this study in patients with rheumatoid factor and anti-cyclic citrullinated peptide antibody positive ocular manifestations occurred frequently in 23, 8% patients versus group of patients seronegative and we found correlation. Rheumatoid factor and ant-cyclic citrullinated peptide antibody has been shown to be predictor of extra-articular manifestations in rheumatoid arthritis, our results seem to suggest that the presence of rheumatoid factor and and-cyclic citrullinated peptide antibody is associated with ocular manifestations, however there was one patients seronegative who were diagnosed with keratoconjuctivitis sicca, which demonstrates that even rheumatoid factor may be absent in Sjögren syndrome related to keratoconjuctivitis sicca and two patients with episcleritis and scleritis. In other study is found that the combined presence of anti-cyclic citrullinated peptide antibody and rheumatoid factor had more severe ocular involvement compared to those who were negative for these antibodies [2]. This indicates that the immune system is implicated in the development of ocular lesions.

5. STUDY LIMITATIONS

The patients in our study were selected from a university hospital center, which could potentially be prone to selection bias by including patients with more severe stages of the disease compared to patients at the community level. However, we tried to minimize this bias by recruiting also all the patients from the hospitals outpatient consultation clinics. Another limitation maybe the small sample size.

6. CONCLUSIONS

Ocular involvement are common in rheumatoid arthrits.v Keratoconjunctivitis sicca, episcleritis and scleritis are ocular manifestations that occur in rheumatoid arthritis. The most common ocular manifestation was keratoconjunctivitis sicca. Immunological alterations are important factors in ocular manifestations.

CONSENT

It is not applicable.

ETHICAL APPROVAL

It is not applicable.

COMPETING INTERESTS

Authors have declared that no competing interests exist.

REFERENCES

1. Turesson C, Jacobsson L, Bergström U. Extra-articular rheumatoid arthritis: prevalence and mortality. Rheumatology. 1999;38(7):668–74.

2. Itty S, Pulido JS, Bakri SJ, Baratz KH, Matteson EL, Hodge DO. Anti-cyclic citrullinated peptide, rheumatoid factor, and ocular symptoms typical of rheumatoid arthritis. Trans Am Ophthalmol Soc. 2008; 106:75–81.

3. Fujita M, Igarashi T, Kurai T, Skane M, Yoshino S, Takahashi H. Correlation between dry eye and rheumatoid arthritis activity. Am J Ophthalmol. 2005;140(5): 808-13.

4. Turesson C, Jacobsson L, Bergström U, Truedsson L, Sturfelt G. Predictors of extra-articular manifestations in rheumatoid arthritis. Scandinavian Journal of Rheumatology. 2000;29(6):358–64.

5. Laura GL, Alberto DR, Manuel PG, Alejandra FC, Mario SP, Arnulfo N, et al. Anti-cyclic citrullinated peptide (anti-ccp) and anti-mutated citrullinated vimentin (anti-mcv) relation with extra- articular manifestations in rheumatoid arthritis. Journal of Immunology Research. 2014;10.

6. Combe B, Landewe R, Lukas C, Bolosiu HD, Breedveld F, Dougados M, et al. EULAR recommendations for the management of early arthritis: Report of a task force of the European Standing Committee for International Clinical Studies Including Therapeutics (ESCISIT). Ann Rheum Dis. 2007;66:34-45.

7. Arthritis and Rheumatism. 2010;62(9): 2569-81.

8. French DD, Margo CE. Postmarketing surveillance rates of uveitis and scleritis with bisphosphonates among a national veteran cohort. Retina. 2008;28(6):889-93.

9. Artifoni M, Rothschild PR, Brézin A, Guillevin L, Puéchal X. Ocular inflammatory diseases associated with rheumatoid arthritis. Nat Rev Rheumatol. 2014;10(2):108-16.

10. Vitali C, Bombardieri S, Jonsson R, Moutsopoulos H, Alexander E, Carsons S, et al. Classification criteria for Sjögren's syndrome: A revised version of the European criteria proposed by the American–European Consensus Group. Ann Rheum Dis. 2002;61(6):554-8.

11. Patel SJ, Lundy DC. Ocular manifestations of autoimmune disease. Am Fam Physician. 2002;66:991–8.

12. Fuerst DJ, Tanzer DJ, Smith RE. Rheumatoid diseases. Int Ophthalmol Clin. 1998;38:47–80.

13. Harper SL, Foster CS. The ocular manifestations of rheumatoid disease. Int Ophthalmol Clin. 1998;38:1–19.

14. Cojocaru M, Cojocaru IM, Silosi I, Vrabie CD, Tanasescu R. Extra-articular Manifestations in Rheumatoid Arthritis. Mædica. 2010;5(4):286-91.

15. McGavin DD, Williamson J, Forrester JV, Foulds WS, Buchanan WW, Dick WC, et al. Episcleritis and scleritis. A study of their clinical manifestations and association with rheumatoid arthritis. Br J Ophthalmol. 1976;60:192–226.

16. Messmer EM, Foster CS. Destructive corneal and scleral disease associated with rheumatoid arthritis. Medical and surgical management. Cornea. 1995;14: 408–17.

17. Tabbara KF, Vera-Cristo CL. Sjogren syndrome. Curr Opin Ophthalmol. 2000; 11:449-54.

18. Anitha B. Ocular manifestations of rheumatoid arthritis: Correlation with disease activity and management protocols. Masters Thesis. Rajiv Gandhi University of Health Sciences, Karnataka, Bangalore; 2011.

29

Third Ventricular Ependymoma Mimicking Foster Kennedy Syndrome- A Case Report

Ee-Ling Tan[1*], Regunath Kandasamy[2,3], Wan-Hitam Wan-Hazabbah[1,3], Thavaratnam Lakana-Kumar[1] and Liza-Sharmini Ahmad Tajudin[1,3]

[1]*Department of Ophthalmology, School of Medical Sciences, Universiti Sains Malaysia, Kubang Kerian, Kelantan, Malaysia.*
[2]*Department of Neuroscience, School of Medical Sciences, Universiti Sains Malaysia, Kubang Kerian, Kelantan, Malaysia.*
[3]*Hospital Universiti Sains Malaysia, Kubang Kerian, Kelantan, Malaysia.*

Authors' contributions

This work is carried out in collaboration of all authors. Authors ELT and RK designed the study, wrote the first draft of the manuscript and managed the literature search. Authors RK, WHWH and LSAT revised it critically for intellectual contents. Authors ELT, RK, WHWH and TLK were involved in the assessment and treatment of the patient. All authors read and approved the final manuscript.

Editor(s):
(1) Rachid Tahiri Joutei Hassani, Ophthalmology Department III, XV – XX National Ophthalmologic Hospital, France.
Reviewers:
(1) Anonymous, Case Western Reserve University School of Medicine, USA.
(2) Anonymous, Kyoto University, Japan.
(3) Anonymous, São Paulo State University, Brazil.

ABSTRACT

Aims: To report a case of a third ventricular tumour mimicking Foster Kennedy Syndrome in a young adult.
Presentation of Case: A 21-year-old female presented with bilateral blurring of vision with preceded by generalized headache, nausea and vomiting. Fundoscopy revealed optic nerve atrophy of the right eye and a swollen optic disc on the left in keeping with features of Foster Kennedy Syndrome. MRI of the brain revealed a third ventricular tumor extending into the suprasellar region with hydrocephalus. Surgical excision of the tumour was done and the subsequent histopathological report confirmed it to be a clear cell ependymoma.
Discussion: Foster Kennedy syndrome is a rare clinical constellation describing a pattern of ocular findings typically related to extraaxial tumours involving the anterior skull base. It is characterized

Corresponding author: E-mail: eeling.tan@gmail.com

by the triad of unilateral optic disc swelling, contralateral optic atrophy and ipsilateral anosmia. The clinical signs of Foster Kennedy syndrome are a result of direct compression of the mass on the optic nerve and an indirect effect from raised intracranial pressure.

Conclusions: We conclude from this report that intraventricular or intraaxial lesions in the vicinity of the optic apparatus may also produce features mimicking Foster Kennedy syndrome in clinical practice.

Keywords: Foster Kennedy syndrome; third ventricle; ependymoma; optic atrophy; optic disc swelling.

1. INTRODUCTION

Foster Kennedy syndrome is a rare clinical entity which was first described in 1911. It is characterized by a triad of unilateral optic atrophy, contralateral optic disc swelling and ipsilateral anosmia [1]. This is a rare clinical syndrome and manifests in only in 1-2% of all intracranial mass lesions [1]. It is believed to have a localizing value which indicates that it arises from the floor of the anterior cranial fossa. The clinical signs are usually caused by tumors related in the frontal lobe, olfactory groove or optic chiasm and are usually meningiomas or gliomas [2]. We therefore report a rare case of third ventricular tumour that resulted in a clinical picture mimicking this syndrome.

2. CASE REPORT

A 21-year-old lady with no prior medical illness, presented with progressive blurring of vision in both eyes for a period of 6 months. The blurring of vision was more profound in right eye and it had worsened over the last one month. The patient's husband noted that she was less aware of objects coming from right side unless she turned her head in that direction. Her visual

symptoms were also preceded by progressively worsening intermittent generalized headaches. The headache was throbbing in nature and more severe in the morning upon awakening and was associated with nausea and vomiting. In the days prior to admission the patient was also noted to be lethargic and withdrawn. She denied any anosmia.

On examination, the patient was alert and conscious and orientated to her surroundings. Her vital signs were normal. Assessment of higher mental function revealed impairment in her short term memory. Ocular examination noted that the right eye was only able to perceive light while the left eye was 6/12. Relative afferent pupillary defect was profound on the right. The anterior segments of both eyes examination were unremarkable and the intraocular pressure was normal bilaterally. There was bilateral sixth nerve palsy. The visual field testing noted temporal field defect in the left eye. Funduscopic examination of the left eye revealed a hyperaemic swollen optic disc with blurred margins, and right eye showed optic atrophy with temporal pallor (Figs. 1A and B). There was no spontaneous venous pulsation noted on both optic discs. Neurological examination was otherwise unremarkable.

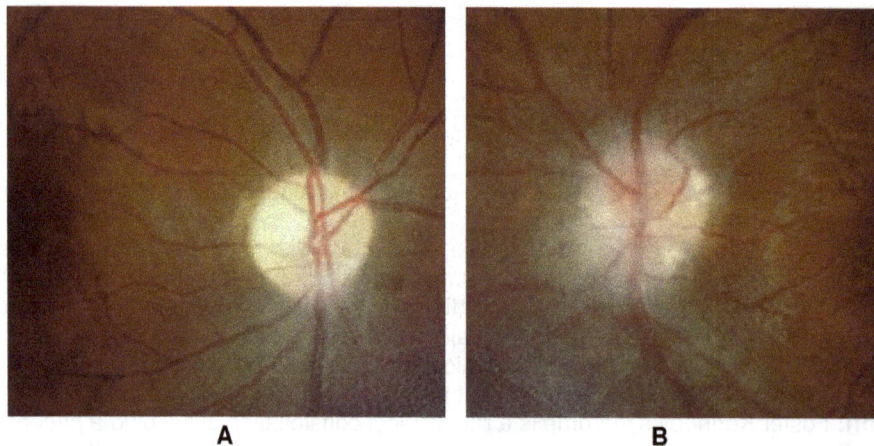

Fig. 1A and B. Right eye optic atrophy and Left optic disc swelling

MRI was done which revealed a heterogeneous enhancing lesion arising within the third ventricle and extending into the suprasellar region. The mass was ill defined, lobulated and measured 3.1 (W) x 3.7 (AP) x 3.7(CC) cm. It appeared hypointense on T1, hyperintense on T2 and was not suppressed by FLAIR. The mass was also noted to be associated with obstructive hydrocephalus Figs. 2A-C).

The patient underwent a frontal craniotomy and excision of her tumour via a subfrontal translamina terminalis approach. Histopathology examination revealed features of clear cell ependymoma (WHO Grade II) (Fig. 3).

One month after surgery, the vision in her eyes remained unchanged but fundoscopic examination noted resolution of the left optic disc swelling. Right eye optic disc remained same. The patient was planned for further MRI imaging, however she defaulted follow up care. The patient presented again after 1 year at which time she suffered from recurrent headaches. An urgent MRI of her brain revealed evidence of tumour recurrence Figs. 4A-B). She was advised for further surgery but refused. Subsequently she was referred to the oncologist who advised a course of Radiation therapy totaling 50Gy in 30 fractions.

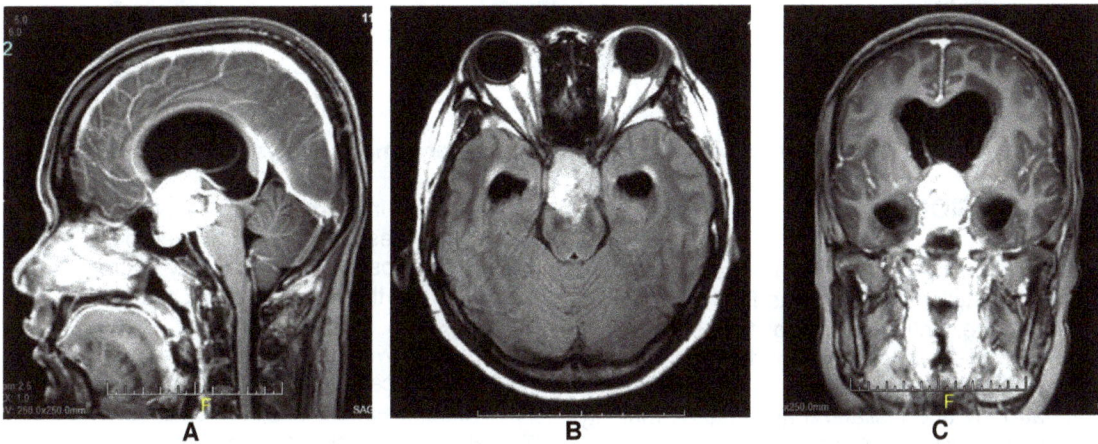

Fig. 2A-C. MRI showing heterogeneous enhanced lesion at the third ventricle extending intosuprasellar region and impinging the right optic nerve with accompanied hydrocephalus

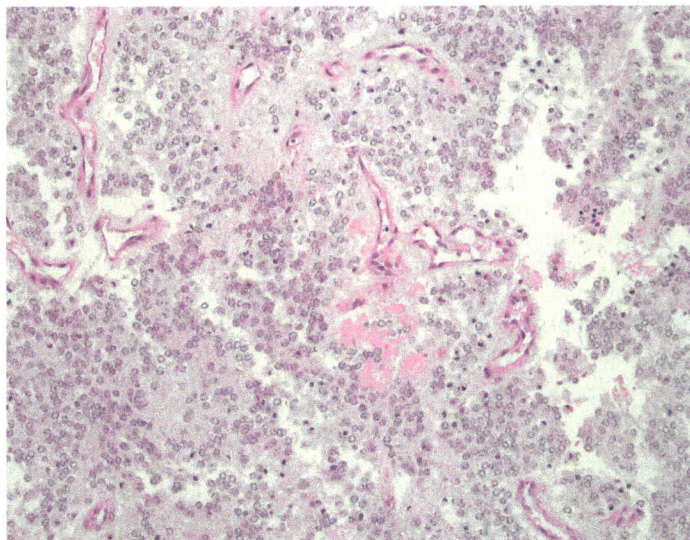

Fig. 3. Histopathological examination revealed clear cell ependymoma (WHO Grade II)

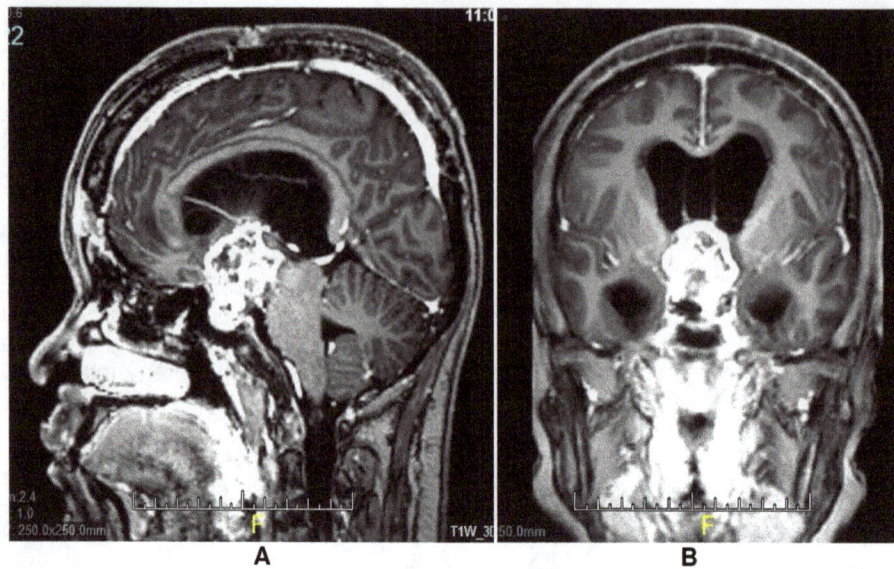

Fig. 4A-B. MRI of the brain showing recurrence of her tumour one year after surgery

3. DISCUSSION

Foster Kennedy syndrome is an uncommon clinical constellation which was first described in 1911 by the British neurologist Robert Foster Kennedy [1-2]. He described the triad of unilateral optic disc swelling with contralateral optic atrophy and ipsilateral anosmia. A majority of patients with features of Foster Kennedy Syndrome have intracranial masses originating from the olfactory groove, frontal lobe or sphenoidal region [1]. There exist some isolated case reports of this syndrome being seen in tumours originating in the sellar or parasellar region, optic nerve or even the occipital lobe. Pseudo Foster Kennedy Syndrome is an alternate term used to describe patients with unilateral optic disc swelling and contralateral optic atrophy in the absence of an intracranial mass [2-3]. It has been reported in patients with bilateral sequential consecutive ischemic optic neuropathy or optic neuritis as well as in conditions such as meningitis, carotid aneurysms, optic nerve hypoplasia, intracranial inflammation and retinitis pigmentosa [3-6]. One case report has even noted optic disc swelling secondary to uncontrolled hypertension with contralateral ischemic optic neuropathy [3].

The exact pathogenesis of Foster Kennedy syndrome has not been well elucidated to date [3,7]. Foster Kennedy himself postulated that the causes of such clinical signs were due to the direct compression of the lesion on the optic

nerve and an indirect cause secondary to raised intracranial pressure [8,9]. However, only 22% of cases of Foster Kennedy Syndrome were supported by this mechanism. Other postulated mechanisms include bilateral optic nerve compression without raised intracranial pressure in 33% of cases, and chronic elevation of intracranial pressure without compression in 5% of cases. In about 40% of cases, the mechanisms of Foster Kennedy Syndrome were unclear [7-10].

In this patient, we are of the opinion that her clinical features mimicking Foster Kennedy syndrome are most explainable by the original hypothesis of direct compression as well as secondarily raised intracranial pressure. From the imaging, the mass at the third ventricle has extended beyond the third ventricle into the suprasellar and sellar region. There was direct compression of the right optic nerve by the mass, leading to right optic nerve atrophy. The contralateral optic disc swelling resulted from the raised intracranial pressure as evidenced by the presence of obstructive hydrocephalus and dilatation of third ventricle. The preceding headache prior to the visual symptoms suggested the chronic elevation of intracranial pressure prior to the direct compression of the optic nerve from the mass. Clinically, there were also bilateral sixth nerve palsies which are likely a false localizing sign from raised intracranial pressure. The presence of memory loss suggested the involvement of the hippocampus.

Anosmia, one of the triad of Foster Kennedy syndrome, which is due to direct compression of olfactory tract, was not elicited in this patient.

We reported this rare case of Foster Kennedy syndrome secondary to ependymoma arising from third ventricle. To our best knowledge, this is the first case of third ventricular ependymomas in young adult leading to clinical features of Foster Kennedy syndrome.

Ependymomas are very rare; they arise from ependymal cells lining the ventricular system, including the spinal cord. They constitute 7% of all intracranial tumors in childrenaged 15 years old or younger [10,11]. It is rarer in adults, accounting for 2-5% of all intracranial tumors [12]. Most of the intracranial ependymoma arise in the posterior fossa, where fourth ventricle being the most common site of occurrence [11]. It can also occur within the brain parenychma. In adults, most of the ependymoma arise in spinal cord [12]. Supratentorial ependymomas are rare; especially those arise from third ventricle [13,14]. The clinical manifestation depends on the structure affected. Surgery remains the mainstay of therapy of ependymomas. However, complete resection is not possible as most of the time it has involved surrounding critical structures.

4. CONCLUSION

Foster Kennedy syndrome may not be necessary due to lesion arising from anterior cranial fossa. Any intraventricular or intraaxial lesions in the vicinity of the optic apparatus may also produce features mimicking Foster Kennedy syndrome in clinical practice.

CONSENT

All authors declare that 'written informed consent was obtained from the patient for publication of this case report and accompanying images.

ETHICAL APPROVAL

Not applicable.

COMPETING INTERESTS

Authors have declared that no competing interests exist.

REFERENCES

1. Lotfipour S, Chiles K, Kahn JA, Bey T, Rudkin S. An unusual presentation of subfrontal meningioma: a case report and literature review for Foster Kennedy syndrome. Int Emerg Med. 2011;6(3):267-269

2. Pastora-Salvador N, Peralta-Calvo J. Foster Kennedy syndrome: papilledema in one eye with optic atrophy in the other eye. CMAJ. 2011;183(18):2135-2135.

3. Bhatnagar KR, Raulji C, Kumar P, Solanki D. Pseudo Foster Kennedy Syndrome secondary to uncontrolled hypertension and diabetes mellitus: A case report. Medical Journal of Dr. DY Patil University. 2014;7(3):385.

4. Liang F, Ozanne A, Offret H, Ducreux D, Labetoulle M. An atypical case of foster kennedy syndrome. Interv Neuroradiol. 2010;16(4):429.

5. Yeh WY, Cheng CK, Peng PH, Huang KH. Foster Kennedy syndrome in a case with retinitis pigmentosa. Ophthalmic Surg Lasers Imaging. 2010;1-3. DOI: 10.3928/15428877-20100216-03.

6. Micieli JA, Al-Obthani M, Sundaram AN. Pseudo-Foster Kennedy syndrome due to idiopathic intracranial hypertension. Can J Ophthalmol. 2014;49(4):e99-e102.

7. DeAngelis LM. General considerations. In: Rowland LP, (ed) Merritt's neurology. Lippincott Williams & Wilkins, USA; 2005.

8. Walia HS, Grumbine FL, Sawhney GK, Risner DS, Palejwala NV, Emanuel ME, et al. An aggressive sphenoid wing meningioma causing Foster Kennedy syndrome. Case Rep Ophthalmol Med. 2012;102365. DOI: 10.1155/2012/102365.

9. Rodríguez-Porcel F, Hughes I, Anderson D, Lee J, Biller J. Foster Kennedy syndrome due to meningioma growth during pregnancy. Front Neurol. 2013;4:183.

10. Mansur DB. Multidisciplinary management of pediatric intracranial ependymoma. CNS Oncology. 2013;2(3):247-257.

11. Maksoud YA, Hahn YS, Engelhard HH. Intracranial ependymoma. Neurosurgical Focus. 2002;13(3):1-5.

12. Metellus P, Barrie M, Figarella-Branger D, Chinot O, Giorgi R, Gouvernet J, et al. Multicentric French study on adult intracranial ependymomas: prognostic factors analysis and therapeutic considerations from a cohort of 152 patients. Brain. 2007;130(5):1338-1349.

13. Feletti A, Marton E, Bendini M, Zanatta L, Valori L, Dei Tos AP, et al. Anaplastic ependymoma of the third ventricle. Brain Tumor Pathol. 2014;1-8.

14. Devadass A, Kirkwood S, Kenwright D. Sudden death from an Ependymoma. Pathology-Journal of the RCPA. 2014;46:S89.

30

Immune Reconstitution Inflammatory Syndrome (IRIS) Presenting as Bilateral Severe Granulomatous Sclerouveitis in a HIV-Infected Patient with Mycobacterium Tuberculosis Infection: A Case Report

Ee-Ling Tan[1,2*], Shelina Oli Mohamed[1], Hanizasurana Hashim[1], Norfariza Ngah[1] and Liza- Sharmini Ahmad Tajudin[2]

[1]Department of Ophthalmology, Selayang Hospital, Selangor, Lebuhraya Selayang-Kepong, 68100, Batu Caves, Selangor, Malaysia.
[2]Department of Ophthalmology, School of Medical Science, Health Campus, Universiti Sains Malaysia, Kota Bharu, 16150, Kubang Kerian, Kelantan, Malaysia.

Authors' contributions

This work is carried out in collaboration of all authors. Author ELT designed the study, wrote the first draft of the manuscript and managed the literature search. Authors SOM and LSAT revised it critically for intellectual contents. Authors ELT, SOM, HH and NN were involved in the assessment and treatment of the patient. All authors read and approved the final manuscript.

Editor(s):
(1) Li Wang, Department of Ophthalmology, Cullen Eye Institute, Baylor College of Medicine, USA.
Reviewers:
(1) Anonymous, Dicle University, Turkey.
(2) Anonymous, Mansoura University, Egypt.
(3) Anonymous, Ardabil University of Medical Sciences, Ardabil, Iran.
(4) Anonymous, Fukushima Medical University, Japan.
(5) Anonymous, University Eye Clinic, Serbia.

ABSTRACT

Aim: To report a case of tuberculosis (TB) associated immune reconstitution inflammatory syndrome (IRIS) presenting as rapid progressive bilateral severe granulomatous sclerouveitis.
Presentation of Case: A 26-year-old Human Immunodeficiency Virus (HIV) -infected male who was on antiretroviral therapy (ART) 3 months prior to presentation complained of left acute painful

Corresponding author: E-mail: eeling.tan@gmail.com

red eye with blurring of vision and floaters. There was severe granulomatous uveitis in both eyes with necrotizing scleritis in the left eye. There was also cervical lymph node that was positive for *Mycobacterium tuberculosis*. He initially responded well to antituberculosis therapy together with topical steroids and antibiotics, oral non-steroidal anti-inflammatory drugs (NSAIDS) and ART. His vision deteriorated after 6 weeks of treatment. He developed bilateral severe sclerouveitis and marked sclera thinning with self-sealed scleral perforation of the left eye. A diagnosis of IRIS was made and systemic steroid was added. Ocular inflammation was controlled, but his left vision remained poor due to perforated extensive necrotizing scleritis, seclusiopupillae and cataract.

Discussion: Intraocular TB may be presented with aggressive, rapid progression of the disease in HIV –infected patients. ART-associated TB is seen in HIV patients who developed TB after initiation of ART. Subset of ART-associated TB could be due to unmasking IRIS. Patients who were treated for opportunistic infection after ART may develop paradoxical IRIS.

Conclusion: Bilateral severe granulomatous uveitis with necrotizing scleritis is a rare manifestation of TB-related IRIS in an HIV patient. It is a potential sight threatening condition. A close monitoring for the development of IRIS during treatment of HIV is essential to minimize the morbidity.

Keywords: Immune reconstitution inflammatory syndrome; tuberculosis; granulomatous uveitis; necrotizing scleritis.

1. INTRODUCTION

Immune reconstitution inflammatory syndrome (IRIS) is an important complication following the management of HIV infected patients on highly active antiretroviral therapy (ART) [1-2]. IRIS is associated with various infections from bacteria, virus and fungi; autoimmune disease and malignancies [1-3]. It could be presented as "unmasked" or "paradoxical" IRIS. Tuberculosis (TB) is commonly associated with IRIS in HIV patients. The incidence ranges from 8 to 45%and is associated with extrapulmonary involvement [2-4]. TB-associated IRIS can lead to substantial morbidity [2,4]. Involvement of central nervous system can lead to high mortality [5,6]. Ocular manifestation of IRIS is rare. Most of the reported ocular cases were immune restoration uveitis or vitritis associated with cytomegalovirus retinitis [7,8]. We report a rare case of IRIS associated with TB presenting as bilateral severe necrotizing granulomatous sclerouveitis.

2. CASE REPORT

A 26-year-old HIV infected man who was recently started at 3 months duration of antiretroviral therapy (ART), presented with sudden left painful red eye for 2 weeks. The ART included Efavirenz 600mg OD, Lamivudine/zidovudine 150/300mg BD. The left painful red eye was associated with blurring of vision and floaters. However, there were no flashes of light. He denied any history of headache, nausea and vomiting. He had no history suggestive of tuberculosis infection prior to ART. He had

recently been treated for herpes varicella infection. His latest CD4 count prior to ART was 104/UL.

On examination, the best corrected right vision was 6/9 and left eye was counting fingers. Both eyes were congested and inflamed. Anterior segment examination of both eyes showed the presence of mutton-fat keratic precipitates, extensive posterior synechiae and anterior chamber cells, which was more severe in left eye. There was active necrotizing anterior scleritis involving the inferonasal quadrant of the left eye (Fig. 1). Both lenses were clear. There was mild vitreous inflammation in right eye. Left eye vitritis was more severe causing poor visualization of fundus. Intraocular pressures were normal in both eyes. Right funduscopy showed hyperemic optic disc with the presence of choroiditis, but there was no evidence of choroidal tubercle. B scan of the left eye revealed moderate vitreous opacities. A fundus fluorescein angiogram of the right eye showed an inflamed optic disc, vasculitis, choroiditis and cystoid macular edema.

Systemic examination revealed normal lung findings. Chest radiography was performed and there was no evidence of cavitation lesion suggestive of tuberculosis infection. At presentation, there was no palpable lymph node noted. Mantoux test was negative and Erythrocyte Sedimentation Rate (ESR) was not raised. Based on the recent history of herpetic infection prior to the onset of ocular symptoms, he was initially diagnosed with bilateral granulomatous panuveitis secondary to herpetic infection. Intravenous acyclovir was then started. Two weeks after intravenous acyclovir, there was no clinical improvement of the ocular condition. A cervical lymph node was then found and was proven positive for *Mycobacterium tuberculosis* following biopsy. Mantoux test was then performed again which was positive and the ESR was raised at 98mm/hour. The diagnosis was revised as presumed intraocular TB. Systemic antituberculous therapy was initiated together with topical steroids [guttae Dexamethasone (Maxidex) 4 hourly both eyes], topical antibiotics [guttae Moxifloxacin (Vigamox) 4 hourly both eyes] and oral NSAIDS (Tab Ibuprofen 400mg BD). ART was continued.

There was remarkable improvement in the ocular inflammation. However, upon review 6 weeks later the ocular condition had deteriorated drastically. He claimed to have maintained compliance to the treatment. His right eye vision was reduced to counting fingers and left eye was only perceptive to light. There was worsening of necrotizing scleritis with scleral thinning in both eyes. There was also intense intraocular inflammation of both eyes with the presence of fibrin in anterior chamber. There was marked scleral thinning with a self-sealed scleral perforation noted on the left eye (Fig. 2). The left eye anterior chamber was shallower with presence of seclusiopupillae. Both corneas were edematous and hazy with raised intraocular pressures, right eye 26mmHg and left eye 30mmHg. There was no view of the fundi. Systemic examination revealed a new lymph node enlargement. Biopsy was done on the new lymph node and yield negative result for *Mycobacterium tuberculosis*. Other septic workout was negative, and there was no evidence suggestive of toxicity to antituberculous therapy. CD4 at this presentation was raised to 243/UL.

In view of the paradoxical worsening of the ocular inflammation, a diagnosis of IRIS was made. Systemic steroids, oral prednisolone 1mg/kg/day, were immediately commenced together with continuation of antiretroviral, antituberculosis and topical medications. The oral prednisolone was slowly tapered based on the clinical responses. At six months of follow up, both eyes ocular inflammation has been controlled. The right eye visual acuity has improved to 6/9. However, the left vision remained hand movements even with well

controlled ocular inflammation (Fig. 3). The left eye anterior chamber remained shallow with presence of seclusiopupillae. There was presence of cataractous lens in the left eye.

3. DISCUSSION

Clinical presentation of intraocular TB varies widely from anterior and posterior segment involvement even to neurophthalmic involvement [9,10]. It is often misdiagnosed due to lack of uniformity of diagnostic criteria, and difficulty in retrieving ocular samples [9,10]. It is even more challenging in HIV patient as in this case [9-11]. The presence of history of herpetic varicella infection masked the potential of intraocular TB. Lack of laboratory evidences further complicates the matters initially.

Moreover, herpetic and TB sclerouveitis are both responsible for the granulomatous type of intraocular inflammation. The differentiation of the clinical presentation was further complicated by poor fundus visualization. Patients with HIV infection may present with aggressive ocular TB infection despite previous adequate antituberculosis therapy [11]. However, in this case there was no history of previous tuberculosis infection. The negative Mantoux test is not surprising in HIV patients. It is reported smear positivity rates in HIV infected patients are poor [12-14].During the treatment of ART, the rapid restoration of the immune system leads to increase immune responses to a specific antigen that may cause positivity in Mantoux test [13,14].

This patient had developed ART associated TB 3 months post ART, which is a term used to define HIV patients who are diagnosed with TB infection after initiation of ART [4]. It is believed to be due to on-going persistent immunodeficiency or due to rapid restoration of the immune response against TB after commencement of antiretroviral therapy [4]. It is reported that it occurred most often within first 3 months of ART initiation [15,16]. A subgroup of ART-associated TB is due to "unmasked" IRIS [4,16]. The rapid aggressive presentation with paradoxical worsening of ocular inflammation after the commencement of anti-TB treatment in this present case leads to the diagnosis of IRIS. To the best of our knowledge, this is the first case of severe granulomatous uveitis and necrotisingscleritis in IRIS. IRIS is postulated to result from rapid restoration of the immune response towards the

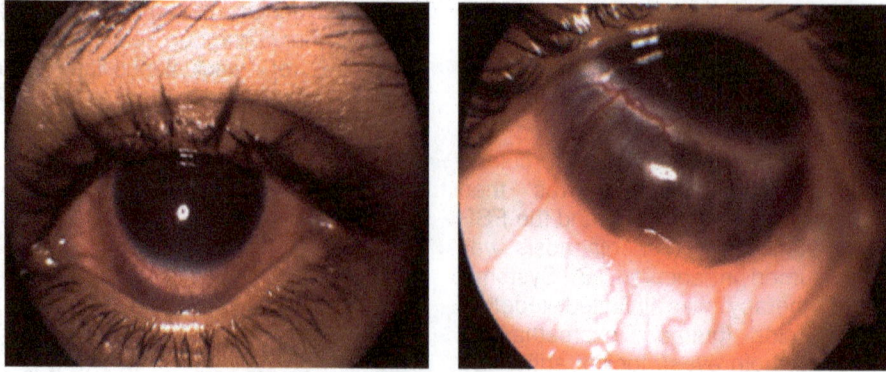

Fig. 1. Severe granulomatous sclerouveitis with inferior thinning in left eye

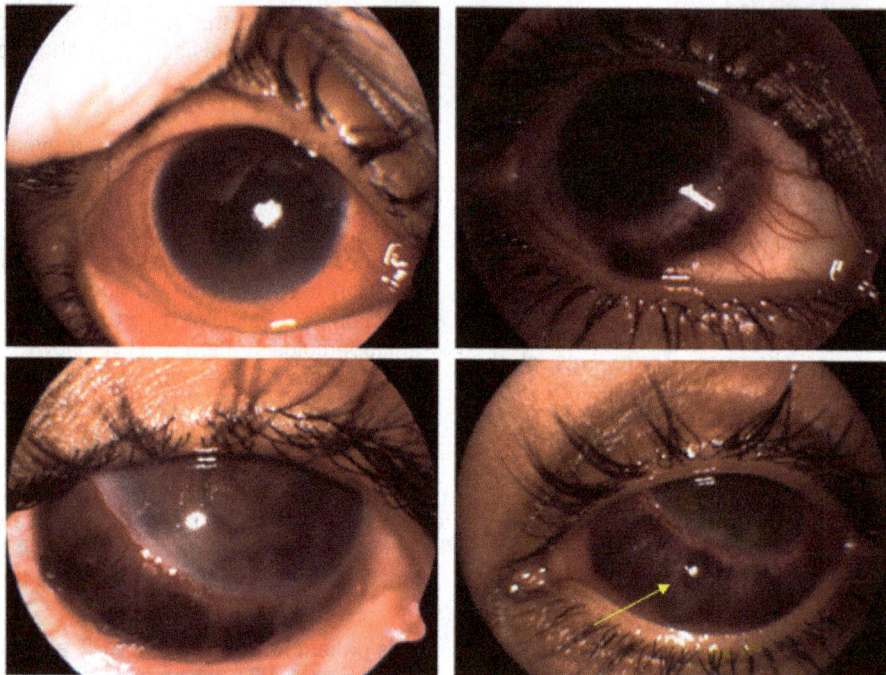

Fig. 2. Worsening of granulomatous sclerouveitis with inferior thinning of bilateral eyes. Upper panels: Right eye. Lower: Left eye with self-sealed perforation and seclusiopupillae

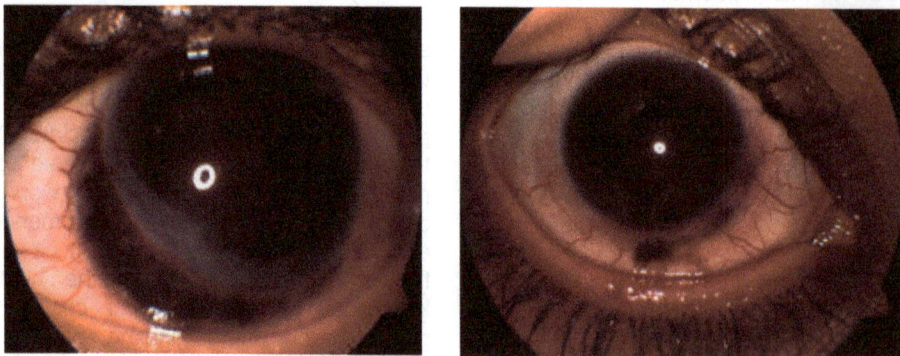

Fig. 3. Improved ocular inflammation after 6 months of follow up. Left: Left eye; Right: Right eye

pathogen and presents with a paradoxical clinical presentation [1,3,4]. It can either present as "unmasking" of an occult opportunistic infection, or "paradoxical" worsening of the symptoms, which can present at the original site or new body site [4,16-19]. Any pathogen which can provoke opportunistic infection can cause IRIS when there is recovery of pathogen specific immune responses during the course of ART [2,3].

These infections may be subclinical prior to commencement of ART and be unmasked after commencement of ART. The restored immune responses often lead to exaggerated inflammation and may be misinterpreted as opportunistic infection [3]. This immune restoration often occurs within first 3 months of ART. In this "unmasked" IRIS, viable pathogens may be isolated from the affected sites [3]. Commencement of ART in recently treated or exposed opportunistic infection can lead to paradoxical worsening of the infection. In this "paradoxical" IRIS, the immune response is against the non-viable pathogen, and cultures often yield sterile result [3]. "Unmasked" and "paradoxical" IRIS was postulated to result from different immunopathogenesis [16].

Following the recent case consensus definition, this patient was diagnosed as "unmasked" TB associated IRIS. The diagnosis of "unmasking" TB associated IRIS is suggested in patients who had not received tuberculosis treatment prior to ART and developed active TB within 3 months of ART, followed by the presence of marked inflammatory clinical manifestation or development of paradoxical responses once patient is established on tuberculosis treatment [4]. Repeated positive Mantoux test in this case supported the evidence of immune restoration as seen in unmasked IRIS in subgroup of ART associated TB [16]. There was also evidence of increment in CD4 count during the course of ART and anti-TB treatment.

The presence of tubercular lymphadenitis also increases the index of suspicious of IRIS. Extrapulmonary TB, for example tubercular lymphadenitis is reported as one of the risk factors of developing IRIS [1,2,19]. In this patient, the latest CD4 count at initiation of ART was slightly more than 100/µl. IRIS is reported to commonly develop in cases with CD4 less than 100µl [1,2,18,19]. This patient had received ART at the age of 26. Greater response to ART seen

in younger age group is a recognized risk factor of IRIS [18]. In this present case, TB was diagnosed at 3 months of ART and TB therapy was then started. Early period of ART and short interval between ART and treatment of opportunistic infection as seen in these patients are another recognized risk factors for IRIS development [1,2,19].

Rapid aggressive ocular presentation with impending ocular perforation is really alarming in this patient. High index of suspicious is important to initiate appropriate treatment and arrest further morbidity for this young HIV patient. Until now, there is no prospective consensus on managing IRIS [1,2,4]. In severe cases, systemic immunosuppressive corticosteroid is recommended with continuation of treatment for opportunistic infection and HAART therapy [1,3,20]. Vision is important to improve quality of life even in HIV patients.

4. CONCLUSION

Detection and management of TB associated IRIS are challenging. The dramatic sight-threatening complications of IRIS may pose a challenge in the management of intraocular TB. High index of suspicion is warranted to minimize the morbidity and mortality due to TB associated IRIS.

CONSENT

All authors declare that 'written informed consent was obtained from the patient for publication of this case report and accompanying images.

ETHICAL APPROVAL

Not applicable.

COMPETING INTERESTS

Authors have declared that no competing interests exist.

REFERENCES

1.   Müller M, Wandel S, Colebunders R, Attia S, Furrer H, Egger M. Immune reconstitution inflammatory syndrome in patients starting antiretroviral therapy for

HIV infection: A systematic review and meta-analysis. The Lancet Infectious Diseases. 2010;10:251-261.

2. Beatty GW. Immune reconstitution inflammatory syndrome. Emergency Medicine Clinics of North America. 2010;28(2):393-407.

3. French MA. Immune reconstitution inflammatory syndrome: A reappraisal. Clinical Infectious Diseases. 2009;48:101-107. DOI: 10.1086/595006.

4. Meintjes G, Lawn SD, Scano F, Maartens G, French MA, Worodria W, et al. Tuberculosis-associated immune reconstitution inflammatory syndrome: Case definitions for use in resource-limited settings. The Lancet Infectious Diseases. 2008;8:516-523. DOI: 10.1016/S1473-3099 (08) 70184-1.

5. Pepper DJ, Marais S, Maartens G, Rebe K, Morroni C, Rangaka MX, et al. Neurologic manifestations of paradoxical tuberculosis-associated immune reconstitution inflammatory syndrome: A case series. Clinical Infectious Diseases. 2009;48(11):e96-e107.

6. Marais S, Meintjes G, Pepper DJ, Dodd LE, Schutz C, Ismail Z, et al. Frequency, severity, and prediction of tuberculosis meningitis immune reconstitution inflammatory syndrome. Clinical Infectious Diseases. 2013;56(3):450-460.

7. Figueiredo L, Rothwell R, Bilhoto M, Varandas R, Fonseca S. Immune recovery uveitis masked as an endogenous endophthalmitis in a patient with active CMV retinitis. Case Reports in Ophthalmological Medicine; 2013.

8. Urban Beata, Alina Bakunowicz-Łazarczyk, Marta Michalczuk. Immune Recovery Uveitis: Pathogenesis, Clinical Symptoms, and Treatment. Mediators of Inflammation; 2014.

9. Gupta V, Gupta A, Rao NA. Intraocular tuberculosis-an update. Survey of Ophthalmology. 2007;52:561-587.

10. Alvarez GG, Roth VR, Hodge W. Ocular tuberculosis: Diagnostic and treatment challenges. International Journal of Infectious Diseases. 2009;13:432-435. DOI: 10.1016/j.ijid.2008.09.018.

11. Sudharshan S, Kaleemunnisha S, Banu AA, Shrikrishna S, George AE, Babu BR, et al. Ocular lesions in 1,000 consecutive HIV-positive patients in India: a long term study. Journal of Ophthalmic Inflammation and Infection. 2013;3(1):1-7.

DOI: 10.1186/1869-5760-3-2

12. Lawn SD, Wood R. Tuberculosis in antiretroviral treatment services in resource-limited settings: Addressing the challenges of screening and diagnosis. J Infect Dis. 2011;204(Suppl):1159-1167. DOI: 10.1093/infdis/jr411.PubMed: 21996698

13. Archi Munawwar, Sarman Singh AIDS associated tuberculosis: A catastrophic collison to evade the host immune system. Tuberculosis. 2012;92:384-387.

14. Nayak Surajit, Basanti Acharjya. Mantoux test and its interpretation. Indian Dermatology Online Journal. 2012;3(1):2-6. DOI: 10.4103/2229-5178.93479

15. Manabe YC, Breen R, Perti T, Girardi E, Sterling T. Unmasked tuberculosis and tuberculosis immune reconstitution inflammatory disease: A disease spectrum after initiation of antiretroviral therapy. The Journal of Infect Dis. 2009;199:437-44.

16. Elliott JH, Vohith K, Saramony S, Savuth C, Dara C, Sarim C, et al. Immunopathogenesis and diagnosis of tuberculosis and tuberculosis-associated immune reconstitution inflammatory syndrome during early antiretroviral therapy. Journal of Infectious Diseases. 2009;200(11):1736-1745.

17. Pornparasert S, Leechanachai P, Klinbuayaem V, Leenasirimakul P, Promping C, Intra P, et al. Unmasking tuberculosis-associated Immune reconstitution inflammatory syndrome in HIV-1 infection after antiretroviral therapy. Asian Pac J Allergy Immunol. 2010;28:206-9.

18. Valin N, Pacanowski J, Denoeud L, Lacombe K, Lalande V, Fongnernie L, et al. Risk factors for "unmasking immune reconstitution inflammatory syndrome" presentation of tuberculosis following combination antiretroviral therapy initiation in HIV-infected patients. AIDS. 2010;24(10):1519-25. DOI: 10.1097/QAD.0b013e3283396007

19. Laureillard D, Marct O, Madec Y, Chea S, Chan S, Borand L, et al. Paradoxical tuberculosis-associated immune reconstitution inflammatory syndrome after early initiation of antiretroviral therapy in a

randomized clinical trial. AIDS. 2013;27(16):2577-2586.

20. Meintjes G, Wilkonson RJ, Morroni C, Pepper DJ, REbe K, Rangaka MX, et al. Randomized placebo-controlled trial of prednisone for paradoxical TB-associated immune reconstitution inflammatory syndrome. AIDS (London, England). 2010;24(15):2381.

31

Delayed Removal of Temporary Non-incisional Silk Suture in Senile Entropion; a Simple Method for Long-time Relief

Gholamhossein Yaghoobi[1*] and Behrouz Heydari[2]

[1]Department of Ophthalmology, Valiasr Hospital, Birjand University of Medical Sciences, Social Determinant Health Research Center, Birjand, Iran.
[2]Department of Ophthalmology, Birjand University of Medical Sceince, Ghafari St, Birjand, Iran.

Authors' contributions

This work was carried out in collaboration between all authors. Author GY designed the study, wrote the protocol, and wrote the first draft of the manuscript. Author BH managed the literature searches. All authors read and approved the final manuscript.

Editor(s):
(1) Ahmad M Mansour, Department of Ophthalmology, American University of Beirut, Lebanon.
Reviewers:
(1) Anonymous, Sevket Yılmaz Resarch and Training Hospital, Turkey.
(2) Elizabeth Awoyesuku, Dept. of Ophthalmology, University of Port Harcourt, Nigeria.

ABSTRACT

Purpose: To assess the long standing effects of transverse lid-everting silk suture in senile entropion.

Methods: Eight patients (9 eyelids) who had only senile entropion participated in this prospective study. The lower lid had retractor laxity and upward migration of the pereseptal orbicularis muscle. The two Quickert-Rathbun silk suture is easily placed under local anesthesia. This is achieved with topical administration of tetracaine drops and subcutaneous infiltration of 2% lidocaine. The patient instilled topical bethamethasone and chloramphenicol every six hour for one week. All patients were followed up regularly at 1 week, 8 weeks, 16 weeks and then, every year for eye lid position (suture was removed after 12 weeks).

Results: Except for one patient, the others had good lid position and no symptoms of corneal discomfort during the three months postoperative period. The other patient developed stitch abscess and responded to medical treatment and early removal of the suture.

Conclusion: Although transverse lid everting suture has been used as a temporary measure in

---

Corresponding author: E-mail: Yaqubig@yahoo.com

treatment of senile entropion, long standing three months silk lid sutures have been shown to have more permanent effect.

The late removal of suture showed long lasting effects and cost-effectiveness as a simple outpatient procedure, especially in debilitated patients.

Keywords: Senile entropion; transverse lid suture; temporary suture.

1. INTRODUCTION

Involutional entropion is the most common phenomenon and by definition occurs as a result of aging. The lower lid is always affected and there is a combination of lower lid retractor laxity and upward migration of the pereseptal orbicularis muscle [1].

Medical management of senile enteropion includes (Emollents, bandage, contact lens, botulinium toxin, ...) which has a temporary effect.But in spite of over a hundred surgical approaches which have been devised to correct involutional entropion, immediate relief can be efficiently brought to the patient with the non-incisional suture technique. Therefore, this should be an ideal and effective operation, with minimum discomfort, rapid recovery and simple enough for trainees, compared with more difficult operations such as a lateral tarsal strip and retractor reattachment [2].

The everting sutures approach in correction of primary or recurrent lower lid involutional entropion was found a simple, successful, long lasting, and cost-effective procedure, by M. Wright et al. [3].

This study was conducted to assess the effects of three months delayed removal of non-incisional silk suture in elderly patients with senile entropion.

2. MATERIALS AND METHODS

A clinical trial treatment was carried out on 9 eyelids (8 patients), undergoing non-incisional lid-everting suture to correct involutional entropion. In this study, patients with only lower lid senile entropion were assessed. The procedure was explained to patients and they signed a consent paper. If they did not accept to participate in the study, they were omitted from the list. Exclusion criteria included a history of previous lower lid surgery other than senile entropion or patients with grade 4 medial canthal tendon laxity by the lateral distraction test.

The main criteria for outcome was lower lid position and changes in lower lid retractor function. In this method, sutures are easily placed under local anesthesia. This is achieved with topical administration of tetracaine drops and subcutaneous infiltration of 2% lidocaine. To place the sutures, the eyelid is pulled from globe with forceps, one needle of double armed suture is passed deep in to the inferior fornix and up through the lid, exiting anteriorly through the skin 2 to 3 millimeters below the lash line. The second needle is passed in the same way, about 5 mm lateral to the first and a knot was tied to correct the lid position. A total of two stitches are placed in each lid, with the most lateral one exiting about 2 mm below the level of the nasal one. The patient instilled topical betamthasone and chloramphenicol every six hour for one week.

To evaluate the immediate results, the patient was asked to look down, which demonstrated appropriate movement of the corrected lid. Suture was removed after three months and the Patients were followed up at 1, 8, 16, week's periods postoperatively and then, they were assessed annually. Successful outcome was long time stability of lid margin without turning in which causes corneal-lash contact. It seems that permanent effect of silk suture was associated with more induced inflammation and scar formation. The data was analyzed by descriptive statistics such as frequency and mean.

3. RESULTS

Most patients had excellent lid position and comfortable eyelid situation as early as post operation or thereafter (Figs. 1,2), except for two patients who developed suture abscess in one case and recurrence of entropion in another one. The stitch abscess responded to oral antibiotics and the recurrence of entropion again underwent repair. (Fig. 3). In Table 1, the other characters and outcomes are also summarized.

The mean age of patients was 69 years old and all patients had lower lid senile entropion. Four eyes had left eyelid entropion and 5 eyes experienced right eyelid entropion. Five patients were male and other three were female. (One male was bilateral).

Only one male patient developed stitches abscess 7 weeks after entropion repair, which responded to oral cephalosporin in one week.

But the patient again managed by other procedures. Between 0.1 to 10 years (average 4.4 years) follow-up for this technique was associated with recurrence of two more senile entropions.

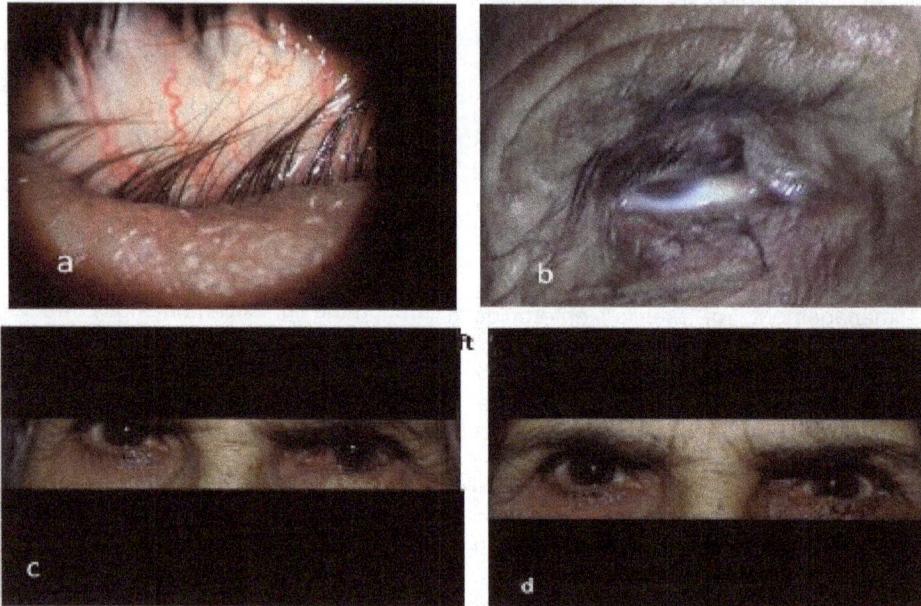

Fig. 1. First case; a, right lower lid entropion before repair, b the day after correction, Second case; c, left lower lid entropion before repair d, post procedure one month thereafter

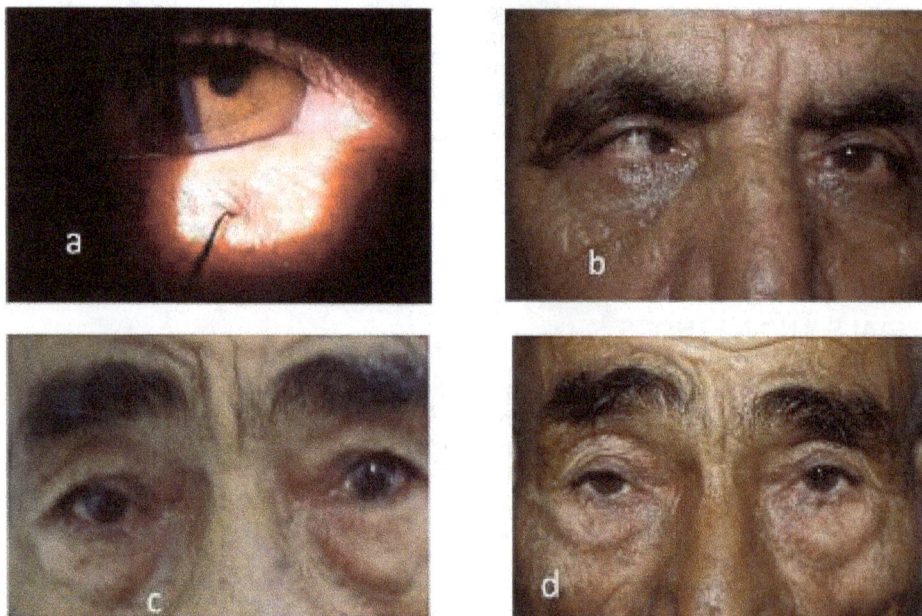

Fig. 2. (Third) case; a, right lower lid enteropion three months after correction, b. 7 years thereafter. Forth bilateral case; c & d before and 5 years after of left lower lid correction

4. DISCUSSION

Non-incisional silk suture has been found to be an effective, easy and temporary procedure which is associated with a high postoperative success rate. The only early complication was stitch abscess in one case that responded to medical treatment. The long term effect was good anatomical and functional corrections which were achieved in 6 eyelides. There are other reports which describe stitch abscess and pyogenic granuloma too [4,5].

Except for one case of reoperation which was managed successfully and one stitch (abscess) which responded to medical treatment and other surgical approach, the lid everting silk suture not only caused temporary relief of symptoms, but also it was associated with long time effects. However, two other cases gradually had late recurrences which again properly managed by this simple approach.

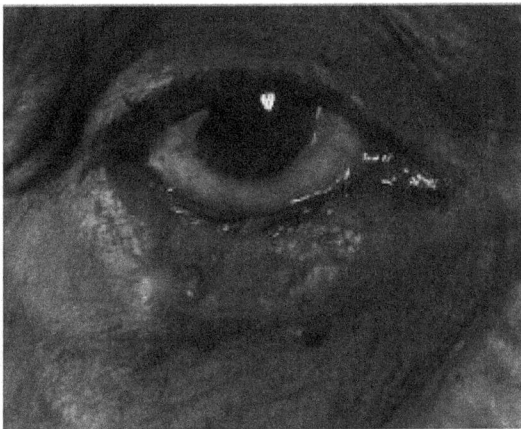

Fig. 3. Stitch indurations and abscess

A study conducted by Scheepers et al. [1] provides strong evidence that success rates at 18 months are higher in patients treated with everting suture and lateral tarsal strip (ES+LTS) procedure compared to ES alone. [2] although many surgical procedures were described with varying long-term success rates for the treatment of entropion, the use of everting sutures alone is advocated by many surgeons because of advantages such as being quick and relatively simple to perform, and also anticoagulation treatment does not need to be omitted compared to more invasive eyelid procedures including anticoagulation.

This study shows long time relief of senile entropion which indicate the important role of the three-month remaining non-incisional silk suture. The surgical approach that Caldato and his colleagues reported, 96.60% success rate was describe in 30 patients with senile entropion who underwent reinsertion of the lower eyelid retractor aponeurosis to the tarsal plate without horizontal shortening or resection of the skin or orbicularis muscle (after 29 months follow-up examination). This study also highlighted the low recurrence rate of senile entropion [6], even though this surgical approach was modified and its results were similar to our study.

Low recurrence rate of entropion is associated with botulinum toxin A. It removes the discomfort symptoms in all patients with improvements in effectivity and acceptability. The mean active duration of the toxin was 70 days. The authors believe that botulinum toxin injection to the lower lid provides a more effective and acceptable interim measurement in relieving lower lid entropion [7].

Table 1. Distribution of age, sex and follow-up outcome

Number	Gender	Age	Lid	Recurrence	Complication	Follow-up Year
1	♀	65	RLL	No	No	5
2	♂	70	RLL	Yes	No	7
3	♂	62	LLL	No	Yes	1
4	♂	60	RLL	No	No	5
5	♀	76	LLL	No	No	5
6	♂	75	LLL	No	No	5
7	♀	75	RLL	No	No	4
8	♀	75	LLL	Yes	No	2.5
9	♂	65	RLL	No	NO	2

RLL=Right Lower Lid; LLL=Left Lower Lid

The other dilemma in the management of involutional entropion was the description provided by Bashour Mounir and Harvey on what John Dalglish and Smith believed that the overriding effect on orbicularis was not an etiologic factor. They conceded that "spasm or over-action of the palpebral orbicularis is a real possibility in cases of entropion, and needs further investigation". The temporary improvement of involutional entropion after botulinium toxin injection could be noted as a supporting evidence for this suggestion [8].

There is a trend to find the ideal approach with minimal expense in any field of management that Wright et al. also assessed the long term efficacy of everting suture [9]. I. Leibovitch introduced a minimally invasive single-stitch lateral wedge technique, Tsang S describe this a simple and effective procedure for repairing involutional lower eyelid entropion which is associated with low recurrence and complication rates [10,11].

The most important result of our research was few complication and recurrences in senile entropion, though our patients were 9 eyelids, but compared to the Tsang study, simplicity and outpatients procedures are other characteristic findings of this procedure.

This conclusion can be clearly reached in a comparative study of Boboridis.K, in which 6 of 37 (16%) eyelids had unsatisfactory results after the tendon plication in contrast to 31 of 65(48%) after the wies procedure (more invasion). [12] These data provide strong evidence that in the absence of horizontal shortening of the lower eyelid, a successful outcome is more likely to result from non-incisional silk suture procedure.

5. CONCLUSION

Among many surgical approaches for repair of senile entropion non-incisional silk suture seems to be the simplest and most repeatable procedure, with minimal manipulation of lower lid. It is also an outpatients' procedure that is associated with high postoperative success rate, in comparison to retractor reinsertion or wies procedure. A reduction on suture number (two sutures) and an increase in the bite of suture may play an important role in our study, even though silk suture induced more inflammation. However, a randomized case control study with a larger number of patients is required to evaluate these results.

ETHICAL APPROVAL

All authors hereby declare that all experiments have been examined and approved by the appropriate ethics committee and have therefore been performed in accordance with the ethical standards laid down in the 1964 Declaration of Helsinki.

ACKNOWLEDGEMENTS

We have acknowledgement of our head nurse Mah Monier Sanaei and the patient who had good coporation in this study.

COMPETING INTERESTS

Authors have declared that no competing interests exist.

REFERENCES

1. Scheepers MA, Singh R, Ng J, Zuercher D, Gibson A, Bunce C, et al. A randomized controlled trial comparing everting sutures with a lateral tarsal strip for involutional entropion. Ophthalmology. 2010;117(2): 352-355.

2. Barnes JA, Bunce C, Olver JM. Simple effective surgery suitable for involutional entropion for the general ophthalmologist, Ophthalmology. 2006;113(1):92-96 .

3. Wright M, Bell D, Scott C, Leatherbarrow B. Everting suture correction of lower lid involutional entropion. Br. J. Ophthalmol. 1999;83(9):1060-3.

4. Erb MH, Uzcategui N, Dresner SC, Efficacy and Compliction of the Transconjunctival Entropion Repair for Lower Eyelid Involutional entropion. Ophthalmology. 2006;113(12):2351-2356.

5. Ben Simon GJ, Molina M, Schwarcz RM, McCann JD, Goldberg RA. Goldberg external (subciliary) vs internal (transconjunctival) iinvolutional entropion repair. American Journal of Ophthalmology. 2005;139(3):482-487.

6. Caldato R, Lauande-Pimentel R, Sabrosa NA, Fonseca RA, Paiva RS, Alves MR, José NK. Role of reinsertion of the lower eyelid retractor on involutional entropion. British Journal of Ophthalmology. 2000; 84(6):606-608

7. Hoh HB, Steel D, Potts MJ , Harrad RA. The use of botulinum toxin for lower lid entropion, Nep J. Oph. 2009;1(1):37-42.

8. Bashour M, Harvey J. Causes of involutional entropion and entropion- age related tarsal changes are the key. Ophthalmic plastic and reconstructive surgery. 2000;16(2):131-141.

9. Wright M, Bell D, Scott C, Leatherbattow B. Everting suture correction of lower lid involutional entropion. Br. J. Ophthalmol. 1999;83(9):1060-3.

10. Leibovitch I, Lateral Wedge Resection: A simple technique for repairing involutional lower eyelid entropion dermatologic surgery. 2010;36(9):1412–1418.

11. Tsang S, Yau GS, Lee JW, Chu AT, Yuen CY. Surgical outcome of involutional lower eyelid entropion correction using transcutaneous everting sutures in Chinese patients. Int Ophthalmol. 2014; 34(4):865-8.
DOI: 10.1007/s10792-013-9893-5. Epub 2013 Dec 31.

12. Boboridi K, Bunce C, Rose GE. A comparative study of two procedures for repaire of iinvolutional lower lid entropion. Ophthalmology. 2000;107(5): 959-61.

The Relationship of HLA-B27 and HLA-B51 on Non-Behcet Uveitis

Ercument Cavdar[1], Abdullah Ozkaya[2], Hande Mefkure Ozkaya[3],
Sınan Bılgın[4*], Ozge Elmastas Gultekin[5] and Mustafa Alparslan Babayigit[6]

[1]*Department of Ophthalmology, Kemalpasa State Hospital, Izmir, Turkey.*
[2]*Department of Ophthalmology, Beyoğlu Eye Training and Research Hospital, Istanbul, Turkey.*
[3]*Department of Ophthalmology, Sisli Etfal Training and Research Hospital, Istanbul, Turkey.*
[4]*Department of Ophthalmology, Sıfa Hospital, Izmir, Turkey.*
[5]*Faculty of Statistics, Ege University, Izmir, Turkey.*
[6]*Department of Public Health, Gulhane Military Medical Academy, Ankara, Turkey.*

Authors' contributions

This work was carried out in collaboration between all authors. Author EC designed the study, wrote the protocol, and wrote the first draft of the manuscript. Authors AO, HMO and MAB managed the literature searches, analyses of the study performed the spectroscopy analysis. Authors SB, EC managed the experimental process and author OEG identified the species of plant. All authors read and approved the final manuscript.

Editor(s):
(1) Tatsuya Mimura, Department of Ophthalmology, Tokyo Women's Medical University Medical Center East, Japan.
Reviewers:
(1) Anonymous, Mansoura University, Egypt.
(2) Luis Fernando Barba Gallardo, Centro De Ciencias De La Salud, Universidad Autónoma De Aguascalientes, México.

ABSTRACT

Aims: The aim of this study was to investigate the relationship of human leukocyte antigen (HLA)-B27 and HLA-B51 on the clinical characteristics, demographic features, localization, laterality, treatment modalities and visual prognosis in non-Behcet uveitis patients

Study Design: Retrospective study.

Place and Duration of Study: Tepecik Eye Training and Research Hospital. January 1999 and March 2009.

Methodology: A total of 143 non-Behcet uveitis patients were included. Socio-demographic data and clinical features of the patients were reviewed. The patients were divided into four groups according to HLA-B27 and B-51 positivity which were as follows; HLA B-27 (-) B-51 (-), HLA B-27

Corresponding author: E-mail: drsinanbilgin@yahoo.com

(+) B-51 (-), HLA B-27 (-) B-51 (+), and HLA B-27 (+) B-51 (+) groups.
Results: Bilateral uveitis and posterior uveitis were more frequent in males in HLA-B27 (+) B51 (+) group, the baseline BCVA values were significantly lower in HLA-B27 (+) B51 (+) group, and also systemic steroid and immunosuppressive treatment were more frequently required to control uveitis attacks in this group. Anterior uveitis was more frequent in the HLA-B27 (-) B51 (-), and HLA-B27 (+) B51 (-) group.
Conclusion: The positivity of both HLA-B27 and HLA-B51 was related with worse visual outcomes in non-Behcet uveitis patients associated with requirement of more aggressive treatment. The negativity of both HLA-B27 and HLA-B51 seemed to be related with better visual outcomes and less number of attacks in non-Behcet uveitis patients.

Keywords: Behcet disease; human leukocyte antigen; uveitis.

1. INTRODUCTION

Uveitis is composed of a diverse group of disease entities and is a cause of significant visual impairment accounting for 10% of blindness in the western world [1]. It refers to intraocular inflammation including the uveal tract, and the adjacent structures including vitreous, retina and, optic nerve [1].

The patients with uveitis should be evaluated in many aspects; including anatomic localization of the inflammation, human leukocyte antigen (HLA) typing, etiologic factors and associated systemic diseases which may primarily affect the clinical course and treatment requirements of the patients [2].

Uveitis is widely classified into anterior, intermediate, posterior and panuveitis based on the anatomical involvement [2]. Also Human Leukocyte Antigens (HLA) are closely associated with disease susceptibility in uveitis patients [3]. HLAs are cell surface proteins involved in immune function. HLA molecules present antigenic peptides to generate immune defense reactions. There are has two classes of HLA antigens, class 1 composed of HLA A, B, C and Class II: HLA-DRB, DQB1 and HLA complex defined by the genes of Major Histocompatibility Complex (MHC) [4].

Uveitis is closely associated with class 1 HLA [3]. HLA- B51 and B27 genes frequently play role in the pathogenesis of uveitis. HLA-B51 is the major gene associated with the pathogenesis of Behcet uveitis [3]. HLA-B27 is usually related to acute anterior uveitis [5]. On the other hand visual prognosis and clinical course is very different between HLA- B27 associated uveitis and HLA-B51 Behcet uveitis [6].

Behcet disease (BD) is a multisystem vasculitic disorder associated with devastating ocular effects, [1] and is dominantly seen on the old silk route between east and west (Korean, Taiwanese, Kuwaiti, Israeli, Turkish, Greek and Tunisian) and associated with HLA-B51. The effects of HLA on BD is well known; however, there is not any data about its effects on non-Behcet uveitis patients [7] Therefore we classified all of the non-infectious uveitis patients who are not diagnosed as Behcet uveitis as non-Behcet uveitis and aimed to investigate the effect of HLA-B27 and HLA-B51 on demographic features, localization, laterality, clinical characteristics, treatment modalities and visual prognosis in this group of uveitis patients.

2. MATERIALS AND METHODS

In this retrospective, comparative study, we reviewed the records of 767 uveitis patients. A hundred and forty-three patients fulfilled the requirements and included in the study. Inclusion criteria were as follows: a minimum follow-up time of 12 months, and a complete laboratory work including HLA typing, and to be in the inactive phase of the disease at the last follow-up visit. Patients were not included in the study, if they were diagnosed as complete or incomplete Behcet disease at any time of the follow-up period. Patients that are contraindicated to start corticosteroids (diabetes, osteoporosis, hypertension, peptic ulcus etc.) are excluded from the study and consulted on the relevant clinics. Diagnosis of Behcet disease was made on the basis of the revised criteria of the Behcet Disease Research Committee of Japan in 2003 [3]. Also the patients who were diagnosed as infectious or traumatic uveitis were excluded from the study since the treatment strategy of them were different from the non-infectious cases and their clinical course did not depend on HLA typing. The study was conducted in accordance with the Declaration of Helsinki and an informed consent was obtained from the patients.

At the initial visit, a comprehensive medical and ophthalmologic history was obtained from each patient. Data collected from the patients' records included age, gender, laterality, follow-up time, associated systemic diseases, best corrected visual acuity (BCVA) at the first uveitis attack, BCVA at the last visit, ophthalmologic examination findings, laboratory tests, treatment regimens. Best corrected visual acuity was measured via Snellen scale and converted to LogMAR scale. At all of the visits, slit lamp biomicroscopy, applanation tonometry, fundus examination with 78 diopter non-contact lens was performed. Laboratory tests and radiologic imagings including complete blood count, Toxoplasmosis, Rubella, CMV, Herpes (TORCH) panel, venereal disease research laboratory, angiotensin-converting enzyme test, chest and pelvis x-ray, liver function tests, C-reactive protein, erythrocyte sedimentation rate, HLA-B51 and HLA-B27 typing were obtained from each patient.

All patients were questioned for systemic diseases and referred to dermatology and neurology clinics. The patients who were not consulted for rheumatologic evaluation prior to the time of admission were referred to a rheumatologist and medical records were reviewed for patients with a previous rheumatologic follow-up. Ankylosing spondylitis and rheumatoid arthritis diagnosis was made by according to previous reports. A questionnaire form was filled at the initial visit by the physician to assess socio-demographic data including gender, age at presentation and any systemic disease according to the patients history and also addressed the clinical features of the uveitis including anatomical location of the uveitis, bilaterality, clinical course, associated ocular findings (hypopyon, papilla edema, papillitis, vasculitis and maculopathy) according to criteria of the standardization of the uveitis nomenclature (SUN) working group [2]. The classification of the uveitis regarding the localization was made according to the whole follow-up period. Previous ophthalmological evaluation and the use of topical and systemic medications (topical steroids, systemic steroids and immunosuppressive agents) for the treatment of uveitis at presentation were recorded. Since BCVA is affected during active inflammation phases of uveitis, baseline BCVA is defined during the initial uveitis attack and last BCVA is defined after the active inflammation episodes, during remission, at the last follow-up visit.

The given treatment regimens depended on the localization, and the severity of the uveitis. For mild AU, topical steroids (prednisolone acetate) were prescribed for the first uveitis attack. If the inflammation was not able to be controlled with topical steroids periocular corticosteroids (dexamethasone) were applied. When the control of the inflammation could not be achieved with topical and periocular steroid treatment, systemic steroid (prednisolone) and/or systemic immunosuppressive agents (cyclosporine, azathiopurine and methotrexate) were also prescribed. If significant cataract or medically intractable glaucoma developed during the follow-up period, appropriate surgical interventions were performed.

The patients were divided into four groups. The first group included HLA-B27 (-) B51 (-) patients, the second group included HLA-B27 (+) B51 (-) patients, the third group included HLA-B27 (-) B51 (+) patients, and the fourth group included HLA-B27 (+) B51 (+) patients. Primary outcome measures of the study were the laterality, localization and visual prognosis of uveitis and the requirement for systemic steroid and/or immunosuppressant treatment among the four groups. Secondary outcomes were to the gender rates, and complications among the four groups and the systemic associations, etiologic factors of uveitis in the whole study group.

2.1 Data Analysis

Conformity of study variables to normal distribution was controlled with Kolmogorov-Simirnov test and as this was not case, non-parametric tests were applied. One-Way ANOVA (with Bonferroni corrected) test was performed for comparison of age means. Evaluations of visual variables of patients were done by Kruskal Wallis test for independent groups, and Wilcoxon Signed Ranks Test for paired groups. Chi-square test was used to evaluate categorical data (gender, uveitis localization of groups etc). All statistical analysis were performed with statistical package for social sciences (SPSS Inc., Chicago, IL, USA) version 15. Two-tailed p value less than 0.05 was accepted to be statistically significant.

3. RESULTS AND DISCUSSION

A total of 143 non-Behcet uveitis patients were included in this study. Mean follow up time was 7.6±2.4 years (ranging between 5 and 10 years). Fifty-eighty patients (40.5%) were HLA-B27 (-) B51 (-), 28 patients (19.5%) were HLA-B27 (+) B51 (-), 37 patients (25.8%) were HLA-B27 (-) B51 (+), and 20 patients (13.9%) were HLA-B27 (+) B51 (+). Mean age of patients at presentation between the groups were similar (p=0.3) (Table 1) and there was no statistically significant difference in terms of male/female ratio between HLA groups (p=0.1) (Table 1).

Ocular damage caused by uveitis depends on several factors like anatomic location, severity, and etiology of the inflammation. Also HLA subgroups are closely associated with disease susceptibility in uveitis patients [8,9].

Anatomic localization of HLA groups were significantly different from each other (p=0.005). Anterior uveitis was more frequent in HLA-B27 (-) B51 (-) (48.6%) and HLA-B27 (+) B51 (-) groups (25.7%). Posterior uveitis was more frequent in HLA-B27 (+) B51 (+) group (40%) (Table 2). There were not any intermediate uveitis cases in the study.

Uveitis laterality was also different among the HLA groups (p=0.02). %64.3 of HLA-B27 (+) B51 (-) group was unilateral and %80.0 of HLA-B27 (+) B51 (+) group was bilateral (Table 3).

During the study period, the mean attack numbers of HLA-B27 (-) B51 (-), HLA-B27 (+) B51 (-), HLA-B27 (-) B51 (+) and HLA-B27 (+) B51 (+) groups were 1.7±1.0, 2.3±1.3, 2.3±1.5 and 2.5±2.0, respectively (p>0.05). Medical management of uveitis patients were summarized in (Table 4).

All patients were treated according to anatomical location of the uveitis, degree of intraocular inflammation and etiology of uveitis. HLA-B27 (-) B 51 (-) and HLA-B27 (+) B51 (-) group usually required only topical steroids (1% prednisolone acetate). On the other hand, in addition to topical and periocular steroid treatment, systemic corticosteroid (prednisolone) and immunosuppressive (cyclosporine, azathioprine and methotrexate) treatment were required more frequently in HLA-B27 (-) B51 (+), and HLA-B27 (+) B51 (+) group. HLA types and medical management had a statistically significant relationship (p< .001) (Table 4).

The visual results of the study were summarized in (Table 5).

The relationship of localization and gender in overall uveitis patients was summarized in (Table 6).

The relationship between localization and laterality of uveitis were summarized in (Table 7).

There was not a statistically significant relationship between localization of uveitis patients and laterality.

Uveitis is commonly diagnosed in the third decade of life [10]. In our study mean age of non-Behcet uveitis patients at presentation was 35.1±24.8 years which was compatible with the previous reports [10,11].

There was no difference in terms of male/female ratio among the HLA groups in this study, and this was consistent with a previous study from Turkey by Tugal-Tutkun et al. [6].

Anterior uveitis accounts for 50% to 92% of uveitis cases in the Western countries and 28% to 50% of uveitis cases in Asian countries, such as, Korea, Japan, and India [10,11]. In Turkey the frequency AU was reported between 28.5% and 90% [7]. In our study AU accounted for 49.0% of total uveitis cases, and this was similar to previous studies [10,12].

There was a statistically significant difference among the HLA groups in regards of anatomic localization and laterality in this study. Unilaterality was statistically frequent in HLA-B27 (+) B51 (-) group (64.3%) and bilaterality was statistically frequent in HLA-B27 (+) B51 (+) group (80.0%). These findings were consistent with previous studies regarding that HLA-B27 (+) B51(-) associated uveitis typically caused a recurrent, dominantly unilateral disease [13,14]. Rosenbaum et al. showed that HLA- B27 was positive in 80% of the patients with unilateral, acute and recurrent uveitis [15]. On the other hand bilaterality was reported to be more frequent in HLA-B27 (+) B51 (+) group of Behcet patients [11]. These data may show that HLA-B27 positivity alone tends to be associated with unilateral uveitis, but when both HLA-27 and HLA-B51 were positive, bilaterality was more frequent. The HLA-B51 (+) cases were associated with posterior segment involvement more frequently than the HLA-B51 (-) cases. In the literature there are some studies supporting this phenomenon [16].

Table 1. Gender and mean age of HLA groups

	HLA-B27 (-) B51 (-)	HLA-B27 (+) B51 (-)	HLA-B27 (-) B51 (+)	HLA-B27 (+) B51 (+)	Total	P
Male	30 (51.8%)	18 (64.3%)	24 (63.8%)	16 (80.0%)	88 (61.5%)	P^1= .1
Female	28 (48.2%)	10 (35.7%)	13 (36.2%)	4 (20.0%)	55 (38.5%)	
Total	58 (100.0%)	28 (100.0%)	37 (100.0%)	20 (100.0%)	143 (100.0%)	
Mean age at presentation	37.3±12.5	37.5±14.7	32.8±13.7	33.4±12.3	35.6±13.3	P^2= .3

HLA, human leukocyte antigen; M, male; F, female, (P1=Chi-square test, P2=One-Way ANOVA (with Bonferroni corrected)

Table 2. Anatomic localization and HLA B27 and B51relationship of the uveitis patients

	Anterior	Posterior	Panuveitis	Total	P^1
HLA B27 (-) B51 (-)	34	3	21	58	.005
% within localization	48.6%	30.0%	33.3%	40.5%	
HLA B27 (+) B51 (-)	18	0	10	28	
% within localization	25.7%	.0%	15.9%	19.6%	
HLA B27 (-) B51(+)	15	3	19	37	
% within localization	21.4%	30.0%	30.2%	25.9%	
HLA B27 (+) B51 (+)	3	4	13	20	
% within localization	4.3%	40.0%	20.6%	14.0%	
Total	70	10	63	143	
% within localization	100.0%	100.0%	100.0%	100.0%	

HLA, human leukocyte antigen, P1=Chi-square test

Table 3. Laterality and HLA B51-B27 relationship of the uveitis patients

	Unilaterality	Bilaterality	Total number of patients	P^1
HLA B27 (-) B51 (-)	30	28	58	.02
% within groups	51.7%	48.3%	40.5%	
HLA B27 (+) B51 (-)	18	10	28	
% within groups	64.3%	35.7%	19.6%	
HLA B27 (-) B51(+)	19	18	37	
% within groups	51.4%	48.6%	25.9%	
HLA B27 (+) B51 (+)	4	16	20	
% within groups	20.0%	80.0%	14.0%	
Total number of patients	71	72	143	
% within groups	49.7%	50.3%	100.0%	

HLA, human leukocyte antigen, P1=Chi-square test

There was also a remarkable difference between the groups in terms of anatomic localization and HLA types. Anterior uveitis was significantly more frequent in HLA-B27 (-) B51 (-), and HLA-B27 (+) B51 (-) group. Posterior uveitis was significantly more frequent in HLA-B27 (+) B51 (+) group.

There was a statistically significant difference among the HLA groups in regards of medical management in the study. While most of the HLA B51 (-) patients could have been treated with only topical steroids, the HLA B51 (+) patients and especially HLA B27 (+) B51 (+) subgroup required systemic steroids and/or immunosuppressives.

In the literature there are few data about the effect of HLA-B51 positivity on visual outcomes in non- Behcet uveitis patients [17,18]. The change in BCVA was found to be statically better in the HLA groups, except in HLA-B27 (+) B51 (+) group. This may be due to heterogeneity and low number of patients.

Male sex and younger age of onset was reported to be negative prognostic factors for Behcet disease and the frequency of HLA-B51 antigen was reported to be higher in male patients with uveitis in Japan [19,20]. These findings were contrast to our findings of non-Behcet uveitis patients.

Table 4. Medical management of uveitis patients

	HLA B27 (-) B51 (-) N=59	HLA B27 (+) B51 (-) N=28	HLA B27 (-) B51 (+) N=36	HLA B27 (+) B51 (+) N=20	Total number of patients	P^1
TOPICAL	38	20	15	0	73	<.001
% within groups	64.4%	71.4%	41.6%	.0%	51.0%	
TOPICAL +PERIOCULAR	9	5	5	1	20	
% within groups	15.2%	17.8%	13.8%	5.0%	14.0%	
TOPICAL +SYSTEMIC STEROID	10	2	10	11	33	
%within groups	16.9%	7.1%	27.7%	55.0%	23.0%	
SYSTEMIC STEROID + TOPICAL + PEROCULAR	0	0	0	2	2	
%within groups	.0%	.0%	.0%	10.0%	1.4%	
SYSTEMIC STEROID+ TOPICAL + IMMUNESUPRESSIVE	1	1	5	4	11	
%within groups	1.6%	3.5%	13.8%	20.0%	7.7%	
SYSTEMIC STEROID+ TOPICAL + IMMUNESUPRESSIVE + PEROCULAR	0	0	2	2	4	
%within groups	.0%	.0%	5.5%	10.0%	2.8%	
Total number of patients	58	28	37	20	143	
% within groups					100.0%	

HLA, human leukocyte antigen, P1=Chi-square test

Table 5. The best corrected visual acuity at baseline and last follow-up visit of the HLA groups

	Baseline BCVA for right eye	BCVA at the last follow-up for right eye	P^1	Baseline BCVA for left eye	BCVA at the last follow-up for left eye	P^1
HLA B27 (-)B51(-) Median	0.80	1.00	.03	0.85	1.00	.008
HLA B27(+)B51(-) Median	0.90	1.00	.002	0.90	1.00	.001
HLA B27 (-)B51(+) Median	0.60	1.00	<.001	0.70	1.00	.004
HLA B27(+)B51(+) Median	0.30	0.50	.052	0.55	0.75	0.2
P^2	.001	0.6		.007	0.1	

BCVA: Best Corrected Visual Acuity, HLA: Human Leukocyte Antigen, P1=Wilcoxon Signed Ranks Test. Balded values shows the significance of the change in BCVA from baseline to the last follow-up within each HLA group for the right and left eye, P2=Kruskal Wallis Test. Balded values shows the significance among the four HLA groups for baseline and last follow-up

In our study bilateral (%80) and posterior uveitis (%40) was found to be frequent in HLA-B27 (+) B51 (+) group. The change in BCVA was significantly lower in this group, and also systemic steroid and immunosuppressives were more frequently required for the treatment. On the other side, AU was more frequent in patients with HLA-B27 (-) B51 (-), and HLA-B27 (+) B51 (-) group.

Table 6. The relationship of localization and gender in overall uveitis patients

	Male	Female	Total number of patients	Male/Female	P^1
Anterior uveitis	36 (51.4%)	34 (48.5%)	70 (49.0%)	1.05	.005
Posterior uveitis	4 (40.0%)	6 (60.0%)	10 (7.0%)	0.66	
Panuveitis	47 (74.6%)	16 (25.3%)	63 (44.0%)	2.93	
Total number of patients	88 (61.5%)	55 (38.5%)	143 (100.0%)	1.6	

P1=Chi-square test

Table 7. Localization of uveitis and laterality relationship

	Unilaterality	Bilaterality	Total number of patients	P^1
Anterior uveitis	43 (61.4%)	27 (38.6%)	70 (49.0%)	.01
Posterior uveitis	2 (20.0%)	8 (80.0%)	10 (7.0%)	
Panuveitis	26 (41.3%)	37 (58.7%)	63 (44.0%)	
Total number of patients	71 (49.7%)	72 (50.3%)	143 (100.0%)	

P1=Chi-square test

In the literature, the relationship between the Behcet Disease and HLA subgroups was evaluated in several studies [1]. However, this study is the first to evaluate the relationship of HLA-B27 and HLA-B51 on non-Behcet uveitis patients in terms of anatomic localization, visual acuity, treatment regimens. Limitations of this study include the retrospective design and the irregularity of follow-up period among the patients. Also we did not perform advanced laboratory tests to exclude the infectious uveitis like aqueous tapping and molecular biology testing for viral uveitis, only serum TORCH panel was performed. Therefore we might have missed some of the infectious anterior uveitis cases. Since there are a few studies about non-Behçet uveitis we could not compare our all results with the literature.

Strengths of the study include the relatively good number of non-Behcet uveitis patients and the center of the study. The study was conducted in a tertiary center which was referred from many state hospitals in Aegean Region of Turkey; therefore the study may reflect the patient characteristics of the non-Behcet uveitis patients in Aegean Region of Turkey

4. CONCLUSION

The relationship between HLA subtypes and Behcet disease was evaluated in previous studies. To our knowledge, this study is the first to investigate the relationship of HLA-B27 and HLA-B51 on Non-Behcet uveitis patients. Bilaterality and posterior uveitis was found to be more frequent in the group of HLA-B27 (+) B51 (+) patients. Also systemic steroid and immunosuppressive requirement was more frequent. Also in contrast to the other three groups, the change in BCVA from baseline to the last follow-up visit was not statistically better in this group. On the other side, anterior uveitis was more frequent in HLA-B27 (+) B51 (-) group.

As a result positivity of both HLA-B27 and B-51 seems to be a negative prognostic factor for non-Behcet uveitis patients. Further studies are required to delineate the prognostic factors for this group of patients.

ETHICAL APPROVAL

Local Ethics Committee approval was obtained for this retrospective study and consent forms were not required.

COMPETING INTERESTS

Authors have declared that no competing interests exist.

REFERENCES

1. Chang JHM, Wakefield D. Uveitis: A global perspective. Ocul Immunol Inflamm. 2002;10:263-79.
2. Jabs DA, Nussenblatt RB, Rosenbaum JT. Standardization of Uveitis Nomenclature Working G. Standardization of uveitis nomenclature for reporting clinical data. Results of the First International Workshop. American Journal of Ophthalmology. 2005;140:509-16.
3. Mizuki N, Ohno S, Tanaka H, Sugimura K, Seki T, Mizuki H. Association of HLA-B51

and lack of association of class II alleles with Behçet's disease. Tissue Antigens. 1992;40:22-30.

4. Flomenberg N, Baxter-Lowe LA, Confer D, et al. Impact of HLA class I and class II high-resolution matching on outcomes of unrelated donor bone marrow transplantation: HLA-C mismatching is associated with a strong adverse effect on transplantation outcome. Blood. 2004;104:1923-30.

5. Ramsay A, Lightman S. Hypopyon uveitis. Survey of Ophthalmology. 2001;46:1-18.

6. Tugal-Tutkun I, Onal S, Altan-Yaycioglu R, Huseyin Altunbas H, Urgancioglu M. Uveitis in Behcet disease: An analysis of 880 patients. American Journal of Ophthalmology. 2004;138:373-80.

7. Sakamoto M, Akazawa K, Nishioka Y, Sanui H, Inomata H, Nose Y. Prognostic factors of vision in patients with Behcet disease. Ophthalmology. 1995;102:317-21.

8. Suzuki Kurokawa M, Suzuki N. Behcet's disease. Clinical and Experimental Medicine. 2004;4:10-20.

9. Frauendorf E, Von Goessel H, May E, Marker-Hermann E. HLA-B27-restricted T cells from patients with ankylosing spondylitis recognize peptides from B*2705 that are similar to bacteria-derived peptides. Clinical and Experimental Immunology. 2003;134:351-9.

10. Rodriguez A, Calonge M, Pedroza-Seres M, et al. Referral patterns of uveitis in a tertiary eye care center. Archives of Ophthalmology. 1996;114:593-9.

11. Bodaghi B, Cassoux N, Wechsler B, et al. Chronic severe uveitis: Etiology and visual outcome in 927 patients from a single center. Medicine. 2001;80:263-70.

12. Mercanti A, Parolini B, Bonora A, Lequaglie Q, Tomazzoli L. Epidemiology of endogenous uveitis in north-eastern Italy. Analysis of 655 new cases. Acta Ophthalmologica Scandinavica. 2001;79:64-8.

13. Tay-Kearney ML, Schwam BL, Lowder C, et al. Clinical features and associated systemic diseases of HLA-B27 uveitis. American Journal of Ophthalmology. 1996;121:47-56.

14. Linssen A, Meenken C. Outcomes of HLA-B27-positive and HLA-B27-negative acute anterior uveitis. American Journal of Ophthalmology. 1995;120:351-61.

15. Rosenbaum JT. Characterization of uveitis associated with spondyloarthritis. The Journal of Rheumatology. 1989;16:792-6.

16. Ahn JK, Park YG. Human leukocyte antigen B27 and B51 double-positive Behcet uveitis. Archives of Ophthalmology. 2007;125:1375-80.

17. Rothova A, Van Veenedaal WG, Linssen A, Glasius E, Kijlstra A, De Jong PT. Clinical features of acute anterior uveitis. American Journal of Ophthalmology. 1987;103:137-45.

18. Tuncer S, Adam YS, Urgancioglu M, Tugal-Tutkun I. Clinical features and outcomes of HLA-b27-positive and HLA-B27-negative acute anterior uveitis in a Turkish patient population. Ocular Immunology and Inflammation. 2005;13:367-73.

19. Yazici H, Tuzun Y, Pazarli H, et al. Influence of age of onset and patient's sex on the prevalence and severity of manifestations of Behcet's syndrome. Annals of the Rheumatic Diseases. 1984;43:783-9.

20. Sakane T, Suzuki N, Nagafuchi H. Etiopathology of Behcet's disease: Immunological aspects. Yonsei Medical Journal. 1997;38:350-8.

Barriers to Free Cataract Surgery in Yaoundé

Kagmeni Giles[1,2*], Domngang Noche Christelle[3] and Noa Noatina Blaise[4]

[1]*Eye Department of the University Teaching Hospital Yaounde (UTHY), Cameroon.*
[2]*University of Yaoundé I, Faculty of Medicine and Biomedical Sciences, Cameroon.*
[3]*Eye Department of the Mountains University Banganté, Cameroon.*
[4]*National Blindness Program, Ministry of Heath, Yaoundé, Cameroon.*

Authors' contributions

This work was carried out in collaboration between all authors. Author KG designed the study and wrote the protocol. Authors KG and DNC analyzed the data and wrote the first draft of the manuscript. Authors KG, DNC and NNB contributed to the writing of the manuscript and were responsible for manuscript results and conclusions. All authors reviewed and approved the final manuscript.

Editor(s):
(1) Li Wang, Department of Ophthalmology, Cullen Eye Institute, Baylor College of Medicine, USA.
(2) Jimmy S. M. Lai, Department of Ophthalmology, The University of Hong Kong, Hong Kong and Honorary Consultant Ophthalmologist, Queen Mary Hospital, Hong Kong, China.
Reviewers:
(1) Anonymous, Mansoura University, Egypt.
(2) Ningli Wang, Beijing Tongren Eye Center, Capital medical University Affiliated Beijing Tongren Hospital, China.
(3) S. K. Prabhakar, Ophthalmology Department, JSS University, India.

ABSTRACT

Purpose: To identifying barriers to massive turnout for free cataract surgery campaigns in Yaoundé
Methods: We prospectively interviewed 68 patients who radically refused free cataract surgery at the University Teaching hospital (UTH) Yaoundé between January 2008 and December 2010. The questionnaire aimed at addressing: the knowledge of the cataract and its surgical treatment, the awareness of government's subvention for free cataract operation, the reasons for refusal. Patient demographic data were also analyzed.
Results: A total of 68 patients (41 males and 27 females), mean age was 57.20 ± 11 years were enrolled in this study. Forty three patients (63.23%) were civil servants with fixed salaries, 25 (36.77%) were workers in the informal sector. 80% of the participants had a good knowledge of cataract and its surgical treatment. 58,82 % of the patients were aware of the ongoing government subsidized campaign. Refusal reasons included: fear 38 (55.88%), awaiting of foreign NGO campaign 20 (29.42%), religious convictions 6(8.82%) wish for surgery abroad 4 (5.58%)
Conclusion: Fear and awaiting for foreign NGO surgery campaign were the main barriers for free

Corresponding author: E-mail: dr.kagmeni@gmx.net

cataract surgery in Yaoundé. Therefore, sporadic free cataract campaigns organized by foreign NGO appear to become a new barrier to cataract surgery.

Keywords: Free cataract surgery; barriers.

1. INTRODUCTION

Cataract remains the most common treatable cause of blindness. In sub Saharan countries the cataract surgical coverage is low and the outcome of cataract surgery is poor because of inadequate human and material resources [1]. To increase the cataract surgery rate (CSR) in Cameroon, the government took some measures such as the subvention of surgical fees in some hospitals; modernisation of equipment in the ophthalmology unit of the Yaoundé Central Hospital; as well as the opening of a specialisation cycle for ophthalmology in the Faculty of Medicine and Biomedical Sciences of the Yaoundé I University. Despite the fact that surgery was free, some patients still declined the offer. The aim of this study was to identify barriers to free cataract surgery in an urban setting and to propose practical solutions to this.

2. PATIENTS AND METHODS

This was a hospital-based prospective study which spanned January 2008 to December 2010 in the ophthalmology unit of the University Teaching hospital in Yaoundé and included all patients who presented with operable cataracts and turned down the offer for free surgery. Written informed consent was obtained from all patients. A simple questionnaire Table 1 was administered. Brevity was the principal objective, since peoples would not will to complete a long questionnaire about something that they don't accept. Moreover, socio-demographic data (age, sex, profession, educational level) and clinical data (ophthalmic history, visual acuity) were also analyzed.

3. RESULTS

Of 756 patients to who free cataract surgery was proposed 68 turned down the offer, giving a refusal rate of 8.99 % and were enrolled in this study. Patient characteristics are presented in Table 2. Our sample consisted of 41 males (60.30%) and 27 females (39.70%). Mean age was 57.20 ± 11.44 years and ranged from 12 to 68 years. Forty three patients (63.23%) were civil servants with fixed salaries, 25 (36.77%) were workers in the informal sector. The mean visual acuity in the eye to be operated was Log MAR 1.15 ± 0.21. Three patients (4.41%) had complications from previous cataract surgery in the other eye. One was a case of aphakic retinal detachment and the two others were pseudophakic bullous keratopathy secondary to anterior chamber lens implantation. Fifty five patients (80%) had the right knowledge about cataract. The idea of cataract surgery subvention by the state was known by 40 patients (58.82%). The main reasons of refusal of free cataract surgery included: fear 38 (55.88%) awaiting of foreign nongovernmental organizations (NGOs) campaigns 20 (29.42%), religious convictions 6(8.82%) wish for surgery abroad 4 (5.58%).

Table 1. Questionnaire

Q01	**In your opinion, what is cataract**	
Q01a	A disease of eye causing progressive blindness 1=Yes 2= No	└─┘
Q01b	A disease of eye causing severe pain 1=Yes 2= No	└─┘
Q02	**In your opinion what is the best treatment of cataract**	
	1= Eye drop; 2= Spectacles; 3= Surgery	└─┘
Q03	**Are you aware of government's subvention for free cataract operation in our hospital?**	└─┘
	1=Yes 2= No	
Q04	**Can you please tell us your reasons for refusing the surgery**	
	1._____	
	2._____	
	3._____	

Data were analyzed using Epi-Info 3.5.1. Qualitative variables were presented as percentages (%) while quantitative ones as mean ± standard deviation.

Table 2. Demographic and interview data of all study participants

Parameters	Number	Percentage (%)
Gender		
- Males	41	60.30
- Females	27	39.70
Occupation		
- Civil servants with fixed salary	43	36.23
- Workers in informal sectors	25	36.77
Interview		
-Right knowledge about cataract and it's surgical treatment	55	80
-Right knowledge about the government subvention	40	58.82
-Reasons of refusal of free cataract surgery		
- Fear	38	55.88
- Awaiting of foreign NGO champagne	20	29.42
- Religious convictions	6	8.82
- Wish for surgery abroad	4	5.58

4. DISCUSSION

The cataract surgery rate (CSR) is defined as total number of cataract surgeries performed / Total population × 1,000,000 [2]. Knowledge on the barriers of cataract surgery is important in any particular setting, as it can be used to devise strategies to increase the CSR. The lack of financial resources, difficult access to eye care service [3] and ignorance [4] are known to be main barriers to cataract surgery in developing word. Government action has led to the removal of such barriers. This study included an urban population, most of them salary-workers, with easy access to eye health care but who refused free surgery, despite low visual acuities. In Nepal, Snellingen et al. [5] reported an acceptance rate to free surgery of less than 60%. In the current study as well as in the series of Ojabo CO et al in Nigeria [6] the majority of the patients has an adequate knowledge on cataract and was also aware that surgery was the answer to their visual dysfunction. This can be explain in our milieu by the numerous mediatised explanation campaigns organised in some institutions to explain the subvention strategy of the ministry of public health and the arrival of foreign NGOs and also the easy access to the internet. In Malawi, Schulze et al. [7] reported that patients who generally refused surgery did not have adequate knowledge about cataract. This difference can be explained by the residence of the study population. More males refused free cataract surgery in the current series, a similar finding reported by Chang et al. [8]. On the contrary, Athanasiov et al. [9] reported a higher acceptance rate for surgery in men. Courtright P et al. [10] found in their study that men with lower socioeconomic status were more likely to accept surgery than men with higher socioeconomic status.

Fear is the most frequent reason for refusal of free cataract surgery in Yaoundé. This reason has been reported in several studies [11]. The origin of fear is multi factorial: the fear of losing the second eye after the loss of vision in the previously operated eye; the fear of blindness following surgery as may have been experienced by a family member or friend. This can be explained by the fact that the techniques of cataract surgery used had not been improved. Intra capsular cataract extraction (ICCE) without implantation or with anterior chamber lens implantation is still the method of choice of most ophthalmologists in Yaoundé. The many complications linked to this technique as seen in tree patients in our series have contributed to creating the phobia of cataract surgery in the population. The negative testimony given by past operated patients constitute a great barrier to the acceptance of cataract surgery in our setting. The desire to be operated during eye camps organised by foreign NGOs is the second most frequent reason for refusal of cataract free surgery. The ministry of public health has signed conventions with some foreign NGOs who organise free cataract surgery camps sporadically in Yaoundé and other towns within the country. Their presence is always highly mediatised and thus has a positive effect in that people are more aware of cataract, its surgical treatment and the expected results. However, these sporadic eye camps pose serious problems: 1) problem of post operative follow up. With most of the camps lasting a week, only immediate post operative follow up is possible. The average and long term post operative complications are not managed. If these complications lead to poor visual outcome, then the euphoria of the first days quickly give rise to phobia of surgery; and these eye camps become a barrier to cataract surgery. 2) These NGOs programme progressively become the reason for increasing cataract backlog. A few of the study population wish to be operated abroad. In most cases, these are high civil servants who know about the outcome of the modern cataract and who can obtain the sponsorship from the state.

To increase the CSR in Yaoundé, local ophthalmologists should conquer the confidence of the population by increasing their surgical success rates According to Yin Q et al. [12], the lack of knowledge about the quality of local services appear to be one of the principal barriers to cataract surgery in rural China. This is only possible through the vulgarisation of newer techniques such as small incision cataract surgery (SICS), an alternative surgical technique which has been shown to yield similar surgical outcomes as phaco emulsification. The adoption of SICS, a cost-effective cataract surgery technique had permitted an exponential increase of CSR in India [13]. This requires political will power with the creation of training and/or reconversion centres. Sensitisation through the media is essential. Programmes should be designed to receive direct testimonies from operated patients and their family members. According to Sapkota et al. [14] in Nepal, good local results lead to a decrease in the demand for surgery abroad.

5. CONCLUSION

In sub Saharan Africa, cataract is a known public health problem. The reduction of the burden of cataract blindness requires effective and sustainable actions. It is therefore important for health policy makers and medical authorities to improve the skills of local ophthalmologists and the quality of ophthalmic services in order to provide cataract patients with the best, most accessible and least expensive services possible. More interesting would be the redrawn of plan of action foreign NGO by putting more emphasis on training with transfer of technology instead of mass surgery on patients.

CONSENT

Written informed consent was obtained from all participants.

ETHICAL APPROVAL

The study was approved by the national ethics committee.

COMPETING INTERESTS

Authors have declared that no competing interests exist.

REFERENCES

1. Tabin G, Chen M, Espandar L Cataract surgery for the developing world urr. Opin Ophthalmol. 2008;19(1):55-9.

2. Foster A. Vision 2020: The Cataract Challenge. Community Eye Health. 2000;13:17–21.

3. Gyasi M, Amoaku W, Asamany D. Barriers to cataract surgical uptake in the upper East region of Ghana. Ghana Med J. 2007;41(4):167-70.

4. Nkumbe HE, Razafinimpanana N, Rakotondrajoa LP. Social marketing to increase the rate of cataract surgery in the Sava region of Madagascar. Med Sante Trop. 2013;23(4):462.

5. Snellingen T, Shrestha BR, Gharti MP, Shrestha JK, Upadhyay MP, Pokhrel RP. Socioeconomic barriers to cataract surgery in Nepal: the South Asian cataract management study. 1998;82(12):142-8.

6. Ojabo CO, Alao O Cataract surgery: limitations and barriers in Makurdi, Benue State. Niger J Med. 2009;18(3):250-5.

7. Schulze Schwerng M, Finger RP, Barrows J, Nyrenda M, Kalua K Barriers to Uptake of Free Pediatric Cataract Surgery in Malawi. Ophthalmic Epidemiol. 2014 Mar 5. [Epub ahead of print].

8. Chang MA, Congdon NG, Baker SK, Bloem MW, Savage H, Sommer A. The surgical management of cataract: barriers, best practices and outcomes. Int Ophthalmol. 2008;28(4):247-60.

9. Athanasiov PA, Casson RJ, Newland HS, Shein WK, Muecke JS, Selva D, Aung T Cataract surgical coverage and self-reported barriers to cataract surgery in a rural Myanmar population. Clin Experiment Ophthalmol 2008;36(6):521-5.

10. Courtright P, Kanjaloti S, Lewallen S Barriers to acceptance of cataract surgery among patients presenting to district hospitals in rural Malawi. Trop Geogr Med. 1995;47(1):15-8.

11. Athanasiov PA, Edussuriva K, Senaratne T, Sennanavake S, Selva D, Casson RJ. Cataract in central Sri Lanka: cataract surgical coverage and self-reported barriers to cataract surgery. 2009;37(8):780-4.

12. Yin Q, HuA, Liang Y, Zhang J, He M, Lam DS, Ge J, Wang N, Frieman DS, Zhao J. A two-site, population-based study of barriers to cataract surgery in rural china. Invest Ophthalmol Vis Sci. 2009;50(3):1069-75.

13. Aravind S, Haripriva A, Sumara Taranum BS. Cataract surgery and intraocular lens manufacturing in India. 2008;19(1):60-5.

14. Sapkota YD, Pokharel GP, Dulal S Byanju RN, Maharjan IM. Barriers to up take cataract surgery in Gandaki Zone, Nepal. Kathmandu Univ Med (KUMJ). 2004;2(2):103-12.

Permissions

List of Contributors

Tarakeswararao Attada and V. V. L. Narasimha Rao
Department of Ophthalmology, Andhramedical College, Govt. Regional Eye Hospital, Visakhapatnam, Andhra Pradesh, India

Bety Yáñez
Department of Ophthalmology, Hospital Nacional Dos de Mayo, Lima, Peru

Mitra Dehghan Harati and Elahe Abbasi Shavazi
Geriatric Ophthalmology Research Center, Shahid Sadoughi University of Medical Sciences, Yazd, Iran

Mohammad Reza Besharati
Department of Ophthalmology, Geriatric Ophthalmology Research Center, Shahid Sadoughi University of Medical Sciences, Yazd, Iran

Mohammad Afkhami Ardekani
Department of Endocrinology, Diabetes Research Center, Shahid Sadoughi University of Medical Sciences, Yazd, Iran

Samira Salimpur
Department of Ophthalmology, Shahid Sadoughi University of Medical Sciences, Yazd, Iran

Sajjad Besharati
Shahid Beheshti University of Medical Sciences, Tehran, Iran

Amandeep Kaur, Vikas Gupta, Ajay Francis Christopher and Parveen Bansal
Division of Herbal Drug Technology, University Centre of Excellence in Research, Baba Farid University of Health Sciences, Faridkot, India

Mafalda Mota, Peter Pêgo, Inês Coutinho, Cristina Santos, Graça Pires and António Melo
Department of Ophthalmology, Hospital Professor Doutor Fernando Fonseca, Lisboa, Portugal

Catarina Klut and Teresa Maia
Departmentof Psychiatry, Hospital Professor Doutor Fernando Fonseca, Lisboa, Portugal

Emmanuel Olu Megbelayin and Stephen Mbosowo Ekpenyong
Department of Ophthalmology, University of Uyo Teaching Hospital, Uyo, Akwa-Ibom State, Nigeria

Chiedozie Kingsley Ojide
Department of Microbiology, Federal Teaching Hospital, Abakaliki, Ebonyi State, Nigeria

Athanasios Karamitsos, Lampros Lamprogiannis and Konstantinos Stamoulas
1st University Eye Clinic, AHEPA Hospital, Thessaloniki, Greece

Kyriakos Gougoulias, Diamantis Almaliotis, Athanasia Skriapa-Manta and Vasileios Karampatakis
Laboratory of Experimental Ophthalmology, Aristotle University of Thessaloniki, Greece

Theofanis Vaseiliadis and Aikaterini Raptou
Department of Nuclear Medicine, "Theageneion" Cancer Hospital of Thessaloniki, Greece

Kelly G. Hoffmann
Neuro Psychology Department, Captain James A Lovell Federal Health Care Center, 3001 Green Bay Road, IL. 60064, North Chicago, USA

Stuart P. Richer
Optometry/Ophthalmology, Captain James A Lovell Federal Health Care Center, 3001 Green Bay Road, IL. 60064,North Chicago, USA

James S. Wrobel
Department of Internal Medicine, University of Michigan Health System, Division of Metabolism, Endocrinology & Diabetes (MEND), USA

Eugenia Chen
Rosalind Franklin University of Medicine and Science, 3333 Green Bay Road, North Chicago, USA

Carla J Podella
Captain James A Lovell Federal Health Care Center, 3001 Green Bay Road, North Chicago, USA

Achyut N. Pandey, Parul Singh, Amit Vikram Raina and Ameeta Kaul
Departement of Ophthalmology, VCSG Medical College and Research Institute, Srinagar Garhwal, Uttarakhand, 246174, India

Anil Kakde
Eye Q Super Speciality Hospital, Gurgaon, India

Miguel Paciuc-Beja and Hugo Quiroz-Mercado
Department of Ophthalmology, University of Colorado School of Medicine, Denver Health Medical Center, USA

Victor Hugo Galicia-Alfaro and Myriam Retchkiman-Bret
Department of Ophthalmology, American British Cowdray Medical Center, Mexico City, Mexico

Ryan Phan
School of Medicine, University of Colorado, USA

Momen Mahmoud Hamdi and Islam Mahmoud Hamdi
Department of Ophthalmology, Ain Shams University, Cairo, Egypt

Brunella Maria Pavan Taffner and Fábio Petersen Saraiva
Departamento de Medicina Especializada/CCS/UFES, Federal University of Espírito Santo, Av. Marechal Campos, 1468, Maruipe, Vitória-ES, Brazil

Patricia Grativol Costa Saraiva
Pesquisa e Extensão AS – Multivix, Rua José Alves, 301, Goiabeiras, Vitória-ES, Brazil

Y. W. Jeremy Hu and Srinivasan Sanjay
Department of Ophthalmology and Visual Sciences, Khoo Teck Puat Hospital, Singapore

Srinivasan Sanjay
Yong Loo Lin School of Medicine, National University of Singapore, Singapore

Lauren R. Hepworth and Fiona J. Rowe
Department of Health Services Research, University of Liverpool, Liverpool L69 3GB, United Kingdom

Ojha Sushil, Tandon Anupama, Saraswat Neeraj and Shukla Dipendra
Department of Ophthalmology, UP RIMS and R, Saifai, Etawah, UP, India

S. Bansal, K. Jasani and K. Taherian
Department of Ophthalmology, Royal Preston Hospital, Preston PR2 9HT, UK

Deborah Buck and Michael P. Clarke
Institute of Neuroscience, Newcastle University, Newcastle Upon Tyne, United Kingdom

Nadeem Ali
Moorfields Eye Hospital, London, United Kingdom

Peter Tiffin
Sunderland Eye Infirmary, Sunderland, United Kingdom

Robert H. Taylor
York Hospitals NHS Trust, York, United Kingdom

Christine J. Powell and Michael P. Clarke
Newcastle Eye Centre, Royal Victoria Infirmary, Newcastle upon Tyne Hospitals NHS Foundation Trust, United Kingdom

Wael A. Ewais, Malak I. El Shazly and Ashraf A. Nossair
Department of Ophthalmology, Cairo University, Egypt

Raşit Kılıç and Abdi Bahadır Çetin
Department of Ophthalmology, Numune Hospital, Sivas, Turkey

Gülay Çetin
Department of Radiology, Numune Hospital, Sivas, Turkey

Rhuen Chiou Chow and Tengku Ain Kamalden
University of Malaya Eye Research Center (UMERC), Malaysia
Department of Ophthalmology, Faculty of Medicine, University of Malaya, Kuala Lumpur, Malaysia

Geoffrey E. Rose
Moorfields Eye Hospital, London, United Kingdom

Saul N. Rajak
The Sussex Eye Hospital, Brighton, United Kingdom
The London School of Hygiene and Tropical Medicine, United Kingdom

Nicolas Cadet and Paul Harasymowycz
Department of Ophthalmology, Université de Montréal, Montreal, Canada

Paul Harasymowycz
Montreal Glaucoma Institute, Montreal, Canada

Hatem M. Marey and Sameh S. Mandour
Ophthalmology Department, Faculty of Medicine Menofia University, Shebin El-Kom, Egypt

Noura A. Semary
Faculty of Computers and Information Menofia University, Shebin El-Kom, Egypt

L. Lamprogiannis, A. Karamitsos, V. Karagkiozaki and S. Logothetidis
Department of Physics, Laboratory for Thin Films Nanosystems and Nanometrology- LTFN, Aristotle University of Thessaloniki, Thessaloniki, Greece

I. Tsinopoulos, L. Lamprogiannis, A. Karamitsos and S. Dimitrakos
Department of Ophthalmology, School of Medicine, Aristotle University of Thessaloniki, "Papageorgiou" General Hospital, Thessaloniki, Greece

Lauren R. Hepworth and Fiona J. Rowe1
Department of Health Services Research, University of Liverpool, Liverpool L69 3GB, United Kingdom

Marion F. Walker
Department of Rehabilitation and Ageing, University of Nottingham, Nottingham NG7 2UH, United Kingdom

Janet Rockliffe
Speakability (North West Development Group), 1 Royal Street, London SE1 7LL, United Kingdom

Carmel Noonan
Department of Ophthalmology, Aintree University Hospital NHS Foundation Trust, L9 7AL, United Kingdom

Claire Howard
Department of Orthoptics, Salford Royal NHS Foundation Trust, Manchester M6 8HD, United Kingdom

Jim Currie
Different Strokes (London South East), 9 Canon Harnett Court, Wolverton Mill, MK12 5NF, United Kingdom

P. Peeush and S. Sarkar
Department of Ophthalmology, M.G.M Medical college Kishanganj, Bihar, India

Lingkun Kong, Sid A. Schechet, David K. Coats and Paul G. Steinkuller
Department of Ophthalmology, Baylor College of Medicine, Houston, Texas, USA

Kimberly L. Dinh
Department of Pharmacy, Baylor College of Medicine, Houston, Texas, USA

Robert G. Voigt and Ann B. Demny
Department of Pediatrics, Baylor College of Medicine, Houston, Texas, USA

Artur Zoto
Department of Rheumatology, University Hospital Center "Mother Teresa", Tirana, Albania

Brikena Selimi
Department of Ophthalmology, University Hospital Center "Mother Teresa", Tirana, Albania

Ee-Ling Tan
Department of Ophthalmology, School of Medical Sciences, Universiti Sains Malaysia, Kubang Kerian, Kelantan, Malaysia

Regunath Kandasamy
Department of Neuroscience, School of Medical Sciences, Universiti Sains Malaysia, Kubang Kerian, Kelantan, Malaysia

Wan-Hitam Wan-Hazabbah, Regunath Kandasamy, Thavaratnam Lakana-Kumar and Liza-Sharmini Ahmad Tajudin
Hospital Universiti Sains Malaysia, Kubang Kerian, Kelantan, Malaysia

Ee-Ling Tan, Shelina Oli Mohamed, Hanizasurana Hashim and Norfariza Ngah
Department of Ophthalmology, Selayang Hospital, Selangor, Lebuhraya Selayang-Kepong, 68100, Batu Caves, Selangor, Malaysia

Liza- Sharmini Ahmad Tajudin and Ee-Ling Tan
Department of Ophthalmology, School of Medical Science, Health Campus, Universiti Sains Malaysia, Kota Bharu, 16150, Kubang Kerian, Kelantan, Malaysia

Gholamhossein Yaghoobi
Department of Ophthalmology, Valiasr Hospital, Birjand University of Medical Sciences, Social Determinant Health Research Center, Birjand, Iran

Behrouz Heydari
Department of Ophthalmology, Birjand University of Medical Sceince, Ghafari St, Birjand, Iran

Ercument Cavdar
Department of Ophthalmology, Kemalpasa State Hospital, Izmir, Turkey

Abdullah Ozkaya
Department of Ophthalmology, Beyoğlu Eye Training and Research Hospital, Istanbul, Turkey

Hande Mefkure Ozkaya
Department of Ophthalmology, Sisli Etfal Training and Research Hospital, Istanbul, Turkey

Sınan Bılgın
Department of Ophthalmology, Sıfa Hospital, Izmir, Turkey

Ozge Elmastas Gultekin
Faculty of Statistics, Ege University, Izmir, Turkey

Mustafa Alparslan Babayigit
Department of Public Health, Gulhane Military Medical Academy, Ankara, Turkey

Kagmeni Giles
Eye Department of the University Teaching Hospital Yaounde (UTHY), Cameroon
University of Yaoundé I, Faculty of Medicine and Biomedical Sciences, Cameroon

Domngang Noche Christelle
Eye Department of the Mountains University Banganté, Cameroon

Noa Noatina Blaise
National Blindness Program, Ministry of Heath, Yaoundé, Cameroon

www.ingramcontent.com/pod-product-compliance
Lightning Source LLC
Chambersburg PA
CBHW080246230326
41458CB00097B/3998